AF830835

HUMAN REPRODUCTIVE GENETICS

HUMAN REPRODUCTIVE GENETICS

EMERGING TECHNOLOGIES AND CLINICAL APPLICATIONS

Edited by

JUAN A. GARCÍA-VELASCO

Rey Juan Carlos University, Madrid, Spain

IVI RMA Madrid, Madrid, Spain

EMRE SELI

Yale University, New Haven, CT, United States

Chief Scientific Officer, IVIRMA Global, Basking Ridge, NJ, United States

ELSEVIER

ACADEMIC PRESS

An imprint of Elsevier

Academic Press is an imprint of Elsevier
125 London Wall, London EC2Y 5AS, United Kingdom
525 B Street, Suite 1650, San Diego, CA 92101, United States
50 Hampshire Street, 5th Floor, Cambridge, MA 02139, United States
The Boulevard, Langford Lane, Kidlington, Oxford OX5 1GB, United Kingdom

British Library Cataloguing-in-Publication Data
A catalogue record for this book is available from the British Library

Library of Congress Cataloging-in-Publication Data
A catalog record for this book is available from the Library of Congress

ISBN: 978-0-12-816561-4

For Information on all Academic Press publications
visit our website at https://www.elsevier.com/books-and-journals

Publisher: Stacy Masucci
Acquisitions Editor: Tari Broderick
Editorial Project Manager: Pat Gonzalez
Production Project Manager: Swapna Srinivasan
Cover Designer: Miles Hitchen

Typeset by MPS Limited, Chennai, India

Contents

C

HOW TO ANALYZE AN EMBRYO

14. Preimplantation genetic testing for monogenic diseases

ANA CERVERO AND JULIO MARTÍN

15. Future technologies for preimplantation genetic applications

NADA KUBIKOVA AND DAGAN WELLS

D

REPRODUCTIVE GENETIC COUNSELING

16. Psychological aspects of reproductive genetic screening and diagnoses

DOROTHY A. GREENFELD

17. Bioethics in human reproduction (human reproductive genetics)

HEIDI MERTES AND GUIDO PENNINGS

18. The role of genetic counseling in the infertile patient

JOSEP PLA-VICTORI

List of contributors

Inmaculada Campos-Galindo Igenomix, Valencia, Spain

Ana Cervero Igenomix, Valencia, Spain

Joshua A. Copel Department of Obstetrics, Gynecology, and Reproductive Sciences, Section of Maternal-Fetal Medicine, Yale School of Medicine, New Haven, CT, United States

Almudena Devesa-Peiró Department of Genomic & Systems Reproductive Medicine, IVI-RMA IVI Foundation, Valencia, Spain; Department of Pediatrics, Obstetrics and Gynaecology, School of Medicine, University of Valencia, Valencia, Spain

Patricia Díaz-Gimeno Department of Genomic & Systems Reproductive Medicine, IVI-RMA IVI Foundation, Valencia, Spain; Biomedical Research Institute Hospital La Fe, Valencia, Spain

Jeffrey S. Dungan Division of Clinical Genetics, Department of Obstetrics & Gynecology, Northwestern University Feinberg School of Medicine, Chicago, IL, United States

Elpida Fragouli IVI RMA Global, Magdalen Centre, Oxford Science Park, Oxford, United Kingdom; Nuffield Department of Obstetrics and Gynaecology, University of Oxford, John Radcliffe Hospital, Oxford, United Kingdom

Juan A. García-Velasco IVI Foundation, Madrid, Spain; IVI RMA Madrid, Madrid, Spain; Rey Juan Carlos University, Madrid, Spain

Dorothy A. Greenfeld Yale University School of Medicine, New Haven, CT, United States

Sun-Wei Guo Shanghai Obstetrics and Gynecology Hospital, Fudan University, Shanghai, P.R. China; Shanghai Key Laboratory of Female Reproductive Endocrine-Related Diseases, Fudan University, Shanghai, P.R. China

Brent M. Hanson RMA New Jersey, Sidney Kimmel Medical College at Thomas Jefferson University, Basking Ridge, NJ, United States

James M. Hotaling Department of Surgery – Urology, University of Utah Center for Reconstructive Urology and Men's Health, Salt Lake City, UT, United States

Amanda N. Kallen Department of Obstetrics, Gynecology and Reproductive Sciences, Yale School of Medicine, New Haven, CT, United States

Katherine Kohari Department of Obstetrics, Gynecology, and Reproductive Sciences, Section of Maternal-Fetal Medicine, Yale School of Medicine, New Haven, CT, United States

Alexander Kotlyar Section of Reproductive Endocrinology and Infertility, Department of Obstetrics, Gynecology, and Reproductive Sciences, Yale School of Medicine, Yale University, New Haven, CT, United States

Nada Kubikova Nuffield Department of Women's and Reproductive Health, John Radcliffe Hospital, University of Oxford, Oxford, United Kingdom

Maria D. Lalioti Department of Translational Genomics, Goldfinch Bio, Cambridge, MA, United States

Joop S.E. Laven Division of Reproductive Endocrinology and Infertility, Erasmus University Medical Center, Rotterdam, The Netherlands

Yvonne V. Louwers Division of Reproductive Endocrinology and Infertility, Erasmus University Medical Center, Rotterdam, The Netherlands

Nick Macklon London Women's Clinic, London, United Kingdom; Zealand University Hospital, Koege, Denmark

Diego Marin IVIRMA New Jersey, Basking Ridge, NJ, United States; Thomas Jefferson University, Philadelphia, PA, United States

Julio Martín Igenomix, Valencia, Spain

Audrey A. Merriam Department of Obstetrics, Gynecology, and Reproductive Sciences, Section of Maternal-Fetal Medicine, Yale School of Medicine, New Haven, CT, United States

Heidi Mertes Department of Philosophy and Moral Science, Bioethics Institute Ghent (BIG), Ghent University, Gent, Belgium

Guido Pennings Department of Philosophy and Moral Science, Bioethics Institute Ghent (BIG), Ghent University, Gent, Belgium

Josep Pla-Victori IVI-RMA Global, Barcelona, Catalonia, Spain

Josefa María Sánchez-Reyes Department of Genomic & Systems Reproductive Medicine, IVI-RMA IVI Foundation, Valencia, Spain; Department of Pediatrics, Obstetrics and Gynaecology, School of Medicine, University of Valencia, Valencia, Spain

Emre Seli IVIRMA New Jersey, Basking Ridge, NJ, United States; Yale School of Medicine, New Haven, CT, United States

Jose Serna IVI RMA Zaragoza, Zaragoza, Spain; IVI Foundation, Madrid, Spain

Elisa Varela IVI Foundation, Madrid, Spain; IVI RMA Madrid, Madrid, Spain

Dagan Wells Nuffield Department of Women's and Reproductive Health, John Radcliffe Hospital, University of Oxford, Oxford, United Kingdom; Juno Genetics, Oxford, United Kingdom

About the editors

Juan A. García-Velasco

Dr. García-Velasco, MD, PhD, is Director of IVI Madrid. He is also a Full Professor of Obstetrics and Gynecology at Rey Juan Carlos University, Madrid, Spain, where he is Director of their Master's Degree Program in Human Reproduction. He graduated from University Medical School, Madrid, in 1990 and received his Obstetrics and Gynecology certification from La Paz Hospital, Madrid, in 1995. He completed his PhD in Medicine from Autonoma University, Madrid, in 1995 and from 1997 to 1998 he studied at Yale University, New Haven, CT, under a Reproductive Endocrinology and Infertility Fellowship. His main research interests have been in IVF and endometriosis. He is the Principal Investigator of projects funded by the Ministry of Education and Ministry of Health, Spain, and has received awards from the Spanish Fertility Society, Spanish Society of Obstetrics and Gynecology, and the European Society of Human Reproduction and Embryology. He has published over 200 peer-reviewed articles as well as 22 book chapters on human reproduction, endometriosis, and difficult cases such as women with hypo- and hyperresponse to ovarian stimulation, and is the author/editor of several books.

Emre Seli

Dr. Seli is Professor of Obstetrics, Gynecology, and Reproductive Sciences at Yale School of Medicine and Chief Scientific Officer at IVIRMA Global. He received his medical degree from the University of Istanbul and completed his Residency in Obstetrics and Gynecology at Yale University. His postdoctoral training included a fellowship in Reproductive Endocrinology and Infertility as well as a research fellowship in Molecular Biology, both at Yale University. As a physician-scientist, his primary focus is to understand and treat infertility. His laboratory characterized the mechanisms regulating translational activation of gene expression in the oocyte. Dr. Seli and his colleagues also made seminal contributions to our understanding of oocyte and embryo competence in IVF and the potential role of noninvasive diagnostic technologies in this context. Dr. Seli is the recipient of many National Institutes of Health (NIH) and pharmaceutical industry-sponsored research grants as well as numerous awards, including the Ira and Ester Rosenwaks New Investigator Award, American Society for Reproductive Medicine (ASRM), and the President's Achievement Award from the Society for Reproductive Investigation (SRI).

Preface

In the last 20 years, treatment of the infertile patient has changed dramatically, and the whole field has evolved rapidly, motivating healthcare professionals to continue their training and education. Although initially described for tubal infertility, in vitro fertilization is now offered to a much wider spectrum of patients that are being treated in assisted reproductive technology units, including fertile couples who are carriers of genetic disorders and want to have a healthy child. Within this context, genetics has advanced tremendously, and the development of new technologies has helped us better understand various medical conditions and offer targeted medical treatment options.

This book aims to present the recent genetic advances and developments that can help us (physicians and scientists committed to infertility treatment) improve the care of our patients.

The first part of the book covers the essentials of genetics for clinicians, establishing the basic understanding of cytogenetics and genetic causes of diseases, including epigenetic regulations. New developments in molecular biology are explained so healthcare providers can understand what these technologies can do for their patients and become aware of their limitations.

The second part focuses on the relationship between genetics and reproductive diseases that may cause infertility, such as endometriosis, polycystic ovary syndrome, mitochondrial diseases, premature ovarian insufficiency, and male factor. The concept of endometrial receptivity and new diagnostic approaches is also covered.

The third part describes the different new genetic tests that can be offered, including prenatal testing, expanded carrier tests, embryo biopsy and preimplantation genetic testing, and newer analysis of embryo viability without the need for a biopsy. Challenges in genetic counseling are also addressed,

This book has put together a wonderful and well-respected group of authors from all across the globe, who are experts in their fields, and their contribution will help us provide better care to our patients.

PART A

Fundamentals Of Genetics

CHAPTER

1

Basic genetics: mitosis, meiosis, chromosomes, DNA, RNA, and beyond

Amanda N. Kallen

Department of Obstetrics, Gynecology and Reproductive Sciences, Yale School of Medicine, New Haven, CT, United States

Introduction

> [The human genome is] a history book: a narrative of the journey of our species through time. It's a shop manual: an incredibly detailed blueprint for building every human cell. And it's a transformative textbook of medicine: with insights that will give health care providers immense new powers to treat, prevent and cure disease. We are delighted by what we've already seen in these books. But we are also profoundly humbled by the privilege of turning the pages that describe the miracle of human life.
>
> ***Francis Collins, Remarks at the Press Conference Announcing Sequencing and Analysis of the Human Genome [1].***

The human genome contains fundamental codes by which heritable information is stored, translated into functional data, and transmitted from one generation to the next. The completion of the Human Genome Project in 2001, an ambitious international undertaking which aimed to map all 3 billion nucleotides of the human genome, ushered in a new era in medicine [2]. Information gleaned from the Human Genome Project has been used to aid our understanding of how those genetic codes can be altered and inherited (as in the case of disease-causing hereditary mutations), manipulated (for example, as biological targets for drug-delivery systems), or utilized for diagnostic purposes (such as to allow for early detection of disease). To understand the enormous potential for advances in human health from this and other discoveries, however, it is first necessary to understand the basic building blocks of the human genome.

DNA, RNA, and protein

Nucleic acids and DNA: the building blocks

Nucleic acids are the building blocks of living organisms. There are two types of nucleic acids: *deoxyribonucleic acid* (DNA) and *ribonucleic acid* (RNA). The discovery of DNA as the "universal genetic material" came in 1953, when James Watson and Francis Crick first presented a three-dimensional, double helical model based on X-ray crystallography observations by Rosalind Franklin [3]. DNA provides the "blueprint" which allows for cellular production of proteins,

DOI: https://doi.org/10.1016/B978-0-12-816561-4.00001-6

and its presence allows for the stable storage of heritable genetic information.

A strand of DNA is composed of thousands of repeating pairs of *nucleotides*, each of which consists of a five-carbon pentose sugar (*deoxyribose*), a *phosphate group*, and a *nitrogen base*. The nitrogen bases are classified as single-ring *pyrimidines* (most commonly, cytosine C and thymine T) and double-ring *purines* (most commonly, adenine A and guanine G). To achieve the characteristic double helix structure of DNA, complementary nitrogenous base pairs (A with T, and G with C) are linked by hydrogen bonds; each nitrogenous base is also attached to an outer pentose sugar-phosphate backbone, with bases pointing inward toward each other in the chain. Nucleotides are linked by joining the phosphate group on the 5′ carbon of one nucleotide to the 3′ hydroxyl group of the next, with the complementary strand running from the 3′ to 5′ direction, conferring polarity to the DNA strand. Although the nitrogenous bases themselves are hydrophobic molecules, the orientation of the sugar-phosphate backbone results in a water-soluble structure [4]. The DNA double helix is also strongly acidic, with a high density of negative charges.

Messenger RNA: the DNA–protein intermediary

Genetic information contained in DNA is not converted directly to protein; rather, this process occurs through a single-stranded messenger RNA (mRNA) intermediary, which is synthesized from one of the two DNA strands in a double helix. Unlike DNA, RNA utilizes *ribose* as its pentose sugar, and contains the base *uracil* (*U*) instead of thymine. Thus, for RNA, A pairs with U, and G pairs with C. The process of RNA synthesis from a DNA template is referred to as *transcription* and is catalyzed by the enzyme *RNA polymerase*. After separation of the intertwined DNA strands, initiation of transcription by RNA polymerase begins on the *template strand* at a specific regulatory sequence of DNA known as a *promoter*. Recognition of the promoter requires the presence of *transcription factors*, which bind to and recognize the promoter, as well as proximal and/or distal DNA sequences known as *enhancers*, to regulate RNA polymerase activity. The presence of cell- and context-specific transcription factors and enhancers allows for cells to express a variety of genes under specific circumstances. Once transcription is initiated, addition of nucleotides continues in a 5′ to 3′ direction along the growing RNA molecule until a nucleotide *termination signal* is reached. The sequence of bases in the RNA molecule is complementary to the DNA strand, except that uracil is substituted in place of thymine [5].

After transcription, the eukaryotic messenger RNA molecule contains a protein coding sequence, as well as an upstream *5′-untranslated region* and a downstream *3′-untranslated region*. This nascent mRNA molecule, known as the *primary transcript*, undergoes further processing prior to transport out of the nucleus, including addition of a *5′ cap* (of GTP residues) and *polyadenylation* [or addition of a *poly(A) tail*], which is required for translation. Upon addition of the 5′ cap and the poly(A) tail, segments of noncoding mRNA known as *introns* are spliced out; mRNA may be spliced in different ways (*alternative splicing*) to allow for a single DNA sequence to code for different proteins [5] (Fig. 1.1).

Protein synthesis: translating the mRNA message into function

The spliced mRNA then exits the nucleus via nuclear pores and enters the cytoplasm, where the genetic information contained in the nucleic acids of mRNA is further decoded into proteins in a process known as *translation*. Proteins are required for a vast array of cellular functions including enzymatic reactions, cellular structure and shape, signaling and immune responses, and cell cycle function. Proteins are assembled from their own subunits, known as

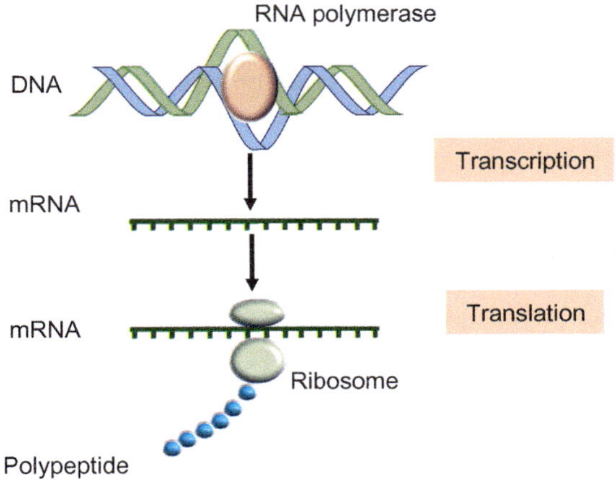

FIGURE 1.1 RNA transcription and translation. Transcription is the process by which DNA is copied to mRNA, which carries the information needed for protein synthesis. During transcription, pre-messenger RNA is formed; the resultant messenger RNA is the reverse-complement of the original DNA sequence. During RNA spicing, the pre-messenger RNA is edited to produce the desired mRNA molecule. The mRNA formed in transcription is transported out of the nucleus, into the cytoplasm, to the ribosome, where protein synthesis (translation) occurs.

amino acids. There are 20 amino acids but only four different nucleotide bases in mRNA; thus, mRNA bases encode proteins in groups of three (known as *codons*). *Ribosomes* (structures composed of *ribosomal RNA* and several proteins) bind and move along the mRNA strand, translating the codon message into a protein chain known as a *polypeptide*. This process is facilitated by a small RNA molecule known as *transfer RNA*, which contains an *anticodon* sequence that is complementary to the mRNA codon as well as the corresponding amino acid [4,6].

Gametes uniquely rely on activation and translation of stored mRNAs

The process of translation is subject to critical regulation by spatiotemporal mechanisms including translational silencing and sequestration; indeed, translational repression of mRNAs plays an important role in gametogenesis. Oocytes are unique in that suppression of transcription occurs during oocyte maturation, fertilization, and early embryo development. Thus, gene expression during this period relies on translational activation of maternally derived mRNAs, which are synthesized in large quantities prior to oocyte maturation. These mRNAs are deadenylated, thus temporarily suppressing their translation, and stored in oocyte cytoplasm, until they are utilized. Upon oocyte maturation, translation of stored mRNAs is mediated via two mechanisms: some mRNAs will undergo further extension of poly(A) tails (*cytoplasmic polyadenylation*), a process specific to gametes, embryos, and neurons; others will undergo translation in a polyadenylation-independent manner. Both of these processes require interaction between the mRNA 3′-UTR and *cis*-acting elements in the 3′-UTR of the mRNA. Likewise, during the sperm maturation process, transcription in mid-spermatogenesis depends on dormant paternal mRNAs. However, in spermatids, removal of poly(A) tails (rather than elongation, as in oocytes) appears to be the primary mechanism by which translation is reactivated [7].

Noncoding RNAs: not "genetic junk"

Noncoding RNAs (ncRNAs) are a diverse group of functional RNA molecules which are transcribed from DNA, but—unlike mRNA—are not translated into protein. For many years, this noncoding portion of the genome was viewed primarily as "genetic junk." Indeed, in a 1957 lecture outlining key ideas about gene function, Francis Crick argued that "the main function of the genetic material is to control...the synthesis of proteins" [8], a concept often referred to as the "Central Dogma" of molecular biology [9]. At that time, only ribosomal RNAs and transfer RNAs were recognized for their roles in protein synthesis. However, it has been gradually recognized that there are vast classes of ncRNAs, and that these molecules play critical roles in numerous biological processes including regulation of other RNA subtypes, gene imprinting, and transcriptional regulation [10]. The Nobel Prize-winning discovery of the concept of "RNA interference," or RNA-dependent gene silencing initiated by small noncoding RNAs was a significant scientific breakthrough [11], and the variety of RNA types, and the complexity of functions encoded in RNA molecules, is now much more complex than was previously believed. While a full review of nonprotein-coding RNA classes and functions is beyond the scope of this chapter, noncoding transcripts can be broadly categorized into "housekeeping" RNAs (a group including transfer RNA, ribosomal RNA, and small nuclear and nucleolar RNA, among others) and regulatory RNAs (which includes long noncoding RNAs (lncRNAs), small interfering RNAs (siRNAs), Piwi-associated RNAS, and microRNAs) [11,12]. ncRNAs can also be classified by size, into small (<200 nucleotides) and long (>200 nucleotides) ncRNAs [13] (Fig. 1.2).

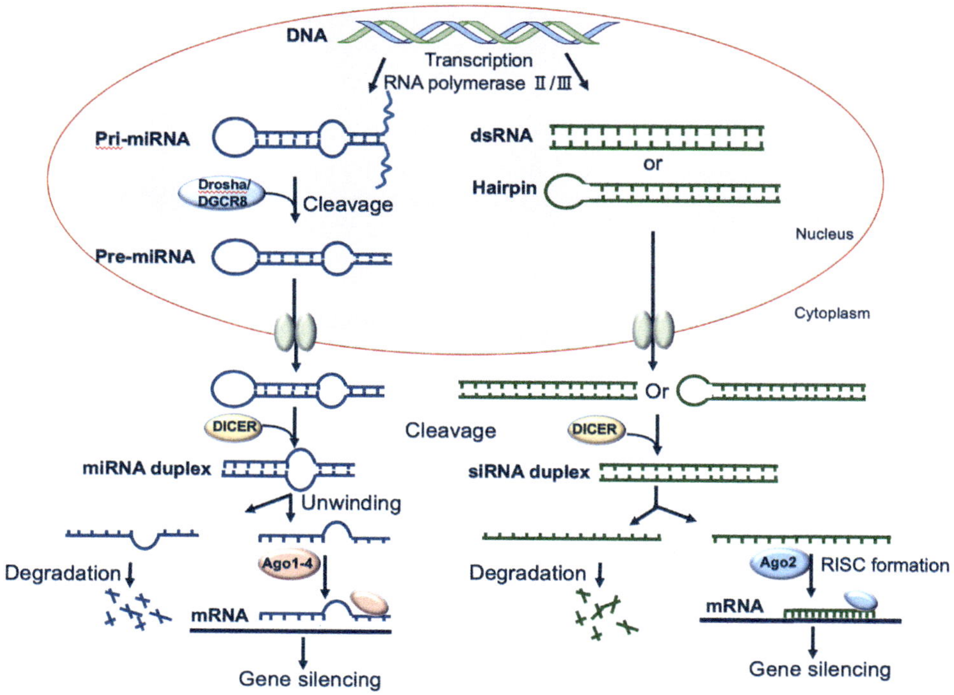

FIGURE 1.2 Coding and noncoding RNAs.Transcription of miRNA genes is carried out by RNA polymerase II in the nucleus to give pri-miRNA, which is then cleaved by Drosha to form pre-miRNA. The pre-miRNA is transported to the cytoplasm where it is processed by Dicer into miRNA. The miRNA is loaded into the RNA induced silencing complex (RISC) where the passenger strand is discarded, and the miRISC is guided by the remaining guide strand to the target mRNA through partially complementary binding. The target mRNA is inhibited via translational repression, degradation or cleavage. For siRNA, dsRNA is processed by Dicer into siRNA which is loaded into the RISC. AGO2, which is a component of RISC, cleaves the passenger strand of siRNA. The guide strand then guides the active RISC to the target mRNA. The full complementary binding between the guide strand of siRNA and the target mRNA leads to the cleavage of mRNA.

Perhaps the best-characterized small ncRNAs are the microRNAs (miRNAs), 21–22-nucleotide ncRNAs that suppress gene expression by silencing mRNA translation or leading to target mRNA degradation. miRNAs recognize their target mRNA 3′-UTR sites by their first eight residues on the 5′-end (the "seed sequence") and form Watson–Crick base pairing [14]. Multiple miRNAs are expressed in human oocytes, including miRNAs targeting genes involved in DNA repair and cell cycle checkpoints [15]. Because oocytes (and embryos) contain higher levels of Dicer (an enzyme required for miRNA biosynthesis) than any other cells or tissues [16,17] and because Dicer-specific knockouts exhibit meiotic defects [16,18,19], it has been postulated that miRNAs are essential in the development of oocytes. However, targeted deletion of DGCR8 (an RNA-binding protein specifically required for miRNA processing) in mice results in oocytes that mature normally and exhibit mRNA profiles which are essentially identical to wild-type oocytes. DGCR8−/− embryos also develop normally to the blastocyst stage (though late embryonic defects are observed and embryonic arrest occurs at E6.5–7.5 postimplantation), and DGCR8-deficient female mice produce healthy (albeit fewer) offspring [20].

Endogenous siRNAs, another class of ncRNAs, function to silence gene expression via cleavage of target mRNAs. Like miRNAs, siRNAs recognize their target mRNA 3′-UTR sites; however, unlike miRNAs, they require full complementarity in order to suppress translation of the target transcript. siRNA processing bypasses DGCR8 but is still subject to cleavage by Dicer [20]. Evidence to support the importance of siRNAs in oocyte development stems from several mouse models. Mice with catalytically inactivated oocyte Ago2 [an Agonaute (AGO) protein family member which mediates siRNA-led target mRNA silencing], exhibit disrupted siRNA function, but intact miRNA processing. These mice display abnormal spindle formation, chromosomal misalignment, and defective oocyte maturation [21]. Given the dramatic effects observed after targeted siRNA pathway disruption in oocytes (in comparison with the minimal effects observed after miRNA suppression), it is becoming increasingly clear that siRNAs, rather than miRNAs, may serve as the primary RNA silencing mechanism during oocyte and early embryo development.

Piwi-interacting RNAs (piRNAs) are a class of small RNAs found almost exclusively in germ cells [22,23]. PiRNAs form RNA–protein complexes by binding to a specific class of proteins known as Piwi proteins; these piRNA–protein complexes are involved in epigenetic and posttranscriptional gene silencing of transposable elements in germ cells (particularly spermatogenic cells). piRNAs are synthesized from long, single-stranded RNA precursor sequences, are larger than miRNAs (26–31 nt), and their processing does not require Dicer; [24] in many respects their mechanism of biogenesis still remains unclear. Female mouse Piwi mutants do not display defective oocytes in contrast to Piwi protein mutant male mice, which exhibit altered spermatogenesis and depletion of spermatogonia [24]. Thus, piRNAs appear to be essential for male gametogenesis.

While the functional small noncoding RNA classes share significant overlap in their processing pathways and molecular interactions, they differ in the mechanism by which they are processed to their mature forms. However, one commonality is that all small ncRNAs utilize the involvement of the AGO family of proteins, which bind different classes of small ncRNAs and their complementary mRNAs and induce cleavage or translational inhibition. Additionally, multiple RNA interference pathways (but not all) utilize the Dicer enzyme, an RNAse III involved in processing double-stranded precursor RNA into mature single-strand RNA fragments [14–19].

The function of lncRNAs, which are more than 200 nucleotides in length, is diverse. lncRNAs can interact with DNA, RNA, and proteins, and act as molecular scaffolds [25], guides to a specific target locus [26], decoys or sponges [27], and enhancers of transcriptional activity [28]. LncRNAs are expressed in a stage-specific manner in human preimplantation embryos [29,30], suggesting involvement of these lncRNAs in preimplantation development. Additionally, in comparison to mouse embryos, lncRNA networks in eight-cell human embryos most closely resemble those of mouse two-cell stage embryos [29], emphasizing the importance of further examination of the functions of lncRNAs in human early embryonic development directly.

Genes and chromosomes

DNA is organized into chromosomes

DNA found in the nucleus (*nuclear DNA*) is organized into linear, functional sequences called *genes*, which carry genetic information. Long, threadlike segments of cellular DNA containing multiple genes are known as *chromosomes*. Genes can be considered as a set of heritable "instructions" for the development and function of an organism, and they allow for the transmission of genetic information from one generation to the next. However, genes are only a small segment of total DNA. The *genome* is the total sum of all genetic sequences in an organism. A notable finding from the Human Genome Project was that the previous guesses at the number of human genes (from 50,000 to 140,000) grossly overestimated the actual number of genes (about 20,500). Another discovery from the Human Genome Project was that the protein-coding portion of the genome accounts for just a fraction of its total length (about 2%). In addition to genes coding for protein, chromosomes have long segments of noncoding DNA, as described in the previous section. Chromosomes, along with their accessory protein molecules which help maintain structure, are known as *chromatin* [5].

In addition to the linear, double-stranded DNA structure, chromosomes also contain a *centromere* (usually located near or at the middle of the chromosome), and a complex of proteins positioned at the centromere known as a kinetochore; these structures join identical *sister chromatids* together and facilitate chromosome separation during cell division. Chromosomes also contain *telomeres* at their ends, which prevent DNA shortening at the time of replication (Fig. 1.3). Humans have two duplicate sets of 23 different chromosomes (for a total of 46) as well as a sex chromosome (either X or Y). These chromosomes are located in the nucleus of the cell, where transcription occurs; mRNA then passes into cytoplasm for translational processing [5].

Because long eukaryotic chromosomes must be packaged into a cell nucleus, they rely on contributions from protein scaffolds to maintain their compact, supercoiled shape. DNA is

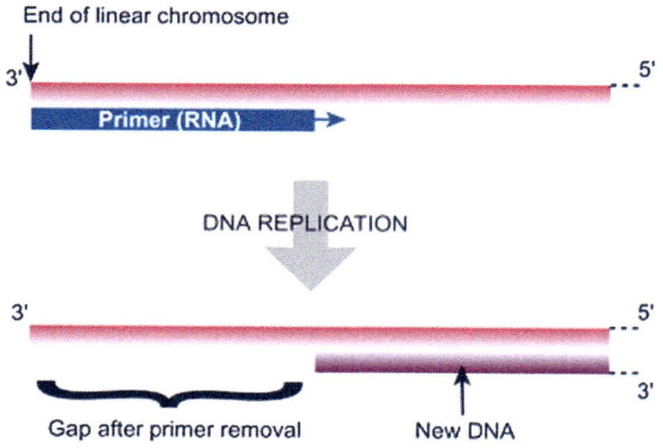

FIGURE 1.3 Ends of linear chromosomes. When an RNA primer is removed after initiating a strand of linear DNA the gap cannot be filled by DNA as there is no upstream 3′-hydroxyl to accept nucleotides. This would result in shortening of linear DNA during each replication cycle. Eukaryotes have solved the problem of replicating linear DNA by using structures known as telomeres.

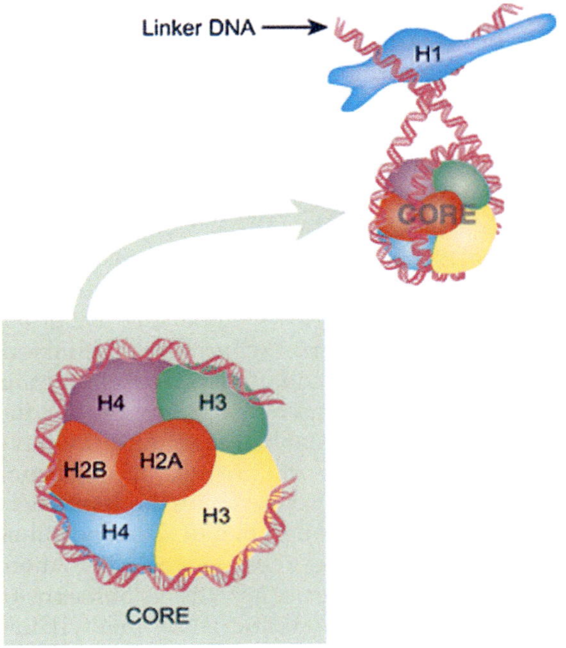

FIGURE 1.4 The basic unit in the folding of eukaryotic DNA is the nucleosome, which consists of a segment of DNA coiled around a specialized protein known as a histone.

wrapped around specialized proteins called *histones*; a segment of DNA coiled around a histone is known as a *nucleosome*. These nucleosomes are further compacted into *fibers* and *loops*. The term *chromatin* indicates DNA and the proteins maintaining its structure (Fig. 1.4) [5].

Mitochondria also contain DNA and chromosomes

While most cellular DNA is located in the nucleus, DNA is also found in mitochondria, the double-membrane-bound intracellular organelles essential for anaerobic metabolism and energy production. Unlike the large, linear structure of nuclear DNA chromosomes, which contain approximately 3 billion base

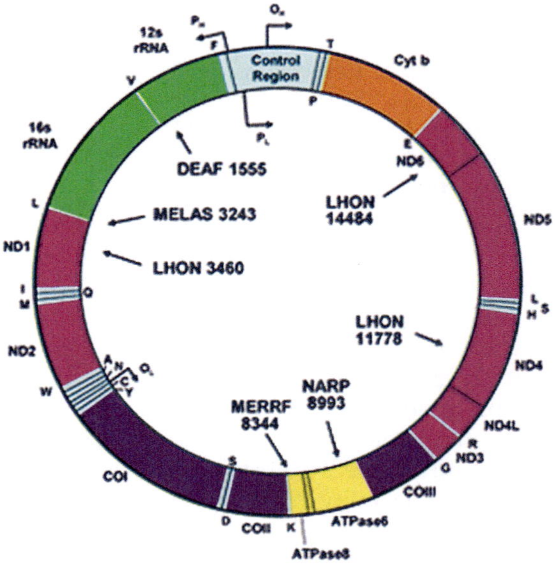

FIGURE 1.5 Mitochondrial DNA structure. Mitochondrial DNA is typically diagrammed as a circular structure with genes and regulatory regions labeled.

pairs, mtDNA chromosomes are small structures (spanning about 16,500 nucleotides) and are packaged in a double-stranded, closed, circular formation (Fig. 1.5). Human mitochondrial DNA (mtDNA) is inherited solely from the mother, except in rare cases of inheritance of both maternal and paternal mtDNA [31,32].

mtDNA encodes 37 genes which are essential for mitochondrial function, including genes encoding tRNA, rRNA, and enzymes involved in oxidative phosphorylation and synthesis of adenosine triphosphate. Mitochondria contain cellular machinery to maintain, replicate, and transcribe their own mtDNA. The mitochondrial genome is polypoid; cells contain thousands of copies of mtDNA. mtDNA mutation rates are on the order of 100-fold higher than those of nuclear DNA, and individuals may harbor a mixture of wild-type and mutant mtDNA (*heteroplasmy*). However, the burden of mutant mtDNA must reach a particular threshold for clinical manifestations of a mitochondrial disorder to occur (the *threshold effect*) [2,31,32].

Regulation of gene expression: posttranslational modifications and imprinting

Gene expression is primarily regulated at the level of transcription; that is, cells can initiate or silence the expression of certain genes by initiating mRNA synthesis from DNA. However, gene expression can also be further modulated in posttranscriptional manner by a number of complex processes. Cells can alter mRNA longevity via a mechanism that promote stability or increase mRNA decay rates. ncRNAs can further modify the stability and expression of target mRNAs. Mature protein products may be synthesized via posttranslational modification of inactive precursor polypeptides.

Most mammalian genes are expressed equally from the maternal and paternal allele (*biallelic* expression). However, a small subset of genes—those that are *imprinted*—are expressed solely from one parental chromosome (*monoallelic* expression), conferring parent-specific origin to a particular gene. The study of *epigenetics* concerns heritable changes in gene expression, such as imprinting, which do not involve alterations in DNA sequence. Imprinted genes (of which about 150 have been identified in the mammalian genome [33]) are essential for normal growth and development. The expression of imprinted genes does not follow the usual rules of inheritance, which would dictate that both parental alleles are equally expressed. Instead, for example, an imprinted gene that is active on a maternally inherited chromosome will be expressed only from the maternal chromosome, and the paternal contribution will be silenced; the expression pattern would be reversed for a paternally imprinted gene. Imprinted genes generally cluster together in regions which also contain a regulatory segment of DNA known as the imprinting control region. A major mechanism for regulation of imprinting is DNA methylation, or the transfer and covalent attachment of a methyl group from *S*-adenosyl-L-methionine to a cytosine residue. DNA methylation frequently occurs along long stretches of cytosine-guanine dinucleotide residues (or *CpG islands*, where the "p" delineates a phosphodiester bond linking C and G), catalyzed by *DNA methyltransferases*. Genomic regions with allele-specific methylation status are known as *differentially methylated regions* [33].

Methylation marks can be maintained through successive cell divisions, propagating specific patterns of gene expression and contributing to the establishment and maintenance of lineage. Following fertilization, maternal and paternal genomes undergo erasure of most methylation marks (*demethylation*); DNA methylation is then reestablished after implantation. In particular, the establishment of correct germline-specific DNA methylation patterns is crucial, as failure to establish appropriate germline methylation marks can have serious consequences for gametogenesis and embryo development. DNA methylation is essential for spermatogenesis; loss of DNMT3A or DNMT3l (two specific DNA methyltransferases) leads to spermatocyte apoptosis and sterility. Mammalian oocytes, in contrast, tolerate loss of methylation until postfertilization, at which point embryos conceived from DNMT3L methyltransferase-deficient oocytes die [34].

DNA methylation is not the only mechanism responsible for the regulation of imprinted genes. Like DNA, histones can undergo modification via methylation, acetylation, and other processes; these regulatory marks allow histones to store epigenetic information and participate in transcriptional activation or repression. Loss of imprinting of specific genes is associated with the development of congenital disorders including Prader–Willi syndrome and Angelman syndrome, and Beckwith–Wiedemann syndrome and Silver–Russell syndrome (the H19/IGF2 domain). Some studies also suggest that the use of assisted reproductive technologies such as *in vitro fertilization* is associated with disorders of imprinting [33].

DNA replication, mitosis, and meiosis: passing on genetic information

DNA replication duplicates cellular DNA

During cellular division, chromosomes divide and distribute from parent to daughter cells. This necessitates that, prior to division, cellular DNA must be duplicated, a process known as *DNA replication*. The process of DNA replication begins with the separation of DNA strands. Because the two helical DNA strands are wound together, separation of the strands without unwinding the entire DNA molecule requires breaking of a strand via *DNA helicase* enzyme. *Single-stranded binding protein* then binds the unwound DNA, preventing re-annealing of the two parent strands. A class of enzymes known as *DNA polymerases* is then responsible for elongation of the new DNA strands. The discovery of one of these polymerases, DNA polymerase I, led to a Nobel Prize for Arthur Kornberg in 1959. Because DNA polymerase cannot initiate new sites of DNA replication from free nucleotides, the process is initiated by a type of RNA polymerase (*RNA primase*), which catalyzes formation of a short RNA primer strand. Upon release of the RNA polymerase, DNA replication proceeds by DNA polymerase via addition of nucleotides to the hydroxyl group at the 3′ end of the elongating chain. DNA replication is initiated at a specific sequence on the *DNA template* (the *origin of* replication), and replication (or *polymerization)* proceeds in both directions at the *replication fork*, producing two elongating, antiparallel DNA strands (one running 5′ to 3′ and the other 3′ to 5′) [4]. However, DNA polymerases can also only catalyze DNA replication in the 5′ to 3′ direction. Thus, synthesis occurs on the *leading strand* in the 5′ to 3′ direction via continuous addition of nucleotides, and occurs on the *lagging strand* via addition of short fragments of DNA (Okazaki fragments) onto new RNA primers. Gaps between Okazaki fragments are filled in by DNA polymerase (which degrades the RNA fragments) and *DNA ligase* (which seals DNA ends together). When mismatches (i.e., incorrect addition of bases to the growing strand) occur, a *3′ exonuclease* removes the incorrect base (the nascent DNA is checked and repaired again at completion of replication by the *mismatch repair* system). Errors during DNA replication which are not repaired can result in alterations within the sequence of the gene; these *polymorphisms* may have no effect on the resulting gene product, or may severely disrupt gene function (*mutations*), depending on the size and location of the variant.

A unique problem arises at the end of the elongating DNA strand. If the terminal (5′) RNA primer were to be removed without replacement, essential genetic information could be lost, because DNA polymerase cannot initiate replacement of this short sequence without an RNA primer. However, the presence of *telomeres* (short nucleotide repeats) at the ends of DNA allow for chromosome shortening without loss of genetic information. Additionally, the enzyme *telomerase*, which carries its own small RNA primer, replaces the lost DNA sequences in cells where it is present.

DNA replication is error-prone

Errors during DNA replication can occur for multiple reasons. Nucleotides may be mismatched (i.e., an A mispaired with a G instead of a T), or a nucleotide base may be added or deleted. While DNA polymerase replicates DNA with high fidelity, errors occur at a rate of about 1 per 100,000 (which roughly translates, in a human cell with 600,000 base pairs, to 120,000 errors per cell division [35]). DNA polymerases can correct these errors through *proofreading* (in which the wrongly positioned or incorrect nucleotide is recognized and removed), which fixes the majority of DNA replication errors. Remaining errors are addressed via *mismatch repair*, during which incorrect nucleotides are excised and replaced with the correct nucleotide. Errors that are not repaired, but persist through cell division, become permanent mutations in the cellular DNA (such as *insertions* and *deletions*).

Mitosis

Mitosis is the process by which a cell nucleus splits in two, and is followed by division of the parent cell. The goal of mitosis is to achieve division of the genetic data contained in somatic cells, generating daughter cells with identical genetic information. At mitosis, disassembly of the nuclear membrane, division of chromosomes, and reassembly of nuclear membranes and division of the mother cell occurs.

Prior to mitosis, the cell undergoes *G1*, a phase of cell growth (Fig. 1.6), the *S-phase*, during which DNA replication occurs, and a second growth phase, *G2*, in preparation for cell division. Collectively, these phases (G1, S, and G2) are known as *interphase*. Mitosis consists of four distinct phases: *prophase, metaphase, anaphase, and telophase*. During prophase, which occurs after the conclusion of the G2 growth phase, nuclear chromosomes begin to compact, and can be visualized under light microscopy as sister chromatids. Each *centrosome* with its associated *centrioles* migrates to an opposite pole of the cell, and the *mitotic spindle*, a microtubule and protein structure that facilitates chromosome alignment and separation, begins to form. During metaphase, chromosomes align along the midpole of the cell (known as the *metaphase plate*). At anaphase, sister chromosomes separate and are pulled toward opposite poles of the cell by fibers of the mitosis spindle. During telophase, the mitotic spindle disassembles and the nuclear membrane reassembles separately around each group of chromosomes. Finally, the parent cell splits in a process known as *cytokinesis*, completing cellular division [5]. Cells undergoing mitosis are subject to errors including *nondisjunction* (failure of sister chromatids to separate, resulting in daughter cells which are *aneuploid* with too few and/or too many chromosomes).

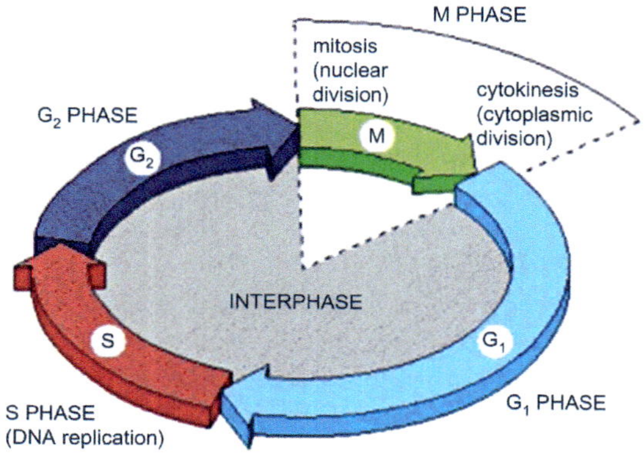

FIGURE 1.6 The cell cycle. The cell grows continuously in interphase, which consists of three phases: DNA replication is confined to S phase; G1 is the gap between M phase and S phase, while G2 is the gap between S phase and M phase. In M phase, the nucleus and then the cytoplasm divide.

Meiosis

In contrast to mitosis, the process of *meiosis* achieves cell division for the purpose of gamete formation (Fig. 1.7). The endpoint of mitosis is the generation of genetically distinct, haploid (n) cells that can fertilize with other gametes. Meiosis consists of two divisions: meiosis I and meiosis II. As in mitosis, a parent cell about to enter meiosis first undergoes DNA replication, resulting in a duplicated set of chromosomes (2n). Meiosis I is a unique process, occurring only in germ cells. First, the cell enters *prophase I*, during which chromatin condenses and homologous chromosomes (each consisting of linked sister chromatids) begin to pair, exchange genetic material, and reseal at points

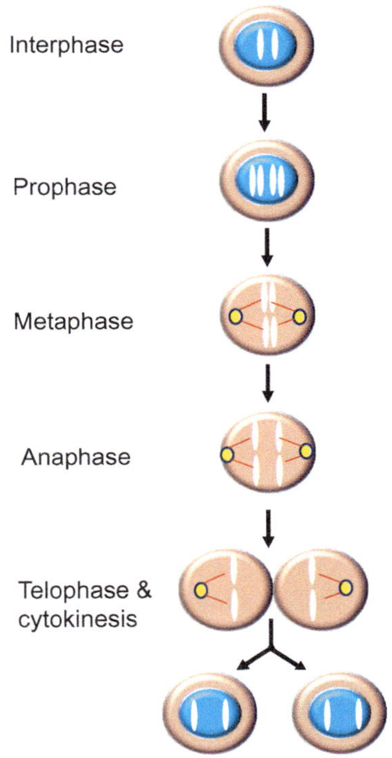

FIGURE 1.7 Principles of Mitosis. Prior to mitosis, the cell undergoes a phase of cell growth and replication known as interphase. During prophase, chromatin in the nucleus begins to condense and becomes visible as chromosomes. The nucleolus disappears. Centrioles begin moving to opposite ends of the cell and fibers extend from the centromeres. Some fibers cross the cell to form the mitotic spindle. In metaphase, spindle fibers align the chromosomes along the middle of the cell nucleus, the metaphase plate. During anaphase, paired chromosomes separate at the kinetochores and move to opposite sides of the cell. In telophase, chromatids arrive at opposite poles of cell, and new membranes form around the daughter nuclei. Cytokinesis results when the center of the cell contracts pinching the cell into two daughter cells, each with one nucleus.

known as *chiasmata*. This process is known as *crossing over* or *homologous recombination*, and the exchange of DNA segments between chromosomes increases the genetic diversity of the resulting gametes, as the end result is paired chromosomes containing genetic material from both oocyte and sperm. During *metaphase I*, the nucleus is no longer visible, and homologous chromosomal pairs align along the metaphase plate. Each chromosome in a pair is equally likely to be found on either side of the midplane of the cell, leading to random assortment of chromosomes in subsequent daughter cells (a process known as *independent assortment*). Genes in close proximity to one another on the same chromosome are considered *linked* and are less likely to become "unlinked" via independent assortment or crossing over. In *anaphase I*, microtubule shortening leads to separation and movement of chromosome pairs to opposite poles of the parent cell. During *telophase I*, chromosomes are separated by the formation of two new nuclei, and *cytokinesis* follows. At completion of meiosis I, chromosome pairs (consisting of linked sister chromatids) have been redistributed to each daughter cell, rendering each daughter cell 1n (one set of chromosomes), 2c (two sister chromatids) [6].

Meiosis II follows meiosis I and is similar to a mitotic division, except that it is not preceded by DNA replication. In *prophase II*, sister chromatids again condense and centrosomes move to opposite poles of the parent cell. During *metaphase II*, single chromosomes align vertically on the metaphase plate (in contrast to *metaphase II*, when pairs of homologous sister chromatids line up in the cell midline). In *anaphase II*, these sister chromatids are separated by the mitotic spindle, and during *telophase II*, complete separation of sister chromatids has occurred and two distinct nuclear membranes form. Meiosis II results in four haploid cells, such that the resulting gametes are 1n, 1c. Each of these cells has one copy each of 43 chromosomes, each with a unique genetic signature. Through this process, germ cells (oocytes and sperm) are produced (Fig. 1.8) [6].

Meiosis differs from mitosis in that two sets of cell division occur, resulting in four unique haploid genomes, and in that the processes of

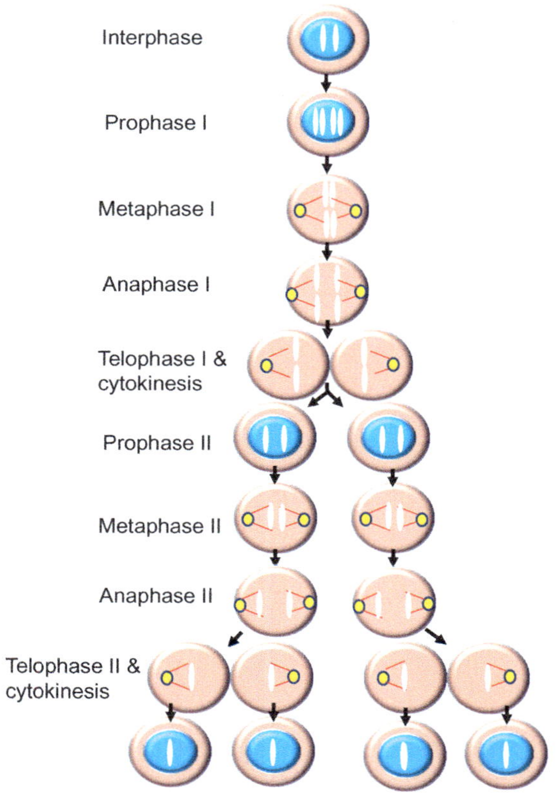

FIGURE 1.8 Meiosis. After interphase, meiosis I (the first meiotic division), begins with prophase I, similar to mitosis. Chromatin in the nucleus begins to condense and becomes visible as chromosomes, and the nucleolus disappears. In metaphase, spindle fibers align along the chromosomes along the middle of the cell nucleus, the metaphase plate. During anaphase, paired chromosomes separate at the kinetochores and move to opposite sides of the cell. In telophase, chromatids arrive at opposite poles of cell, and new membranes form around the daughter nuclei. The cell now undergoes cytokinesis that divides the cytoplasm of the original cell into two daughter cells. Each daughter cell is haploid and has only one set of chromosomes, or half the total number of chromosomes of the original cell. Meiosis II is a mitotic division of each of the haploid cells produced in meiosis I. At the conclusion of meiosis, there are four haploid daughter cells that go on to develop into either sperm or egg cells.

recombination and independent assortment add genetic diversity. Cells undergoing meiosis are subject to error during both meiosis I and meiosis II. Errors may involve failure of division of either whole chromosomes or sister chromatids. Such errors can include *nondisjunction* (the failure of chromosomes or sister chromatids to separate), *nonhomologous recombination* between chromosomes, or *premature homologue* or *sister chromatid separation* (early loss of connections between homologous chromosomes or sister chromatids), all of which can result in gametes with a missing or extra chromosome or sister chromatid.

And beyond—is the human genome “editable”?

Genome editing occurs also as a natural process—via insertions, deletions, or modifications of cellular DNA. However, genome editing (also called gene editing) can also be achieved via several scientifically engineered approaches. These technologies allow genetic material to be added, removed, or altered at particular locations in the genome. Several approaches to genome editing have been developed. Among the available methods, *Crispr/Cas9*, a method which utilizes endonucleases to generate targeted double-stranded DNA breaks (resulting in activation of cellular DNA repair machinery via nonhomologous end joining or homologous recombination), appears promising due to its efficiency, cost, and ease of use. However, major concerns exist regarding the use of this technology, especially if used to perform germline and/or embryo editing (which would result in genomic changes that would be passed on to future generations). These concerns include the possibility for off-target effects at other genomic locations, and lack of efficiency or inaccurate repair resulting in mosaic embryos [36]. While many countries have discouraged or banned research on germline editing at this time, ongoing public deliberation and debate can be expected to keep this issue at the forefront of scientific discussion.

References

[1] Remarks at the Press Conference Announcing Sequencing and Analysis of the Human Genome [Internet]. Available from: <https://www.genome.gov/10001379/february-2001-working-draft-of-human-genome-director-collins/>.

[2] The Human Genome Project: Frequently Asked Questions [Internet]. Available from: <https://www.genome.gov/11006943/human-genome-project-completion-frequently-asked-questions/>.

[3] The Francis Crick Papers: The Discovery of the Double Helix, 1951-1953 [Internet]. Available from: <https://profiles.nlm.nih.gov/SC/Views/Exhibit/narrative/doublehelix.html>.

[4] K.B. Ahluwalia, Genetics, New Age International, 2009, ProQuest Ebook Central, <https://ebookcentral.proquest.com/lib/yale-ebooks/detail.action?docID = 437721>.

[5] Clark DP, Pazdernik NJ, McGehee M. Molecular Biology. Academic Cell; 2018.

[6] Powar C. Genetics. Himalaya Publishing House; 2006.

[7] Esencan E, Kallen A, Zhang M, Seli E. Translational activation of maternally-derived mRNAs in oocytes and early embryos and the role of embryonic poly(A) binding protein. Biol Reprod 2019;100(5):1147–57.

[8] Crick F. Central dogma of molecular biology. Nature 1970;227:561–3.

[9] Cobb M. 60 years ago, Francis Crick changed the logic of biology. PLoS Biol 2017;15(9):1–8.

[10] Cech TR, Steitz JA. Review The noncoding RNA revolution—trashing old rules to forge new ones. Cell [Internet] 2014;157(1):77–94. Available from: https://doi.org/10.1016/j.cell.2014.03.008. Available from.

[11] A.Z. Fire, C.C. Mello, The Nobel Prize in Physiology or Medicine 2006 [Internet]. Nobel Media AB. Available from: <http://www.nobelprize.org/nobel_prizes/medicine/laureates/2006/>, 2014 (cited 21.06.18).

[12] Szymanski M, Erdmann V, Barcizewski J. Riboregulators: an overview. Noncoding RNAs: Molecular Biology and Molecular Medicine. Kluwer Academic/Plenum Publishers; 2003. p. 1–6.

[13] Brosnan CA, Voinnet O. The long and the short of noncoding RNAs. Curr Opin Cell Biol 2009;21(3):416–25.

[14] Bartel DP. Review MicroRNAs: target recognition and regulatory functions. Cell. 2009;136(2):215–33.

[15] Tulay P, Naja RP, Cascales-Roman O, Doshi A, Serhal P, SenGupta SB. Investigation of microRNA expression and DNA repair gene transcripts in human oocytes and blastocysts. J Assist Reprod Genet 2015;32(12):1757–64.

[16] Eisenberg I, Kotaja N, Goldman-Wohl D, Imbar T. microRNA: medical evidence. Adv Exp Med Biol [Internet] 2015;888:353–87. Available from: http://link.springer.com/10.1007/978-3-319-22671-2.

[17] Su AI, Cooke MP, Ching KA, Hakak Y, Walker JR, Wiltshire T, et al. Large-scale analysis of the human and mouse transcriptomes. Proc Natl Acad Sci USA 2002;99(7):4465–70.

[18] Imbar T, Eisenberg I. Regulatory role of microRNAs in ovarian function. Fertil Steril [Internet] 2014;101(6):1524–30. Available from: https://doi.org/10.1016/j.fertnstert.2014.04.024. Available from.

[19] Lei L, Jin S, Gonzalez G, Behringer RR, Woodruff TK. The regulatory role of Dicer in folliculogenesis in mice Mol Cell Endocrinol [Internet] 2010;315(1–2):63–73 [cited 2017 Aug 22] Available from. Available from: http://ac.els-cdn.com/S0303720709005048/1-s2.0-S0303720709005048-main.pdf?_tid = dc244350-8778-11e7-953a-00000aab0f01&acdnat = 1503434061_0d32b51ec283744433c540a6504e0e46.

[20] Suh N, Baehner L, Moltzahn F, Melton C, Shenoy A, Chen J. Report microRNA function is globally suppressed in mouse oocytes and early embryos. Curr Biol [Internet] 2010;20(3):271–7. Available from: https://doi.org/10.1016/j.cub.2009.12.044. Available from.

[21] Stein P, Rozhkov NV, Li F, Cárdenas FL, Davydenk O, Vandivier LE, et al. Essential role for endogenous siRNAs during meiosis in mouse oocytes. PLoS Genet 2015;11(2):1–19.

[22] Grivna ST, Beyret E, Wang Z, Lin H. Research communication. A novel class of small RNAs in mouse spermatogenic cells. Genes Dev 2006;20(13):1709–14.

[23] Embryos E, Roovers EF, Rosenkranz D, Roelen BAJ, Roovers EF, Rosenkranz D, et al. Piwi proteins and piRNAs in mammalian oocytes and resource piwi proteins and piRNAs in mammalian oocytes and early embryos. Cell Rep 2015;10(12):2069–82.

[24] Ketting RF. Review. The many faces of RNAi. Dev Cell 2011;20(2):148–61.

[25] Guttman M, Rinn JL. Modular regulatory principles of large non-coding RNAs. Nature. 2012;482(345):1240–1.

[26] Schorderet P, Duboule D. Structural and functional differences in the long non- coding RNA hotair in mouse and human. PLoS Genet 2011;7(5):1–10.

[27] Kallen AN, Zhou XB, Xu J, Qiao C, Ma J, Yan L, et al. The imprinted H19 lncRNA antagonizes Let-7 microRNAs. Mol Cell 2013;52(1):101–12.

[28] Ørom UA, Shiekhattar R. Minireview long noncoding RNAs Usher in a new era in the biology of enhancers. Cell [Internet] 2013;154(6):1190–3.

[29] Qiu J, Ren Z, Yan J. Identification and functional analysis of long non-coding RNAs in human and mouse

early embryos based on single-cell transcriptome data. Oncotarget 2016;7(38):61215–28.
[30] Yan L, Yang M, Guo H, Yang L, Wu J, Li R, et al. Single-cell RNA-Seq profiling of human preimplantation embryos and embryonic stem cells. Nat Struct Mol Biol [Internet] 2013;20(9):1131–9. Available from: https://doi.org/10.1038/nsmb.2660.
[31] Parr RL, Martin LH. Mitochondrial and nuclear genomics and the emergence of personalized medicine. Hum Genomics 2012;6(1):1–8.
[32] Chial H, Craig J. MtDNA and mitochondrial diseases. Nat Educ 2008;1(1):217.
[33] Weaver J, Bartolomei M. Chromatin regulators of genomic imprinting. Biochim Biophys Acta Mol Basis Dis 2014;1839(3):169–77.
[34] Stewart K, Veselovska L, Kelsey G. Establishment and functions of DNA methylation in the germline. Epigenomics 2016;8(10):1399–413.
[35] Pray L. DNA replication and causes of mutations. Nat Educ 2008;1(1):214.
[36] Doudna JA, Charpentier E. The new frontier of genome engineering with CRISPR-Cas9. Science (80–) 2014;346(6213):1258096.

CHAPTER

2

Identification of genetic causes of gynecologic disorders

Alexander Kotlyar[1] *and Maria D. Lalioti*[2]

[1]Section of Reproductive Endocrinology and Infertility, Department of Obstetrics, Gynecology, and Reproductive Sciences, Yale School of Medicine, Yale University, New Haven, CT, United States

[2]Department of Translational Genomics, Goldfinch Bio, Cambridge, MA, United States

Introduction

Since the discovery of the double helix in 1953, the genetic causes of human disease have become increasingly understood. This has not only influenced our diagnostic approaches to disease, but has also led to treatments targeting the resultant defect. One prime example is identification of the BCR-ABL fusion gene in chronic myelogenous leukemia and the use of a specific kinase inhibitor, Imatinib, to curtail the function of this aberrant protein. This has led to dramatic improvements in treatment of this disease. Similar approaches have been undertaken in the field of gynecology for both benign and malignant disease. This text will focus on the methods used to discover numerous key genetic causes of gynecologic disease, understand the pathogenesis, and improve the diagnostic potential. Advanced genetics methods discussed below have revealed the absolutely fascinating complexity of the genome and the interplay of regulatory mechanisms that safeguard homeostasis and health.

The Human Genome Project, Mendelian and complex genetic inheritance

The Human Genome Project is one of the most ambitious and influential projects undertaken in genetics and provided a wealth of information that benefits science and medicine today [1]. As a result of this effort, the precise position of genes and polymorphic elements in humans have been precisely mapped, and open the way for studying regulatory elements. The human genome contains 3 billion base pairs and has the estimated 20,000–25,000 genes that code for proteins and numerous noncoding regions that modulate the expression of genes or noncoding RNAs. These include promoters that are crucial in initiating gene expression, enhancers which increase expression, splicing modulators, and

Human Reproductive Genetics
DOI: https://doi.org/10.1016/B978-0-12-816561-4.00002-8

noncoding RNA elements leading to the production of small RNAs including but not limited to microRNAs, snoRNAs, and others, which modulate gene expression.

Genetic diseases can be categorized into monogenic or polygenic. Monogenic or Mendelian are those diseases caused by defects in one or a handful of genes, following roughly the mode of inheritance that Mendel observed in the 19th century. Polygenic or complex diseases are those that have a less well-defined mode of inheritance and may be caused by variation in several genomic regions. Polygenic, more than Mendelian diseases, are often subject to incomplete penetrance, in other words not all individuals that carry the genetic risk factors will develop the disease. In addition, the natural environment and life habits, including diet and exercise, have substantial interactions with the genome in promoting or preventing disease. Cystic fibrosis and spinal muscular atrophy are examples of Mendelian diseases, while several neurological diseases, such as Alzheimer's and Parkinson's, and most cancers including gynecologic ones, are genetically complex. Interestingly, there are gynecologic cancers that follow both modes of inheritance in different individuals. For example, breast cancer can be caused by *BRCA1* or *BRCA2* mutations in an autosomal dominant mode of inheritance, however, in the majority of patients, the inherited genetic defect is unknown [2,3].

Difference between mutations and polymorphisms

Since the development of DNA sequencing, our desire to understand the effects of single base-pair changes in DNA on disease development has been ever-present. Throughout the literature the designation of these base-pair changes in DNA has been somewhat fluid with the interchangeable use of terms such as "mutation" and "polymorphism." The classic definitions of these terms can be traced back to two papers from 1993 [4,5]. These papers recommended that any change in the nucleotide sequence can be called a "mutation" even if it leads to disease. This notion is no longer valid for the reasons explained below. In contrast, a polymorphism is a variation in the DNA sequence that occurs in at least 1% of the population [6]. The most common polymorphism is a single-nucleotide polymorphism (SNP) which is calculated to occur every 1000 base pairs in the human genome. These variants can occur in both coding and noncoding sequences [7].

The terms mutation and polymorphism imply a clear distinction of pathogenicity of the change. However, none of the two can account for genetic risk factors and incomplete penetrance. Recently, with the expansion of next-generation methods which have allowed the sequencing of thousands of genomes of diverse ethnic backgrounds, the use of mutation and polymorphism was somewhat abandoned and substituted by the terms rare and common variants.

The variation in the genome can be inherited (germline transmission) from the parents or acquired (somatic) and can arise from DNA damage, replication errors, repair errors, or modification from mobile genetic elements. During evolution some variants have become more prominent, and others disappeared, presumably because they conferred a disadvantage to the environment or disease. On the other hand, variants providing a survival advantage have been maintained, such as the sickle cell anemia rare mutation protecting from malaria. Variants can be a single base change or whole regions of genes and even chromosomes can be deleted, duplicated, inverted, or translocated [8].

Approaches for identifying the genetic cause of a disorder

Dramatic advances have been made in investigating the role of variants in monogenic disorders. Despite genome-wide association studies (GWAS) of thousands of patient genomes, understanding of many polygenic gynecologic disorders remains elusive. A sea of DNA variants were associated with common gynecologic disorders such as polycystic ovary syndrome (PCOS) and endometriosis [9,10]. Methods for consolidating this plethora of data to determine the causal genetic variants responsible for disease continue to improve. Multimodal types of analyses that combine genomics with additional types of data such as transcriptomics, functional characterization, clinical, and even artificial intelligence have been developed.

The followings sections discuss the different approaches that can be used in the quest to find the genetic cause of reproductive disorders.

Candidate gene approach

Candidate gene approach has been used extensively to find associations between disease state and genetic variations, well before the Human Genome Project (HGP) was conceptualized. This method requires in-depth knowledge of the function of an organ, secretion and function of hormones, and interactions between several systems. It also depends on the available clinical and molecular assays in order to accurately characterize the disease phenotype. Direct Sanger sequencing of the candidate gene has been used to find the molecular defect, sometimes in conjunction with reverse transcription polymerase chain reaction (RT-PCR) of the cDNA. The main disadvantage of this method is that it is not high throughput as it examines one gene at a time. It is only recommended when the phenotype allows an educated guess of the affected gene.

Many disease genes have been discovered using this approach, including genes of reproductive disorders. For example, the follicle-stimulating hormone (FSH) units and follicle-stimulating hormone receptor (FSHR) have been of particular interest in studies of hypogonadotropic hypogonadism. FSH is a protein hormone that binds to FHSR, a G-protein-coupled receptor in granulosa cells, which is essential for driving oocyte development and maturation [11]. Mutations in the FSH and FSHR have been discovered by direct Sanger sequencing genes in patients presenting with hypogonadism [12,13]. Recessive inheritance by compound heterozygous mode of transmission, as well as functional characterization of the variants in vitro, was deemed necessary to prove the pathogenicity of these variants.

Premature ovarian insufficiency (POI) is a condition which affects approximately 1%–2% of reproductive-age women globally. It involves the spontaneous cessation of menstrual cycles before age 40 [14]. Several mechanisms are thought to play a role in POI. These include chromosomal abnormalities, either of the autosomal chromosomes or the X-chromosome, autoimmune conditions, toxin exposure from the environment, or iatrogenic causes such as chemotherapy or radiation therapy [15]. No single mutation has been associated with POI, with any one mutation accounting for no more than 10% of incident cases [16,17]. One of these candidate genes is premutation of the *FMR1* gene. Other genes that have since been identified include *FSHR*, *POF1B*, *FOXL2*, and *BMP15* with functional studies providing a causative relationship for each of these candidate genes [18–20]. Missense mutations and polymorphisms have also been found: *GDF9*, *FOXO3A*, *FOXO1A*, and *INHA* [21–23].

In 2007 Aleksander Rajkovic's group used sequencing of the *NANOS3* gene in Chinese and Caucasian women with POI and found one SNP, rs2016163, in exon 1 [24]. *NANOS3* is the gene encoding an RNA-binding protein which was first identified in *Drosophila* and is activated during germ cell development. In the same year, this group studied the Newborn ovary homeobox gene (*NOBOX* gene) in 96 Caucasian women with POI. They detected seven known SNP s and four new variants, two of which led to missense mutations of this gene. These two mutations, p.Arg355His and p.Arg360Gln, led to missense mutations that disrupted NOBOX homeodomain binding to its DNA-binding element based on electrophoretic mobility shift assays [25]. This group further investigated the role of the *FSHR* in two Indian sisters with POI. This sequencing led to the discovery of a new pathogenic variant of the *FSHR* gene, c.1253 T > G, leading to a single amino acid substitution, Ile418Ser. This single change leads to loss of functions for *FSHR* in an exon which has been previously associated with a gene variant in a patient with primary amenorrhea [26].

Male and female *NANOS3* knockout mice were both found to be infertile. The mouse genes' high degree of homology to its human analogue made it a possible candidate gene for POI. Sufficient conservation of ovarian function between humans and mice has permitted using animal models to study the effects of gene knockouts in mice and better understand ovarian function with possible implications to improve the treatment of human conditions [11,27]. Recapitulating the phenotype in animal models provided additional support for the identification of the causal human gene for the disorder.

However, except for recessive disorders with a clear mode of transmission, investigators using candidate gene approaches to study the genetic basis of a gynecologic disease have often met with mixed success. This suggests that our ability to determine an exact genetic cause is dependent on the precision of the phenotypic diagnosis.

Single-nucleotide variants of the *FSHR* have been studied in patients undergoing controlled ovarian stimulation (COI), since patients are treated with several formulations that contain FSH [28,29]. Two common *FSHR* variants in exon 10 (dbSNP; rs6165 and rs6166) result in two amino acid changes in the intracellular domain of the receptor, giving rise to two polymorphic proteins that contain threonine or asparagine in position 307, and alanine or serine in position 680. Clinical data indicated less favorable associations of the least common $Ala^{307}Ser^{680}$ variant with relevant endpoints of ovarian stimulation, including basal FSH, number of oocytes, pregnancy rate, and maximum E2 [30]. In in-vitro studies the least common variants appear to lead to decreased sensitivity of the FSHR [31].

Additionally, splicing variants of the FSHR receptor lacking exon 2 have been discovered using RT-PCR from granulosa cell mRNA of patients undergoing COI [28,32]. Although the variants cannot completely explain the extent of the variability, the variants were consistent with the phenotype in subsets of patients.

PCOS and POI are two gynecologic conditions which have been studied using a candidate gene approach with mixed results. PCOS affects up to one in five women of reproductive age. It can lead to irregular periods and is the most common cause for anovulation [33]. POI is a condition in which lack of ovarian function manifests as amenorrhea, increased gonadotrophin secretion, and estrogen deficiency in women younger than 40. Numerous studies have shown an association between inhibition of FSH production or signaling and the arrest of ovarian folliculogenesis seen in PCOS [34–36]. However, associations with FSHR mutations or polymorphisms and either of these diseases have not yet shown any significant relationship, despite several studies being conducted. For example, Conway et al. looked at 49 women with POI and 93 women with PCOS compared to 51 controls using sequencing of restriction fragments from the *FSHR* gene and found no variant associated with either disease [37]. Tong et al. looked at FSHR receptor polymorphisms in 16 patients with

POI, 124 patients with PCOS, and 236 control subjects using both direct sequencing and analysis of restriction fragment length polymorphisms (RFLPs) and no associated FSHR variants [38]. Simoni et al. examined an array of promoter and coding variants of the FSHR gene and did not find any associations [30].

The candidate gene approach can be confused with linkage analysis, a technique that will be described in the next section. While linkage analysis takes advantage of familial transmission to find genetic variations, candidate gene analysis seeks to associate a gene across a population. Association over a whole population, in a sense, represents an extreme form of linkage in which genetic variations can be identified in unrelated individuals with a common disease or syndrome [39].

Linkage analysis

The distribution of chromosomes, and subsequently to genes during meiosis, is believed to follow the idea of "independent assortment of genes." This means that genes are allocated to offspring without any relation to one another. However, as the location of genes on chromosomes became known, it was clear that physical proximity of the genes influenced their coinheritance. It was as if the genes were "linked," in a sense. This was first demonstrated by T. H. Morgan in *Drosophila*, who showed that certain genes were not allocated independently, but rather tended to associate with other genes. Using the paradigm he was able to show how the genes of the *Drosophila* fly exist in four "linkage groups" which corresponds to the four chromosomes in this fly [40].

As a result, linkage analysis could be used to follow the pattern of inheritance of a genetic disease within families and examine which parts of the genome are shared by all affected individuals, while being absent from all unaffected ones. The existence of families with several affected members is necessary to perform linkage analysis. A family, the disease status, and genetic information segregation can be graphically assessed using a pedigree. This is done by outlining the affected and unaffected individuals over a series of generations with different symbols. Using this graphical representation, dominance and whether a gene is autosomal or X-linked can be deduced [41]. In Fig. 2.1, we show a simple pedigree of an autosomal recessive gene which spans two generations. Note how both the parents (F1) are carriers, but are unaffected. However, of their

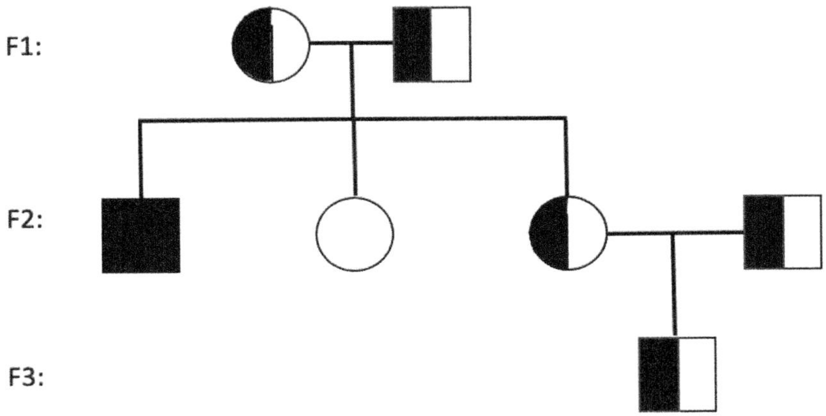

FIGURE 2.1 A three-generation family carrying a monogenic disease of recessive inheritance is shown. *Boxes* indicate males and circles females. *Half-shaded shapes* indicate non-affected carriers. *Fully shaded shapes* indicate homozygous affected. *Open spaces* indicate not carriers. Hypogonanotrohic hypogonadism due to follicle-stimulating hormone receptor (FSHR) mutations, cystic fibrosis, and spinal muscular atrophy show this model of inheritance.

four offspring, two have two copies of the disease and are affected.

Linkage analysis used the typing of polymorphic markers that were distributed across the genome to discover the parts of the genome that contained the causal gene, which was shared by all affected individuals. Once a chromosome location has been found, genetic linkage analysis can be done to determine if the disease stems from one gene or numerous genes. Systematic Sanger sequencing of the coding regions of all included genes followed and many disease genes have been identified this way, and some examples are discussed below.

The most common type of polymorphisms used in linkage analysis were variable number tandem repeat and RFLPs that are sequences that show allelic differences among individuals. A mathematical algorithm was used to calculate the results at a genome-wide level. Linkage between a disease and a chromosomal location is quantified by the logarithm of odds (LOD) score. The LOD score, Z, is the logarithm of the odds that certain loci are linked to a disease divided by the odds that certain loci are unlinked. A LOD score greater than 3.0 is considered indicative of linkage, whereas a LOD score of −2 is indicative that linkage is not present. Although the markers used in linkage analysis were more polymorphic than SNPs they were not as dense as SNPs. The reason why SNPs were not used as extensively in linkage as microsatellite repeats is purely historical. SNPs were not discovered until the late 1990s, while a large number of linkage studies were performed before that date.

The genes for many monogenic diseases have been discovered using linkage analysis including the genes for breast and ovarian cancer, *BRCA1* and *BRCA2* [2,42]. They were both identified in the 1990s by analyzing families at high risk of ovarian and breast cancer. Together they comprise 15%−20% of all cases of familial breast cancer. Loss of one *BRCA* gene leads to an enhanced predisposition to cancer, whereas loss of two copies is consistently seen in tumor cells [43,44]. As in the candidate gene approach, studies in animal models and in vitro systems are necessary to confirm gene causality for a disease, as well as help the identification of therapies. For diseases like breast cancer, identifying mutations in the *BRCA* genes is pivotal for the choice of therapeutic management in the case of cancer, disease prevention, and family counseling.

Besides monogenic diseases, linkage analysis has been successful in identifying genes of familial types of polygenic diseases, such as autosomal dominant spinocerebellar ataxia, amyotrophic lateral sclerosis, and Parkinson's disease [45−48]. Although a disease can be linked to a gene in only a fraction of affected individuals, identification via linkage allowed studies into the pathophysiology of the disease. This technique allowed for insight into disease mechanisms many years before the availability of more complex genetic methods such as GWAS were available.

Another benefit of early linkage studies, in the era before the completion of the HGP, was the valuable information it provided about chromosomal size, distance between genes, and rates of meiotic recombination. The basic unit of linkage is a Morgan, which was defined as the chromosomal length over which one recombination event occurs during one meiosis. Two loci are 1 centiMorgan (cM) apart if they are segregated away from each other in 1% of meiotic transmissions to offspring. One centiMorgan is roughly 1 million base pairs of DNA, although recombination rates differ between male and female meiosis even for the same chromosome [40,49].

Despite the substantial success of linkage analysis in identifying disease-associated genes and opening the road to therapies, it is limited by the need for families with several affected members. Therefore for reproductive disorders that preclude from having large families, linkage analysis cannot be effectively deployed. Instead, GWAS, described in the next section, are more appropriate.

Genome-wide association studies (polycystic ovary syndrome)

The discovery of the SNPs was a major inflection point in genetic analysis, as it allowed the development of association studies with a case–control study design, without the requirement of families [50,51]. The study design is based on gathering representative populations affected and unaffected by the disease in question. Then the DNAs are SNP-genotyped using arrays. GWAS attempt to detect an association between a SNP and a certain disease, by examining the allele frequency between the cases and the controls. The greater the frequency of a certain SNP in a group of unrelated individuals with a specific disease condition, the greater the chance that this SNP may directly or indirectly underlie the condition (Mitjans and Arias, n.d.). A SNP is considered significantly associated with a disease/trait when the P value is less than 5×10^{-8}.

Gene association studies are especially effective for polygenic disease. The technological explosion that allowed screening of thousands of SNPs on an array simultaneously and the advancement of computational algorithms to analyze the data mapped a very large number of diseases and traits to chromosomal locations. By 2019 there were 7796 GWAS publications and 159,202 associations! The GWAS catalog is a repository of all associations detected to date (https://www.ebi.ac.uk/gwas/) (Fig. 2.2).What is very important to emphasize here is that GWAS use the analysis of common variants (SNPs) to pinpoint the chromosomal locus that is causal for a disease, but in most cases cannot indicate which of the genes in the area is causal. Often the closest gene to the SNP is considered the causal gene; however, this is not always the case. Sophisticated statistical genetics methods, as well as a combination of additional evidence of gene expression, can be used to provide supportive evidence for the causal gene.

Since the development of array-based genotyping techniques and their complementary software tools to assess the results of these arrays, GWAS have become an increasingly relied-upon tool to determine the genetic causes for gynecologic diseases. GWAS rely on comparing the genotyping results from large homogeneous affected and unaffected patient populations to determine a genetic association. Ovarian physiology, especially in relation to folliculogenesis, has been a pivotal focus of GWAS, particularly in the setting of PCOS [52]. One of the hallmarks of PCOS is hyperandrogenemia. This is thought to be due to contributions from ovarian theca cells and adrenal cells from the zona reticularis. The link between these cells is indicated by the concomitant suppression of androgen production from these cells with the use of combined oral contraceptives and insulin-sensitizing agents [53,54]. Since 2011 five studies have been published which have identified 16 loci associated with this condition. In a study by Day et al., this group looked at 5128 subjects with PCOS and 82,759 controls and found six loci at genome-wide statistical significance, near the genes *ERBB4/HER4*, *YAP1*, *THADA*, *FSHB*, *RAD50*, and *KRR1* (Fig. 2.3) [55]. Chen et al. looked at 744 PCOS patient and 895 controls and found three loci associated with PCOS, namely on chromosome locations 2p16.3 (rs13405728), 2p21 (rs13429458), and 9q33.3 (rs2479106) [56]. Shi et al. found seven signal loci indicative genes involved in insulin signaling, sex hormone function, and type two diabetes mellitus. These included *DENND1A*, *INSR*, *YAP1*, *C9orf3*, *RAB5B*, *HMGA2*, *TOX3*, *SUMO1P1/ZNF217*, *THADA*, *FSHR*, and *LHCGR* [57]. Several subsequent GWAS

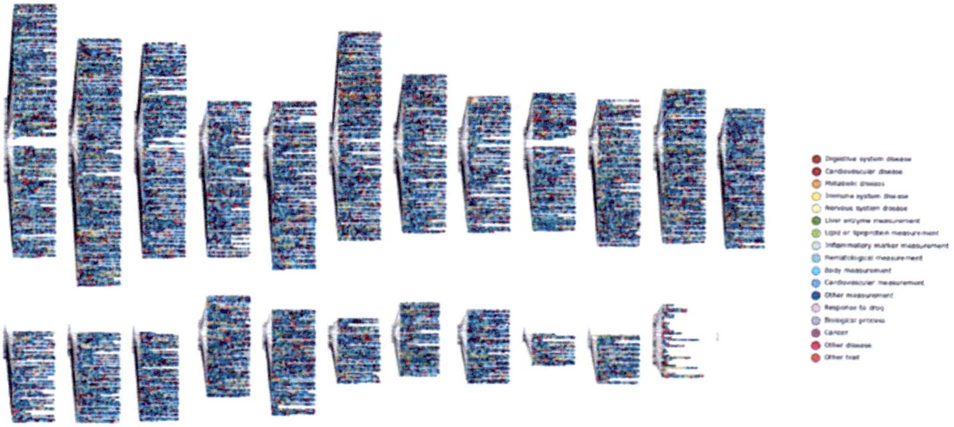

FIGURE 2.2 Genome-wide association studies (GWAS) map of all disease-associated single-nucleotide polymorphisms (SNPs) for each of the 23 chromosomes. Each *color dot* corresponds to the physiologic system studied. Source: *Derived from the GWAS catalog, https://www.ebi.ac.uk/gwas/diagram.*

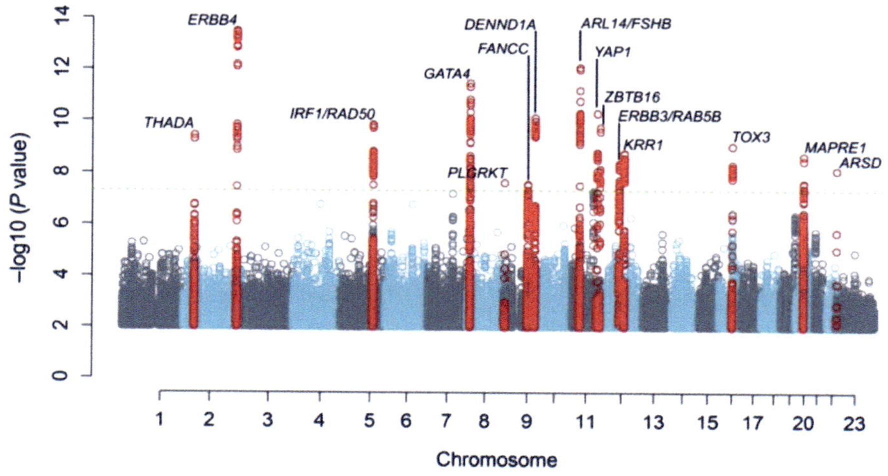

FIGURE 2.3 Example of a Manhattan plot outlining significant genes identified in metaanalysis of genome-wide association studies (GWAS). Source: *From Day F, Karaderi T, Jones MR, Meun C, He C, Drong A, et al. Large-scale genome-wide meta-analysis of polycystic ovary syndrome suggests shared genetic architecture for different diagnosis criteria. PLoS Genet 2018;14(12): e1007813.*

further confirmed the association of *DENND1A* and *THADA* genes with PCOS, with the study by Louwers et al. also confirming the association with *FSHR*, *C9orf3*, *LHCGR*, *SUMO1P1*, and *YAP1* [9,58,59].

Although the association of several of the GWAS candidate genes such as *FSHR* and *LHCGR* (LH receptor) are expected based upon the known pathophysiology of PCOS, it has yet to be determined the exact role of many of the genes found in GWAS of PCOS. Inactivating mutations of FSHR have been shown to halt follicle development at the preantral stage as is seen in PCOS. Numerous mutations in FSH have been tested in cell culture systems; however the mutations tested have shown similar FSH binding and signal transduction [31,60]. The LH receptor, like FSHR, is a G-protein-coupled receptor. It allows the preovulatory follicle to be receptive to the LH surge in the middle of the menstrual cycle. Inactivating mutations of LHCGR have been associated with increased ovarian size, increased LH levels, and oligomenorrhea [61]. Conversely, numerous mutations thought to activate the LH receptor have not been associated with the hyperandrogenemia that is thought to arise from ovarian thecal cell dysfunction [62].

A major limitation to this approach is the risk of confounding at the very least by ethnicity. Therefore stratification of populations via ethnic or racial divides could help mitigate, but likely not completely eliminate, this confounding effect. This limitation leads to a high false-positive rate for case–control studies, which is exacerbated by a lack of possible causal relationships. In contrast, when a causal relationship is possible, such as variants in human leukocyte antigen antigens and autoimmune disease, consistent associations can be found [63].

Despite the statistical power of GWAS, polygenic diseases remain hard to comprehend fully. In recent years additional statistical methods have been developed to harness the full power of GWAS. Metaanalysis of GWAS is a way to add statistical power by combining many studies together. In PCOS, this was performed by Day et al., and clearly showed the genomic areas involved in this disease [64].

Another statistical tool aims to calculate the risk of inheriting several disease loci discovered in GWAS. This is called a polygenic risk score (PRS) and takes into consideration the population frequency of an allele multiplied by the effect size found in GWAS. A high PRS signifies that an individual has inherited a large percentage of the risk alleles, or some alleles that confer more risk than others. PRS has been calculated in PCOS by Lee et al. [65].

Whole-genome sequencing/whole-exome sequencing

Although significant progress has been made using indirect genetic markers to discover genes associated with disease, DNA sequencing and, in particular, next-generation sequencing (NGS) has brought a new level of investigative power [66]. The big advantage of NGS versus GWAS is the potential to screen rare and common variants simultaneously and to pinpoint the causal gene with higher confidence. The biggest disadvantages are cost and a very large volume of data that require specialized analysis methods.

Many years ago, Sanger sequencing provided the means for genomics advancement with the development of DNA sequencing using dideoxynucleotides by Prof. Frederick Sanger's lab at Cambridge University in the early 1970s [67]. This technique was further refined with the advent of fluorescently labeled dideoxynucleotides and capillary electrophoresis in 1986 and 1999, respectively. However, in approximately 2005, a revolution in sequencing arose with the introduction of massively parallel sequencing. Briefly, this method involved tagging fragments of DNA to oligonucleotide primers which are unique to a respective sequencing platform. These primers bind in complementary fashion to oligonucleotides on a bead or flat glass microfluidic channel. Each bound length of DNA is termed an amplification locus. Then DNA amplification is tracked digitally at each amplification locus. This allows for amplification and sequencing to happen nearly simultaneously [68]. NGS is constantly evolving, both in the chemistry and hardware used.

The current Illumina protocol leads to reads approximately 150 bp with error rates in the range of 0.1%–0.5%. Second is the long-read method of NGS using single molecule techniques from Pacific Biosciences which yields 10–100 kilobase (kb) reads. Unfortunately, with the longer read length comes a higher error rate of 10%–15%. Finally, the third method, called linked-read WGS, uses barcoded short-reads synthesized from longer lengths. Given this wide disparity in error rates and cost, the majority of genetic studies have utilized short-read WGS.

To decrease the chance for error in WGS, repeated reads over multiple randomly fragmented DNA targets is needed to ensure that a mutation is genuine and not an error. The greater the number of targets the deeper the sequencing needs to be. For rare mutations, approximately 30 reads or more (30 × coverage) are needed to detect a mutation or de novo heterozygous variant. To detect somatic mutations in tumors much deeper sequencing of 100 × or more is necessary, because not all cells will contain the same variants. Upon completion of sequencing, the task then becomes to reassemble and interpret the DNA reads. The first step in reassembling a genome from millions of sequences is to align it to a reference genome [69,70].

The two main types of NGS are whole-exome sequencing (WES) and whole-genome sequencing (WGS). WES and WGS refer to sequencing the entire gene or coding regions of the gene by NGS and not by Sanger sequencing. WES is a variation on WGS in which only the portion of the genome that codes for proteins is sequenced. Therefore only 1%–1.5% of the whole genome undergoes sequencing. The first step in identifying the exome or region of interest in the exome is by hybridizing fragmented DNA to an array or solution-based system of oligonucleotides specific to the coding regions of DNA, deemed direct genomic selection [71].

The biggest hurdle of WGS/WES is to assign pathogenicity to the identified variants. The American College of Medical Genetics has published a suggested method of variant evaluation, to help classifying variants [72]. The incidence of variants in the population scale remains one of the best indications of pathogenicity. The Exac and gnomAD databases developed by the Broad Institute provide a valuable resource for variant frequency in different populations [73].

Urbanek et al. utilized WGS to analyze genetic variants in PCOS. They sequenced the genomes of 80 patients with PCOS and 24 controls without PCOS. They found 24 rare variants of the AMH gene among both groups with 18 of the variants specific to women with PCOS. Seventeen of these variants showed significant decreases in AMH signaling based upon dual luciferase assays [74].

Exome sequencing has been applied to gynecology in the setting of POI. A recent study by a Colombian-French collaboration using WES demonstrated the polygenic nature of POI. This group extracted DNA from 69 women with POI. Fifty-five gene variants were identified in 49 candidate genes in 48% of the patients. The presence of a minimum of two mutations in separate genes in 42% of the patients supported the polygenic basis for POI. Several mutations in the genes *BMPR1B* and *GREM1* were validated using computational modeling tools to simulate the molecular interactions of the amino acid changes these mutations led to. These simulations showed all of these mutations to have some pathogenic consequence [75]. Additional pathogenic variants in the *PMM2*, *MCM9*, and *PSMC3IP* genes were identified in French POI patients, demonstrating the polygenic architecture of this disease [76].

Multimodal approaches and systems biology

According to Kirschner, systems biology involves the analysis of the interaction of biological processes through its molecular components [77]. Systems biology seeks to determine possible connects between genotype and phenotype. It does this by using physical principles and data from molecular biology to determine the interactions underlying various physiologic and disease states. The four aspects of this method are quantitative measurement, theory, modeling, and reconstruction. Although the theoretical basis for systems biology comes from the disciplines used to model component behavior in physics and engineering, biological systems provide a far greater degree of variation. Admittedly, this has led to an occasional inconsistency and incomplete picture of how some model systems may work. Nonetheless, the role of combining mathematical modeling to better understand the ever-expanding fund of genomics is being increasingly accepted [78].

Several gynecologic conditions have been investigated using systems biology. One of these is endometriosis, where Matthew et al. used data from human endometrial microarrays to show that FOXD3 is an essential regulator of gene expression of secretory phase endometrium and endometriosis. They then confirmed the role of FOXD3 by measuring protein and RNA levels in endometrial stromal cells and demonstrating downregulation of the FOXD3 with Levonogestrel treatment [79].

Since GWAS results still remain the richest database of disease associations, the need to identify the causal gene is important. Association of different alleles of significant SNPs with expression of nearby genes is deployed. These SNPs are called eQTL or pQTL, for expression quantitative trait loci and protein quantitative trait loci, respectively [80]. Protein–protein interaction networks are also used to identify the gene from within the GWAS locus that forms complexes with other proteins relevant to disease [81]. To our knowledge, these methods have not been applied to reproductive disorders yet.

Genetic architecture of multifactorial diseases—area of artificial intelligence

With the profound advances in DNA sequencing, genomics, transcriptomics, and studies of the epigenome, the amount of genetic information available has vastly expanded. To utilize this information to determine new associations and patterns, machine learning had emerged as a new tool. The area of machine learning deals with the application of computer algorithms that adapt and develop with increasing iterations of data processing. This process generally involves three stages. The first involves algorithm development. Second, the algorithm is given a bank of data such as a list of variants for a given gene/disease and other complementary data, clinical, spatial, and temporal gene expression, and protein–protein interactions. From this list a model is developed and stored. Third, other types of data, for example, a list of unlabeled sequence variants, are provided to the algorithm which then attempts to predict which of the sequences has a pathogenic variant. The percentage of correct predictions is the measure of success for the algorithm [82]. Machine learning has been applied to identify enhancers, splice sites, and promoters [83,84]. In addition, machine learning has been used to analyze other genomic data such as microarray, RNA-sequencing expression data, and even chromatin accessibility assays such as DNase-seq and ChiP-seq. The applications of machine learning even extend to gene ontology and determining functional relationships between various genes [85].

PCOS has also become a focus for machine learning technologies. Shen et al. in 2013 used genome-wide methylated DNA immunoprecipitation (MeDIP-chip) to characterize the PCOS methylome compared to controls. Seventy-nine genes were found to be differentially methylated between insulin-resistant and insulin-sensitive patients and 40 genes were differentially methylated between PCOS patients and controls. Gene ontology analysis indicated differential methylation in immune response genes and various genes involved in RNA and DNA replications and nucleotide metabolism [86]. A case–control study was also carried out in China using MeDIP-chip and showed methylation was higher outside of gene bodies in women with PCOS. Furthermore, machine learning analysis of microarray data predicted numerous genes such as *SLC2A8, NRIP1, IGF2BP2, CYP19A1,* and *AMHR2* to be hypermethylated. This degree of hypermethylated and decreased gene expression was confirmed using methylation-specific polymerase chain reaction [87].

Determining a genetic basis for endometriosis has been one of the tasks for machine learning. Endometriosis is a disease characterized by the presence of endometrial tissue outside the endometrium and affects 5%–10% of all reproductive-age women [88]. The risk of endometriosis is greater in patients who have a family history of the condition [10,89]. Fassbender et al. looked at the mRNA expression data in eutopic endometrium in patients with and without endometriosis. These groups showed a difference in mRNA expression between the menstrual endometrium and luteal endometrium in patients with endometriosis. Furthermore, they used proteomic analysis to identify four protein peaks that are differentially expressed in luteal phase endometrium (used as the training set) that have a sensitivity of 91% and specificity of 95% for endometriosis [90]. An enhancement of machine learning is the use of an artificial neural network which attempts to mimic the processing strategy of neurons in order to enhance selective and predictive power when interpreting a data set [91]. This approach was combined with proteomics in similar fashion by Wang et al. in two papers using surface-enhanced laser desorption/ionization time-of-flight mass spectrometry protein chip array methods. In each study, the group was able to find a novel set of biomarkers for endometriosis [93].

Summary

Determining the genetic basis for gynecologic conditions ranging from endometriosis to POI has been both elusive and fruitful. Older techniques such as linkage analysis have resulted in some successes such as the discovery of the *BRCA1* and *BRCA2* genes, and hereditary breast and ovarian cancers. However, with the advancement of sequencing technologies and the additional data coming from RNA sequencing and epigenetics, the potential for discovering new target genes has vastly expanded. The development of techniques to better interpret and model the relevance of these genetic targets has concomitantly improved. They have enhanced our ability to discover the genetic basis for gynecologic disease beyond our capabilities even a decade ago. The impact of genetic discoveries on patient care, including better understanding of pathophysiology, diagnostics, disease prevention, and drug development, has grown exponentially. During the last decade, fascinating genetic discoveries are being deployed to realize the aspirations of precision medicine.

References

[1] Hood L, Rowen L. The Human Genome Project: big science transforms biology and medicine. Genome Med 2013;5:79.

[2] Hall JM, Lee MK, Newman B, Morrow JE, Anderson LA, Huey B, et al. Linkage of early-onset familial breast cancer to chromosome 17q21. Science (New York, NY) 1990;250:1684–9.

[3] Wu L, Shi W, Long J, Guo X, Michailidou K, Beesley J, et al. A transcriptome-wide association study of 229,000 women identifies new candidate susceptibility genes for breast cancer. Nat Genet 2018;50(7):968–78.

[4] Beaudet AL, Tsui LC. A suggested nomenclature for designating mutations. Hum Mutat. 1993;2:245–8.

[5] Beutler E. The designation of mutations. Am J Hum Genet 1993;53:783–5.

[6] Brookes AJ. The essence of SNPs. Gene 1999;234:177–86.

[7] Aerts J, Wetzels Y, Cohen N, Aerssens J. Data mining of public SNP databases for the selection of intragenic SNPs. Hum Mutat 2002;20:162–73.

[8] Vissers LELM, de Vries BBA, Osoegawa K, Janssen IM, Feuth T, Choy CO, et al. Array-based comparative genomic hybridization for the genomewide detection of submicroscopic chromosomal abnormalities. Am J Hum Genet 2003;73:1261–70.

[9] Louwers YV, Stolk L, Uitterlinden AG, Laven JSE. Cross-ethnic meta-analysis of genetic variants for polycystic ovary syndrome. J Clin Endocrinol Metab. 2013;98:E2006–12.

[10] Stefansson H, Geirsson RT, Steinthorsdottir V, Jonsson H, Manolescu A, Kong A, et al. Genetic factors contribute to the risk of developing endometriosis. Hum Reprod (Oxford, Engl) 2002;17:555–9.

[11] Kumar TR, Wang Y, Lu N, Matzuk MM. Follicle stimulating hormone is required for ovarian follicle maturation but not male fertility. Nat Genet 1997;15 (2):201–4.

[12] Layman LC, Lee EJ, Peak DB, Namnoum AB, Vu KV, van Lingen BL, et al. Delayed puberty and hypogonadism caused by mutations in the follicle-stimulating hormone beta-subunit gene. N Engl J Med 1997;337 (9):607–11.

[13] Layman LC, Porto AL, Xie J, da Motta LA, da Motta LD, Weiser W, et al. FSH beta gene mutations in a female with partial breast development and a male sibling with normal puberty and azoospermia. J Clin Endocrinol Metab 2002;87(8):3702–7.

[14] Coulam CB, Adamson SC, Annegers JF. Incidence of premature ovarian failure. Obstet Gynecol 1986;67:604–6.

[15] Toniolo D. X-linked premature ovarian failure: a complex disease. Curr Opin Genet Dev 2006;16:293–300.

[16] Vegetti W, Grazia Tibiletti M, Testa G, Yankowski de Laurentis, Alagna F, Castoldi E, et al. Inheritance in idiopathic premature ovarian failure: analysis of 71 cases. Hum Reprod (Oxford, Engl) 1998;13:1796–800.

[17] Woad KJ, Watkins WJ, Prendergast D, Shelling AN. The genetic basis of premature ovarian failure. Aust N Z J Obstet Gynaecol 2006;46:242–4.

[18] Aittomäki KLJ, Pakarinen P, Sistonen P, Tapanainen J, Gromoll J, Kaskikari R, et al. Mutation in the follicle-stimulating hormone receptor gene causes hereditary hypergonadotropic ovarian failure. Cell 1995; 82:959–68.

[19] Lacombe A, Lee H, Zahed L, Choucair M, Muller J-M, Nelson SF, et al. Disruption of POF1B binding to non-muscle actin filaments is associated with premature ovarian failure. Am J Hum Genet 2006;79:113–19.

[20] Gersak K, Harris SE, Smale WJ, Shelling AN. A novel 30 bp deletion in the FOXL2 gene in a phenotypically normal woman with primary amenorrhoea: case report. Hum Reprod (Oxford, Engl) 2004;19:2767–70.

[21] Laissue P, Christin-Maitre S, Touraine P, Kuttenn F, Ritvos O, Aittomaki K, et al. Mutations and sequence variants in GDF9 and BMP15 in patients with premature ovarian failure. Eur J Endocrinol 2006;154:739–44.

[22] Watkins WJ, Umbers AJ, Woad KJ, Harris SE, Winship IM, Gersak K, et al. Mutational screening of FOXO3A and FOXO1A in women with premature ovarian failure. Fertil Steril 2006;86:1518–21.

[23] Harris SE, Chand AL, Winship IM, Gersak K, Nishi Y, Yanase T, et al. INHA promoter polymorphisms are associated with premature ovarian failure. Mol Hum Reprod 2005;11:779–84.

[24] Qin Y, Zhao H, Kovanci E, Simpson JL, Chen Z-J, Rajkovic A. Mutation analysis of NANOS3 in 80 Chinese and 88 Caucasian women with premature ovarian failure. Fertil Steril 2007;88:1465–7.

[25] Qin Y, Choi Y, Zhao H, Simpson JL, Chen Z-J, Rajkovic A. NOBOX homeobox mutation causes premature ovarian failure. Am J Hum Genet 2007;81:576–81.

[26] Katari S, Wood-Trageser MA, Jiang H, Kalynchuk E, Muzumdar R, Yatsenko SA, et al. Novel inactivating mutation of the FSH receptor in two siblings of Indian origin with premature ovarian failure. J Clin Endocrinol Metab 2015;100:2154–7.

[27] Dierich A, Sairam MR, Monaco L, Fimia GM, Gansmuller A, LeMeur M, et al. Impairing follicle-stimulating hormone (FSH) signaling in vivo: targeted disruption of the FSH receptor leads to aberrant gametogenesis and hormonal imbalance. Proc Natl Acad Sci U S A 1998;95(23):13612–17.

[28] Karakaya C, Guzeloglu-Kayisli O, Hobbs RJ, Gerasimova T, Uyar A, Erdem M, et al. Follicle-stimulating hormone receptor (FSHR) alternative skipping of exon 2 or 3 affects ovarian response to FSH. Mol Hum Reprod 2014;20(7):630–43.

[29] Lalioti MD. Impact of follicle stimulating hormone receptor variants in fertility. Curr Opin Obstet Gynecol 2011;23(3):158–67.

[30] Simoni M, Nieschlag E, Gromoll J. Isoforms and single nucleotide polymorphisms of the FSH receptor gene: implications for human reproduction. Hum Reprod Update 2002;8:413–21.

[31] Sudo S, Kudo M, Wada S-i, Sato O, Hsueh AJW, Fujimoto S. Genetic and functional analyses of

polymorphisms in the human FSH receptor gene. Mol Hum Reprod 2002;8:893–9.
[32] Gerasimova T, Thanasoula MN, Zattas D, Seli E, Sakkas D, Lalioti MD. Identification and in vitro characterization of follicle stimulating hormone (FSH) receptor variants associated with abnormal ovarian response to FSH. J Clin Endocrinol Metab 2010;95(2):529–36.
[33] Teede H, Deeks A, Moran L. Polycystic ovary syndrome: a complex condition with psychological, reproductive and metabolic manifestations that impacts on health across the lifespan. BMC Med 2010;8:41.
[34] Beau I, Touraine P, Meduri G, Gougeon A, Desroches A, Matuchansky C, et al. A novel phenotype related to partial loss of function mutations of the follicle stimulating hormone receptor. J Clin Invest 1998;102:1352–9.
[35] Guo Q, Kumar TR, Woodruff T, Hadsell LA, DeMayo FJ, Matzuk MM. Overexpression of mouse follistatin causes reproductive defects in transgenic mice. Mol Endocrinol 1998;12:96–106.
[36] Matthews CH, Borgato S, Beck-Peccoz P, Adams M, Tone Y, Gambino G, et al. Primary amenorrhoea and infertility due to a mutation in the β–subunit of follicle–stimulating hormone. Nat Genet 1993;5:83–6.
[37] Conway GS, Conway E, Walker C, Hoppner W, Gromoll J, Simoni M. Mutation screening and isoform prevalence of the follicle stimulating hormone receptor gene in women with premature ovarian failure, resistant ovary syndrome and polycystic ovary syndrome. Clin Endocrinol 1999;51:97–9.
[38] Tong Y, Liao WX, Roy AC, Ng SC. Absence of mutations in the coding regions of follicle-stimulating hormone receptor gene in Singapore Chinese women with premature ovarian failure and polycystic ovary syndrome. Horm Metab Res 2001;33:221–6.
[39] Cordell HJ, Clayton DG. Genetic association studies. Lancet 2005;366:1121–31.
[40] Pulst SM. Genetic linkage analysis. Arch Neurol 1999;56:667–72.
[41] Griffiths AJ, Gelbart WM, Miller JH, Lewontin RC. Human pedigree analysis. New York: W. H. Freeman; 1999.
[42] Kent P, O'Donoghue JM, O'Hanlon DM, Kerin MJ, Maher DJ, Given HF. Linkage analysis and the susceptibility gene (BRCA-1) in familial breast cancer. Eur J Surg Oncol 1995;21:240–1.
[43] Venkitaraman AR. Cancer susceptibility and the functions of BRCA1 and BRCA2. Cell 2002;108:171–82.
[44] Venkitaraman AR. Linking the cellular functions of BRCA genes to cancer pathogenesis and treatment. Annu Rev Pathol Mech Dis 2009;4:461–87.
[45] Elden AC, Kim HJ, Hart MP, Chen-Plotkin AS, Johnson BS, Fang X, et al. Ataxin-2 intermediate-length polyglutamine expansions are associated with increased risk for ALS. Nature 2010;466(7310):1069–75.
[46] Huynh DP, Del Bigio MR, Ho DH, Pulst SM. Expression of ataxin-2 in brains from normal individuals and patients with Alzheimer's disease and spinocerebellar ataxia 2. Ann Neurol 1999;45(2):232–41.
[47] Rosen DR, Bowling AC, Patterson D, Usdin TB, Sapp P, Mezey E, et al. A frequent ala 4 to val superoxide dismutase-1 mutation is associated with a rapidly progressive familial amyotrophic lateral sclerosis. Hum Mol Genet 1994;3(6):981–7.
[48] Lees AJ, Hardy J, Revesz T. Parkinson's disease. Lancet 2009;373(9680):2055–66.
[49] Tanzi RE, Watkins PC, Stewart GD, Wexler NS, Gusella JF, Haines JL. A genetic linkage map of human chromosome 21: analysis of recombination as a function of sex and age. Am J Hum Genet 1992;50(3):551–8.
[50] Wellcome Trust Case Control Consortium. Genome-wide association study of 14,000 cases of seven common diseases and 3,000 shared controls. Nature 2007;447(7145):661–78.
[51] Auton A, Brooks LD, Durbin RM, Garrison EP, Kang HM, Korbel JO, et al. A global reference for human genetic variation. Nature 2015;526(7571):68–74.
[52] Laisk-Podar T, Lindgren CM, Peters M, Tapanainen JS, Lambalk CB, Salumets A, et al. Ovarian physiology and GWAS: biobanks, biology, and beyond. Trends Endocrinol Metab 2016;27:516–28.
[53] De Leo V, Di Sabatino A, Musacchio MC, Morgante G, Scolaro V, Cianci A, et al. Effect of oral contraceptives on markers of hyperandrogenism and SHBG in women with polycystic ovary syndrome. Contraception 2010;82:276–80.
[54] Azziz R, Ehrmann DA, Legro RS, Fereshetian AG, O'Keefe M, Ghazzi MN, et al. Troglitazone decreases adrenal androgen levels in women with polycystic ovary syndrome. Fertil Steril 2003;79:932–7.
[55] Day FR, Hinds DA, Tung JY, Stolk L, Styrkarsdottir U, Saxena R, et al. Causal mechanisms and balancing selection inferred from genetic associations with polycystic ovary syndrome. Nat Commun 2015;6:8464.
[56] Chen Z-J, Zhao H, He L, Shi Y, Qin Y, Shi Y, et al. Genome-wide association study identifies susceptibility loci for polycystic ovary syndrome on chromosome 2p16.3, 2p21 and 9q33.3. Nat Genet 2011;43:55–9.
[57] Shi Y, Zhao H, Shi Y, Cao Y, Yang D, Li Z, et al. Genome-wide association study identifies eight new risk loci for polycystic ovary syndrome. Nat Genet 2012;44:1020–5.

[58] Goodarzi MO, Jones MR, Li X, Chua AK, Garcia OA, Chen Y-DI, et al. Replication of association of DENND1A and THADA variants with polycystic ovary syndrome in European cohorts. J Med Genet 2012;49:90–5.
[59] Welt CK, Styrkarsdottir U, Ehrmann DA, Thorleifsson G, Arason G, Gudmundsson JA, et al. Variants in DENND1A are associated with polycystic ovary syndrome in women of European ancestry. J Clin Endocrinol Metab 2012;97:E1342–7.
[60] Huhtaniemi I. The Parkes lecture. Mutations of gonadotrophin and gonadotrophin receptor genes: what do they teach us about reproductive physiology? J Reprod Fertil 2000;119:173–86.
[61] Toledo SP, Brunner HG, Kraaij R, Post M, Dahia PL, Hayashida CY, et al. An inactivating mutation of the luteinizing hormone receptor causes amenorrhea in a 46, XX female. J Clin Endocrinol Metab 1996;81:3850–4.
[62] Latronico AC, Lins TS, Brito VN, Arnhold IJ, Mendonca BB. The effect of distinct activating mutations of the luteinizing hormone receptor gene on the pituitary-gonadal axis in both sexes. Clin Endocrinol 2000;53:609–13.
[63] Risch NJ. Searching for genetic determinants in the new millennium. Nature 2000;405:847–56.
[64] Day F, Karaderi T, Jones MR, Meun C, He C, Drong A, et al. Large-scale genome-wide meta-analysis of polycystic ovary syndrome suggests shared genetic architecture for different diagnosis criteria. PLoS Genet 2018;14(12):e1007813.
[65] Lee H, Oh JY, Sung YA, Chung HW. A genetic risk score is associated with polycystic ovary syndrome-related traits. Hum Reprod 2016;31(1):209–15.
[66] Lappalainen T, Scott AJ, Brandt M, Hall IM. Genomic analysis in the age of human genome sequencing. Cell 2019;177:70–84.
[67] Sanger F, Coulson AR. A rapid method for determining sequences in DNA by primed synthesis with DNA polymerase. J Mol Biol 1975;94:441–8.
[68] Mardis ER. Next-generation sequencing platforms. Annu Rev Anal Chem 2013;6:287–303.
[69] Li H. Aligning sequence reads, clone sequences and assembly contigs with BWA-MEM. 2013. https://arxiv.org/abs/1303.3997
[70] Tetreault M, Bareke E, Nadaf J, Alirezaie N, Majewski J. Whole-exome sequencing as a diagnostic tool: current challenges and future opportunities. Expert Rev Mol Diagn 2015;15:749–60.
[71] Bashiardes S, Veile R, Helms C, Mardis ER, Bowcock AM, Lovett M. Direct genomic selection. Nat Methods 2005;2:63–9.
[72] Richards S, Aziz N, Bale S, Bick D, Das S, Gastier-Foster J, et al. Standards and guidelines for the interpretation of sequence variants: a joint consensus recommendation of the American College of Medical Genetics and Genomics and the Association for Molecular Pathology. Genet Med 2015;17(5):405–24.
[73] de Andrade KC, Frone MN, Wegman-Ostrosky T, Khincha PP, Kim J, Amadou A, et al. Variable population prevalence estimates of germline TP53 variants: a gnomAD-based analysis. Hum Mutat 2019;40(1):97–105.
[74] Gorsic LK, Kosova G, Werstein B, Sisk R, Legro RS, Hayes MG, et al. Pathogenic anti-Müllerian hormone variants in polycystic ovary syndrome. J Clin Endocrinol Metab 2017;102:2862–72.
[75] Patiño LC, Beau I, Carlosama C, Buitrago JC, González R, Suárez CF, et al. New mutations in non-syndromic primary ovarian insufficiency patients identified via whole-exome sequencing. Hum Reprod 2017;32:1512–20.
[76] Yang X, Touraine P, Desai S, Humphreys G, Jiang H, Yatsenko A, et al. Gene variants identified by whole-exome sequencing in 33 French women with premature ovarian insufficiency. J Assist Reprod Genet 2019;36(1):39–45.
[77] Kirschner MW. The meaning of systems biology. Cell 2005;121:503–4.
[78] Macilwain C. Systems biology: evolving into the mainstream. Cell 2011;144:839–41.
[79] Mathew D, Drury JA, Valentijn AJ, Vasieva O, Hapangama DK. In silico, in vitro and in vivo analysis identifies a potential role for steroid hormone regulation of FOXD3 in endometriosis-associated genes. Hum Reprod 2015;31:dev307.
[80] Zhernakova DV, Deelen P, Vermaat M, van Iterson M, van Galen M, Arindrarto W, et al. Identification of context-dependent expression quantitative trait loci in whole blood. Nat Genet 2017;49(1):139–45.
[81] Pollack S, Igo Jr. RP, Jensen RA, Christiansen M, Li X, Cheng CY, et al. Multiethnic genome-wide association study of diabetic retinopathy using liability threshold modeling of duration of diabetes and glycemic control. Diabetes 2019;68(2):441–56.
[82] Libbrecht MW, Noble WS. Machine learning applications in genetics and genomics. Nat Rev Genet 2015;16:321–32.
[83] Degroeve S, De Baets B, Van de Peer Y, Rouzé P. Feature subset selection for splice site prediction. Bioinformatics (Oxford, Engl) 2002;18(Suppl. 2): S75–83.
[84] Heintzman ND, Stuart RK, Hon G, Fu Y, Ching CW, Hawkins RD, et al. Distinct and predictive chromatin

signatures of transcriptional promoters and enhancers in the human genome. Nat Genet 2007;39:311–18.

[85] Fraser AG, Marcotte EM. A probabilistic view of gene function. Nat Genet 2004;36:559–64.

[86] Shen H-r, Qiu L-h, Zhang Z-q, Qin Y-y, Cao C, Di W. Genome-wide methylated DNA immunoprecipitation analysis of patients with polycystic ovary syndrome. PLoS One 2013;8:e64801.

[87] Yu Y-Y, Sun C-X, Liu Y-K, Li Y, Wang L, Zhang W. Genome-wide screen of ovary-specific DNA methylation in polycystic ovary syndrome. Fertil Steril 2015;104:145–153.e6.

[88] Bulun S. Endometriosis. N Engl J Med 2009;360.

[89] Simpson JL, Bischoff FZ. Heritability and molecular genetic studies of endometriosis. Ann N Y Acad Sci 2002;955:239–51 discussion 93–5, 396–406.

[90] Fassbender A, Verbeeck N, Börnigen D, Kyama CM, Bokor A, Vodolazkaia A, et al. Combined mRNA microarray and proteomic analysis of eutopic endometrium of women with and without endometriosis. Hum Reprod 2012;27:2020–9.

[91] Han S-H, Kim KW, Kim S, Youn YC. Artificial neural network: understanding the basic concepts without mathematics. Dement Neurocogn Disord 2018;17:83.

[92] Wang L, Zheng W, Yu J-k, Jiang W-z, Mu L, Zhang S-z. Artificial neural networks combined with surface-enhanced laser desorption/ionization mass spectra distinguish endometriosis from healthy population. Fertil Steril 2007;88:1700–2.

CHAPTER

3

Cytogenetics techniques

Inmaculada Campos-Galindo

Igenomix, Valencia, Spain

Introduction

Cytogenetics is the study of chromosome structure and properties, including chromosomal behavior during somatic cell division in growth and development, mitosis, germ cell division in reproduction, meiosis, chromosomal influence on phenotypes, and factors that cause chromosomal changes [1]. **Chromosomal analysis** provides valuable information about a person's genetic constitution because normal chromosomes have constant morphology and size. Furthermore, chromosomal anomalies result in numerous genetic diseases and are responsible for gestational losses, implantation failures, and congenital malformations.

Early cytogenetic analysis techniques, such as Casperson's fluorescent stains [2–4], uniformly stained chromosomes so that they could not be distinguished from one other. Differential staining techniques subsequently improved cytogenetic analysis. Pardue and Gall developed the first nonfluorescent banding technique, Giemsa stain [5]. Banding was further improved by Yunis's development of high-resolution banding, a technique that synchronizes lymphocyte cultures to obtain higher numbers of cells in stages called prometaphase or prophase, increasing the resolution from 500 to over 1000 bands in a haploid genome [6].

Chromosomes are divided by a primary constriction called the **centromere** between the short or *p* arm (*p* from the French word *petite*) and long or *q* arm (*q* from the French *queue,*). The centromere is a reference point of a chromosome. Metaphasic chromosomes are classified according to the length of the *p* and *q* arms and position of the centromere (metacentric, submetacentric, acrocentric, or telocentric). Chromosome ends are called **telomeres**. Each arm of the chromosome is divided into **regions**, which are divided into **bands**. A band is defined as part of a chromosome, that is, clearly distinguishable from adjacent segments by appearing darker or lighter with one or more banding techniques [7].

Bands contain approximately 5–10 megabases of DNA and reflect the functional organization of the genome to regulate DNA replication, repair, transcription, and genetic recombination. Regions and bands are numbered from the centromere to the telomeres. The centromere does not form a band and is designated as 10 but is not shown on idiograms (the diagrammatic chart of chromosomes). The two regions adjacent to the centromere are

Human Reproductive Genetics
DOI: https://doi.org/10.1016/B978-0-12-816561-4.00003-X

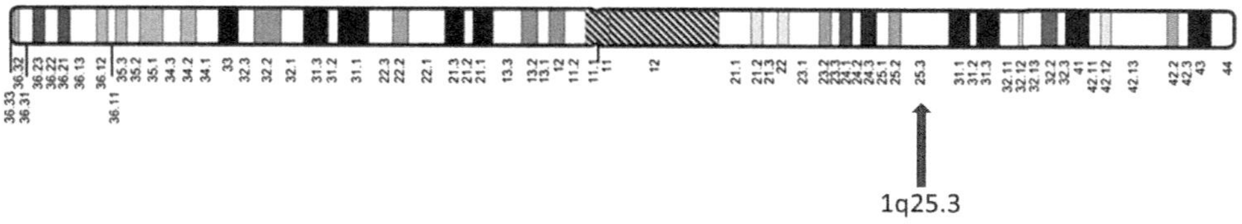

FIGURE 3.1 Localization of cytoband 1q25.3 [7].

labeled 1 in each arm, the next more distal regions are labeled 2, and so on. If a band is subdivided, a decimal point is placed after the name of the band, followed by the number assigned to the sub-band. Sub-bands are numbered sequentially from the centromere to the telomere. A band is usually subdivided into three sub-bands. A specific band is designated by chromosome number followed by arm symbol (*p* or *q*), region number, band number, and subband number, without spacing or punctuation [7]. For example, the name of sub-band 3, band 5, region 2 of the *q* arm of chromosome 1 is 1q25.3 (Fig. 3.1).

Karyogram, karyotype, and idiogram

The terms karyogram, karyotype, and idiogram are often used indiscriminately. However, ***karyogram*** refers to a systematized array of chromosomes prepared either by drawing, digitized imaging, or photography, with the extended meaning that chromosomes of a single cell can typify chromosomes of an individual or even species. ***Karyotype*** describes the normal or abnormal chromosomal complement of an individual, tissue, or cell line. ***Idiogram*** is a diagrammatic representation of a karyotype [7].

At the 1971 Paris Conference, an international nomenclature system for human chromosomes was established based on G-band patterns. These standards, known as the **International System of Chromosome Nomenclature** (ISCN), have been updated over the years and have allowed standardized descriptions of normal and pathological karyotypes. The Paris Conferences of 1971 and 1975 proposed to organize the 46 human chromosomes in pairs numbered from 1 to 22 (autosomes) in order of decreasing length, except for chromosome 21, which is shorter than chromosome 22, and the two sex chromosomes X and Y (Fig. 3.2).

The **chromosomal formula** summarizes a detailed description of an individual's karyotype using a series of abbreviations and symbols (Table 3.1). A chromosomal formula begins with the total number of chromosomes followed by sex chromosome constitution, separated by a comma without spaces (normal male: 46,XY and normal female: 46,XX). If there are structural abnormalities, chromosomal alterations are formulated after the sex chromosomes, such as: translocation 46,XX,t(11;16)(q13;q22); deletion 46,XY,del(22)(q11.2); and inversion 46,XX,inv(7)(p13q22.1).

A **standard karyotype** has around 400 ± 500 bands per haploid genome, and deletions or duplications of >10 Mb can be detected. **High-resolution karyotype** can achieve up to 1000 bands per haploid genome; at this level of resolution, an alteration of 3 ± 5 Mb can be detected [8]. Cytogenetic laboratories evaluate resolution by identifying and scoring landmarks on chromosome images (Table 3.2). At least three landmark criteria are needed to indicate band-level resolution [9], which laboratories specify in karyotype reports (Fig. 3.3).

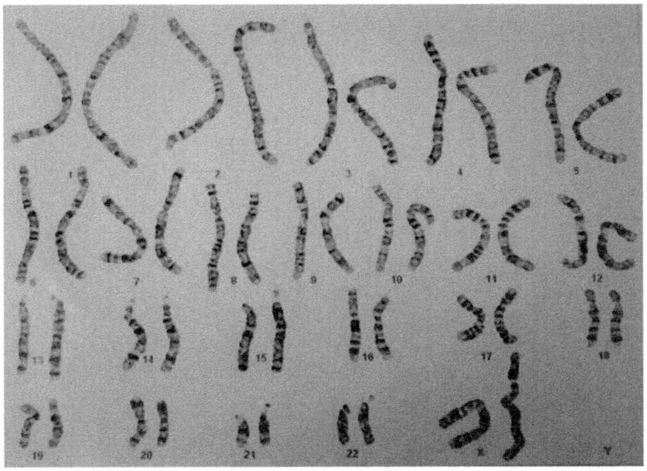

FIGURE 3.2 High-resolution karyotype of peripheral blood showing a normal female karyotype (46,XX). Source: *IVIRMA Murcia*.

TABLE 3.1 Abbreviations and symbols most frequently used by International System of Chromosome Nomenclature [7].

add	Additional material of unknown origin	**fra**	Fragile site	**Minus sign (−)**	Loss, decrease in length, locus absent from a specific chromosome	**r**	Ring chromosome
cen	Centromere	**i**	Isochromosome	**mos**	Mosaic	**rob**	Robertsonian translocation
chr	Chromosome	**ins**	Insertion	**p**	Short arm of chromosome	**s**	Satellite
del	Deletion	**inv**	Inversion	**pat**	Paternal origin	**stk**	Satellite stalk
der	Derivative chromosome	**ish**	In situ hybridization	**Plus sign (+)**	Additional normal or abnormal chromosome, increase in length, locus present on a specific chromosome	**subtel**	Subtelomeric
dic	Dicentric	**male**	Male	**pter**	Terminal end of short arm	**t**	Translocation
dup	Duplication	**mar**	Marker chromosome	**q**	Long arm of chromosome	**ter**	Terminal
fem	Female	**mat**	Maternal origin	**qter**	Terminal end of short arm		

Most frequent karyotype abnormalities

Ploidy is the number of chromosome sets in a cell. In humans, a normal somatic cell has two sets of chromosomes, one inherited from the mother and one inherited from the father, and is called diploid. Gametes with a single set of chromosomes (normal sperm or normal oocyte) are denoted as **haploid**. Chromosomal abnormalities can be caused by changes in chromosome number or structure.

1. ***Numerical abnormalities*** are defined as an abnormal number of chromosomes and are subclassified as follows.

TABLE 3.2 Giemsa banding (G-banding) evaluation score [9].

300 band	Two dark bands on 8p (8p12 and 8p22) Three dark bands on 10q (10q21, 10q23, and 10q25) 20p12 visible 22q12 distinct
400 band	Three dark bands on mid-4q (q22–28) Three dark bands mid-5q (5q14, 5q21, and 5q23) Two dark bands on 9p (9p21 and 9p23) 13q33 distinct
500 band	7q33 and 7q35 distinct Three dark bands on 11p (11p12, 11p14, and 11p15.4) 14q32.2 distinct Four dark bands on 18q (18q12.1, 18q12.3, 18q21.2, and 18q22)
550 band	5q31.2 distinct 8p21.2 visible Two dark bands on 11pter (11p15.2 and 11p15.4) 22q13.2 distinct
700 band	2p25.2 distinct 2q37.2 distinct 10q21.1 and 10q21.3 resolve 17q22–24 resolves into three dark bands
850 band	4p15.31 and 4p15.33 distinct 5p15.32 distinct 11q24.1 and 11q24.3 distinct 19p13.12 and 19p13.2 distinct

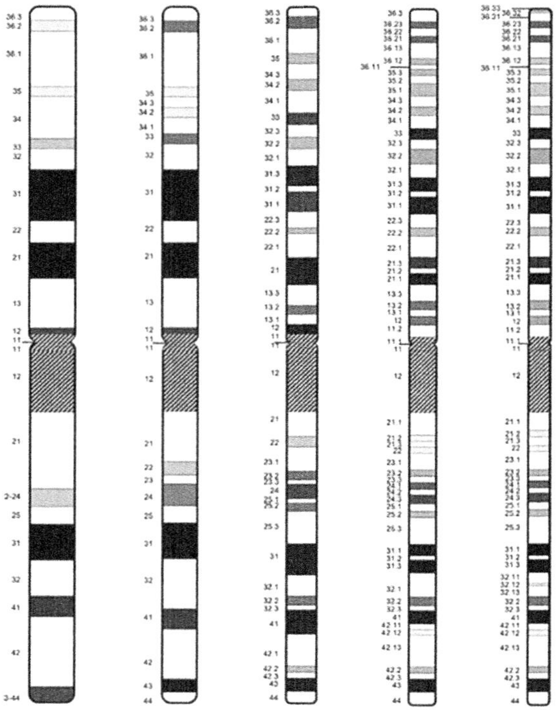

FIGURE 3.3 Idiograms of Giemsa banding (G-banding) patterns for normal human chromosome 1 at (left to right), approximately 300-, 400-, 550-, 700-, and 850-band level resolutions [7].

a. *Aneuploidies* are gains (**trisomies**) or losses (**monosomies**) of one or more chromosomes. Viability of a trisomic embryo depends of the chromosome involved. Most trisomic embryos finish as early pregnancy loss. Trisomies of chromosomes 13, 18, and 21 are the only nonmosaic viable autosomal trisomies in humans. All other nonmosaic trisomies that affect autosomes are generally nonviable. Chromosomes 13, 18, 21 and chromosomes 8, 9, 20, and 22 may be viable in a mosaic form. However, most fetuses with sexual trisomies survive up to birth. Full monosomies are extremely rare in liveborns. Monosomy X (Turner syndrome) is a single viable monosomy (45,X0) in mosaic and nonmosaic forms. Aneuploidy (trisomy or monosomy) is the most common chromosome abnormality, occurring in at least 5% of all clinically recognized pregnancies. About 1 in 3 miscarriages is aneuploid, with monosomy X (45,X) and trisomy 16 the most common [10].
b. ***Mosaicism*** is defined as two or more different genetic cell lines in one individual. The presence of more than one cell line confined to the gonads is called germinal mosaicism, in which chromosomal abnormality occurs only in gametes. In preimplantation embryos,

mosaicism rates are 6%–8.5%, although some groups report up to 21%. Mosaic embryos are characterized by decreased implantation and pregnancy potential, as well as increased risk of miscarriage and adverse perinatal outcomes [11]. This result is consistent with cytogenetic analysis of products of conception (POC) that shows that embryonic mosaicism is ~6% in natural conception and ~5% in pregnancies from Assisted Reproductive Treatment (ART) [12].

c. ***Polyploidy*** is an abnormality in the number of a full set of chromosomes, and polyploid fetuses are usually nonviable. **Triploidy** is characterized on extra haploid set of chromosomes that occurs in up to 3% of recognized human conceptuses and in ~20% of chromosomally abnormal first-trimester spontaneous miscarriages [13]. Triploidy is estimated to occur in 1 of 3,500 pregnancies at 12 weeks, 1 in 30,000 at 16 weeks, and 1 in 250,000 at 20 weeks of gestation [13]. The majority of fetuses with triploidy are spontaneously miscarried at 7–17 weeks of gestation [14,15]. **Tetraploidy** is the presence of four haploid sets of chromosomes, and is generally observed in ~2% of first-trimester miscarriages, although some studies report higher incidences due to diploid/tetraploid mosaicism [16]. Most tetraploid gestations arrest spontaneously, although a few cases of liveborns have been reported [17].

2. ***Structural abnormalities*** are rearrangements within or between chromosomes and can be classified as follows:

   a. ***Balanced rearrangements*** occur when there is a rearrangement with no loss or gain of genetic material, and they usually do not lead to phenotypic abnormalities. The most common balanced rearrangements are as follows:

      i. ***Translocations*** refer to interchange of a chromosomal fragment between two or more chromosomes. There are two types of translocations, Robertsonian and reciprocal translocations. **Robertsonian translocations** involve two acrocentric chromosomes (13, 14, 15, 21, and 22) joined at the centromere. Loss of the short arm of acrocentric chromosomes does not result in phenotypic alterations because they only contain rRNA genes. The incidence of Robertsonian translocations is 0.1% in the general population, 1.1% in patients with Recurrent Pregnancy Loss (RPL), and 3% in infertile men [18,19]. **Reciprocal translocations** involve nonacrocentric chromosomes and are one of the most common chromosome structural abnormalities, with an incidence of 0.2% of human newborns [20,21]. Both types of translocations can be inherited or *de novo*. In de novo translocations, an apparently balanced rearrangement can disrupt genes located near the breakpoints and have clinical consequences. Inherited balanced translocations are commonly innocuous for the carrier, although the carrier is at risk of producing offspring with unbalanced gametes. The risk of the imbalance depends on the size of the involved chromosomal regions and which parent is the carrier. The risk of having abnormal offspring is specific for each translocation event.

      ii. ***Inversions*** are rearrangements that occur when a single chromosome breaks at two points and rotates 180 degrees. In a **pericentric inversion**, the inverted region contains the centromere; in a **paracentric inversion**, the inverted region does not contain the centromere. Excluding variant forms, pericentric inversions are estimated to have a frequency of ~0.12%–0.7% [22], and paracentric inversions are estimated to have a frequency of 0.1%–0.5% [21,23,24]. Carriers of inversions are at risk of having offspring with unbalanced karyotypes. This risk depends of the implicated chromosome and the length of the inverted segment [27–29].

iii. ***Fragile sites*** are specific loci that preferentially exhibit gaps and breaks on metaphase chromosomes following partial inhibition of DNA synthesis [30]. Fragile sites can be classified in three categories according to their behavior under different culture conditions [31,32]: folate-sensitive fragile sites (2q11, 2q13, 6p23, 7p11, 8q22, 9p21, 9q32, 10q23, 11q13, 11q23, 12q13, 16p12, 20p11, 22q13, and Xq27); fragile sites at 16q22 and 17p12, which are not affected by folate concentration but their expression can be enhanced by distamycin A or bromodeoxyuridine (BrdU) [33,34]; and fragile site 10q25, which can be induced by BrdU [35,36].

b. ***Unbalanced rearrangements*** occur when there is a rearrangement with loss or gain of genetic material, causing an abnormal phenotype. The most common unbalanced rearrangements are as follows.

i. ***Deletions*** are structural abnormalities consisting of loss of chromosomal fragments that produce partial chromosomal monosomies. Cytogenetically visible deletions occur in 1 in ~7000 live births [36]. Another study showed 4.7% of all reported chromosome abnormalities are deletions, including microdeletions, giving a prevalence of 1.99 per 10,000 births [37].

ii. ***Duplications*** are structural abnormalities consisting of gain of chromosomal fragments that produce partial chromosomal trisomies. Duplications are less common, with a prevalence of 0.7 per 10,000 births and representing 1.6% of all reported chromosome abnormalities [37].

iii. ***Insertions*** occur when a chromosomal segment is moved and inserted, directly or inverted, into the same or another chromosome. Insertion events are frequent, with an reported incidence of 0.2% [38] or 0.18% [39]. Another study demonstrated that ~2.1% of apparently *de novo* interstitial copy number variations (CNVs) are actually consequences of imbalances resulting from parents with balanced insertions [40].

iv. ***Isochromosomes*** are chromosomes with two equal arms, in which one arm is duplicated and the other is deleted.

v. ***Ring chromosomes*** originate when there is a break in a chromosome at two points followed by rejoining in a ring structure. Phenotypes associated with ring chromosomes are highly variable. If there is an addition to the primary deletion associated with ring formation, then a loss or gain may occur due to ring chromosome instability [41]. There are also reports of ring chromosomes without clinical consequences apart from possible infertility [42]. Constitutional ring chromosomes are a rare type of intrachromosomal structural abnormality with an estimated occurrence of 1 in 50,000 newborns [43].

xvi. ***Small supernumerary marker chromosomes (sSMC)*** are structurally abnormal chromosomes that are smaller than a normal chromosome, and they are rarely identifiable by conventional banding cytogenetic analysis [44]. Phenotypic effects of sSMCs depend on factors such as size, genetic content, and level of mosaicism [45]. The presence of an sSMC can cause partial trisomy or tetrasomy [46]. Frequency in the general population is estimated at ~0.04% [47].

Heteromorphisms, polymorphisms, or normal variants

There are heritable variants in specific chromosomal regions that have no proven impact on the patient's phenotype. These variants are called heteromorphisms, polymorphisms, or normal variants [48], and are generally inherited but can occur *de novo*. In some published studies, chromosome heteromorphisms are reported to be more frequent in infertile couples than the normal population [49–51], especially on chromosomes 1, 9, 16, and Y [49]. An increased frequency of polymorphic variants has been shown among infertile patients (19.4% vs. 13.4% in controls; $P < .01$) [52]. The most normal variants are listed in Table 3.3.

TABLE 3.3 Most common normal variants.

Heteromorphism	Nomenclature	Examples
Large heterochromatin	**qh +**	1qh + , 9qh + , and 16qh +
Pericentric inversion	**inv**	inv(9)(p12q13) and inv (9)(p11q13)
Variant satellite region	**stk + /stk−**	13pstk + and 14pstk −
	s + /s−	15ps + , 21ps − , and 22ps +
Variant Yqh	+ /−	Yqh + and Yqh−

- ***Large heterochromatin*** refers to a variable amount of heterochromatin below the centromere in the proximal q arm of chromosomes 1, 9, and 16. In general, there is no clinical consequence.
- ***Variant Yqh*** indicates that part of the Y chromosome contains only heterochromatin in the distal long arm (Yqh). The Yqh region has variable size, a small Yqh is designated Yqh−, while a large Yqh is designated Yqh + .
- ***Pericentric inversions***: Generally, they have no clinical consequence. One of the most common is pericentric inversion of chromosome 9, including inv(9)(p12q13) and inv(9)(p11q13) [53]. The most common is inv (9)(p11q12)/(p11q13), which is present in 1%–3% of the population [54].
- ***Variant satellite regions*** indicate that stalk and satellite regions of acrocentric chromosomes can be larger or smaller than normal, or satellites may appear as double satellites. If no euchromatin is affected, they are considered normal variants.

Tissue culture techniques and chromosome preparation

To perform chromosomal analysis, cells should be grown and divided in culture. Metaphase chromosomes are then collected and stained with specific dyes for microscopic analysis. Chromosome analysis can be performed on a variety of specimen types.

TABLE 3.4 Typical acceptable failure rates by specimen type (Modified table from [55]).

Specimen type	Accepted culture failure rate (%)
Amniotic fluid and chorionic villus sampling	5–10
Products of Conception (POC)	5–42
Peripheral blood	1–5

The most common specimens in reproductive medicine are amniotic fluid and chorionic villus sampling for prenatal studies, peripheral blood for postnatal studies, and fetal tissue from POC [55]. Protocols for sample processing differ according to the sample type.

Cell cultures can be contaminated by the presence of bacteria or fungi in the specimen itself, at the time of collection, during transport, or in the laboratory [56]. Usually, antibacterial and antifungal products are used in the laboratory to minimize contamination. Some protocols also can reduce or remove contamination to enable successful karyotyping. However, contamination is sometimes the cause of culture failure. In other cases, chromosomal abnormalities themselves or the status of the sample can cause culture failure (Table 3.4).

Cell culture for standard karyotypes in peripheral blood

The most common cytogenetic analysis is karyotype of **T lymphocytes** from peripheral blood. Culturing lymphocytes for cytogenetic analysis is a relatively simple technique that was initially reported by Moorhead *et al.* [45] (Table 3.5) [57]. Peripheral blood is collected in a tube with heparin to avoid coagulation, and then a blood sample is cultured with culture medium and antibiotics to avoid microbial contamination. T lymphocytes in culture are stimulated with mitogens for a few days and then treated with mitotic spindle inhibitors to arrest dividing cells at metaphase. Cells are lysed with a hypotonic solution to release chromosomes from cell nuclei and separate chromosomes for counting. Chromosomes are

TABLE 3.5 Cell culture protocol for standard karyotype.

Cell culture
Blood collected in sterile tubes containing anticoagulant **heparin**
Whole blood leukocytes separated from red blood cells or purified lymphocytes put in a tube with **culture medium** supplemented with serum and antibiotics
Mitogen [**phytohemagglutinin (PHA)**] added to induce mitosis [58]. PHA is a lectin extracted from *Phaseolus vulgaris* that interacts with glycoproteins present on the surface of T cells and stimulates proliferation
Cultures incubated at **37°C for 72 or 96 hours in an incubator**, shaken at least twice daily to increase mitosis
Colchicine or **colcemid** added to cultures a few hours before harvesting to arrest cells in metaphase. Colcemid is a synthetic analogue of colchicine, an alkaloid derived from *Autumn crocus*, that exerts an antimitotic effect by blocking formation of the mitotic spindle, preventing cells from advancing to anaphase
Harvest
Tubes centrifuged after incubation for 72 hours
Supernatant discarded and cells resuspended
Hypotonic treatment of fresh potassium chloride solution (KCl, 0.075 M) added. Osmosis causes inflammation of cells, dispersing chromosomes [25,26]
Tubes centrifuged, supernatant discarded, and pellet resuspended
Fixation
Carnoy's solution (3:1 methanol and glacial acetic acid) used for fixation and several washings
Extension
Cell suspension dropped on a clean slide to fix chromosomes
Slides aged at room temperature for a few daysor in an oven
Prepared slides are stained (banding)

then fixed and spread on a slide, air-dried, and stained [57]. The number of chromosomes and presence of whole and/or partial chromosomes are analyzed on a microscope. The cell culture protocol for a standard karyotype is summarized in Table 3.5.

Cell culture for high-resolution karyotypes in peripheral blood

The level of resolution of a karyotype is determined by the number of bands visualized in a haploid set of chromosomes (22 autosomes, X and Y) [7]. Resolution of chromosome analysis in a conventional karyotype remained relatively limited to 400–550 bands per haploid set until the development of high-resolution karyotyping [6]. This technique synchronizes lymphocyte cultures to obtain chromosomes in early stages of mitosis, such as prophase or prometaphase, when chromosomes are less condensed. In a high-resolution karyotype, prometaphase chromosomes are obtained by incubating the culture with methotrexate (MTX) and then restarting cell division by adding thymidine **to synchronize** the culture [59]. The protocol then continues as a standard karyotype. Chromosomes in prometaphase have a band resolution of 550–850 bands or more in a haploid complement, so more bands can be observed with staining of G or R bands. High-resolution karyotypes are useful to confirm conventional karyotype results, to detect small structural anomalies in a chromosome, and to more precisely define the breakpoints of a chromosomal rearrangement. However, abnormalities detected in the karyotype must be confirmed by Fuorescent *In Situ* Hybridization (FISH) with specific probes or with another molecular cytogenetic technique.

Chromosome banding techniques

Until 1970, chromosomes were uniformly stained and ordered in pairs by size and morphology. In 1971, new techniques were developed that stained chromosomes in light and dark bands [60,61]. These bands showed different patterns that were consistent in each pair of paternal and maternal chromosomes. In metaphase chromosomes, banding techniques produce a series of landmarks that allow recognition of individual chromosomes and identification of specific segments of each chromosome. These landmarks allow assessment of normal chromosomes and identification of breakpoints if there is a rearrangement [62].

Different banding techniques with specific properties and applications have been developed [63]. The banding pattern of a chromosome is identical in all cells from an individual. In polymorphic regions, the banding pattern can differ from one individual to another. These banding patterns behave like a barcode that cytogeneticists can recognized to identify numerical and structural abnormalities, such as translocations, inversions, deletions, duplications, fragile sites, and other more complex rearrangements, and refine breakpoints. For routine analysis, Giemsa banding (G-banding) is the most accepted banding technique and most commonly evaluates 20–25 metaphase cells [64].

Banding techniques fall into the following two groups [7].

Bands distributed along the length of the whole chromosome

- *Giemsa banding (G-banding, GTG)* is the most commonly used technique for cytogenetic diagnosis [65]. GTG-banding uses the proteolytic enzyme trypsin as a pretreatment, followed by staining with Giemsa. G-banding can be visualized with a brightfield microscope. In general, Giemsa-positive bands (dark bands) are AT-rich, late replicating, and gene-poor, whereas Giemsa-negative bands (light bands) are CG-rich, early replicating, and relatively gene-rich [65]. Abnormalities detected by G-banding are whole chromosome aneuploidies, balanced rearrangements, deletions, duplications, >20% mosaicism, sSMC (nonmosaic), and polyploidy.

- ***Quinacrine banding (Q-banding, QFQ)*** was the first chromosome banding technique developed [3,66,67]. Q-banding exposes slides of metaphase chromosomes to the fluorescent DNA intercalating agent quinacrine, and chromosomes are viewed with a fluorescence microscope with UV illumination [1,62]. Fluorescent and bright bands are observed in contrast with other nonfluorescent bands. Bright Q-bands correspond to dark G-bands.
- ***Reverse banding (R-banding, RHG)*** produces a pattern of bands that are the reverse of the Q- and G-banding pattern. R-banding is useful for visualization of telomeric ends of chromosomes. R-banding can be obtained with different methods, including one based on heating slides at 88°C in a buffer and then staining with Giemsa [60,62].

Bands that stain specific chromosome structures

- ***Centromeric heterochromatin staining (C-banding, CBG)*** uses mild alkali treatment and Giemsa dyes to stain centromeric regions of each chromosome and other heterochromatin-containing regions: acrocentric chromosomes 1q, 9q, and 16q adjacent to the centromere, and the distal portion of Yq. This banding is viewed with a brightfield microscope [62]. Polymorphic regions can be distinct yet not clinically significant in different individuals.
- ***Nucleolar-organizer-region staining (NOR staining)*** is a technique that stains NOR regions [68] that contain genes for ribosomal RNA. NOR are located in the satellite stalks of acrocentric chromosomes 13, 14, 15, 21, and 22. Acrocentric chromosomes have long and short arms with stalks and satellite regions without euchromatic regions. This stain uses a silver nitrate solution and is viewed with a brightfield microscope [62]. NOR banding is useful to study some chromosome polymorphisms and to identify satellite stalks in nonacrocentric chromosomes.
- ***T-banding*** stains telomeric regions of chromosomes. It is an R-banding variant developed by Dutrillaux [69] that only deeply stains telomeres.
- ***FISH*** is a combination of a molecular technique and a cytogenetic technique that uses a fluorescent signal to identify a chromosomal region containing a determined sequence. This technique can be performed on conventional preparations used for karyotypes. A sequence localized in the region of interest is hybridized with a complementary DNA probe labeled with fluorescence [70–72]. There are DNA probes for specific centromeres, subtelomeric regions of each chromosome, and locus-specific probes. Subtelomeric probes allow identification of cryptic structural rearrangements that are not detected with a karyotype.

Clinical indications for cytogenetic analysis

Cytogenetic analysis in parents

Genetic analysis has allowed identification of genetic changes that are responsible for ***chromosomopathies***. Although conventional cytogenetic techniques have been in existence for almost half a century, they continue to provide valuable clinical information. Since the introduction of karyotyping, reproductive problems have been associated with chromosomal abnormalities [73], so karyotyping has been recommended for infertile couples [74].

Chromosomal abnormalities are an important cause of infertility. Patients with abnormal karyotypes can have gametogenesis failure, leading to reproductive failures or congenital birth anomalies. Karyotype analysis allows detection of chromosomal anomalies in infertile patients who are phenotypically normal [75]. Identification of chromosomal abnormalities is crucial to detecting the etiology of infertility and thus facilitating counseling and management of the case. Consequently, conventional cytogenetic analysis has been recommended in infertile patients before starting treatment, specifically for the following conditions.

- *Recurrent Pregnancy Loss (RPL)*: The frequency of chromosomal abnormalities among couples with RPL is 2%–8% ([76,77]; [18,78,79]), which is higher than in the general population (0.2%) [80]. Balanced translocations are the most frequent abnormalities [81,82]. Preimplantation Genetic Testing For Structural Rearrangements (PGT-SR) allows selection of normal/balanced embryos for transfer in structural rearrangement carriers. Breakpoints of the rearrangement, and thus the resulting fragment sizes, determine the PGT-SR strategy. For this reason, it is very important to know the precise karyotype formula of the parents to select an accurate methodology. In couples with a normal karyotype, an abnormal embryonic karyotype is often the cause of recurrent miscarriages [83]. The prevalence of abnormal embryonic karyotypes is reported to be 25.4%–44.1% [83–87]. The difference depends on the woman's age and the number of miscarriages. The abnormality rate increases as a woman's age increases and the previous number of miscarriages decreases [88].
- *Repetitive implantation failure (RIF)*: Aneuploidies also have been largely associated with implantation failure. Carriers of a balanced translocation can produce unbalanced gametes, which can result in implantation failure, mainly due to autosomal monosomies [89]. An increased prevalence of chromosome structural abnormalities has been documented in RIF patients [90,91]. The incidence of karyotype anomalies in RIF patients is only about 2%, and most abnormalities found in embryos arise *de novo* during meiosis or mitosis [92].
- *Male factor infertility (MF):* Genetic abnormalities are thought to account for 15%–30% of MF [93]. Abnormal male karyotypes account for ~5% of infertility in males, and the prevalence increases to 15% in azoospermic males [94]. Severe MF is associated with an increased occurrence of sex chromosome abnormalities in embryos compared to embryos derived from men with normal semen [95]. One of the most common cytogenetic abnormalities related to MF is Klinefelter syndrome (47,XXY), which affects hormone levels, testicular volume, and sperm count [96]. In fact, elevated chromosomal abnormalities for both sex chromosomes and autosomes have been found in embryos from males with Klinefelter syndrome [97].

When a karyotypic abnormality is found in the parents or in cases of normal karyotype but high risk of *de novo* aneuploidies, Preimplantation Genetic Testing (PGT) is a powerful tool to improve reproductive outcomes. PGT-SR is used for carriers of abnormal karyotypes, while PGT-A is used for aneuploidies. PGT-A has been extensively applied in couples of advanced female age; in couples with a history of RPL, RIF, or MF; and carriers of numerical chromosomal abnormalities (e.g., sex chromosome aneuploidies and mosaic karyotypes).

Cytogenetic analysis in Product Of Conception(POC)

Traditional POC studies using cell culture followed by conventional karyotyping have shown an incidence of chromosomal abnormalities in the general population of 40%–80%, depending on the culture method used [98,99–101]. Proper chromosomal analysis of POC samples by karyotyping is not always feasible for cell **culture growth failure** (5%–42% failure rate in POC samples cultured after curettage), suboptimal chromosome preparations, and maternal cell contamination (MCC). Culture-independent molecular biology techniques can avoid such limitations [102]. The incidence of fetoplacental aneuploidies increases significantly with advancing female age [37]. A higher rate of abnormal POC also has been found in ART patients using their own oocytes (62.7%) compared to natural conceptions (40.6%). These results could be explained by differences in female age, which is higher in ART patients than natural conceptions [102].

Prenatal diagnosis

Karyotyping in prenatal samples requires invasive procedures (amniocentesis and chorionic villi biopsy), which are associated with a 0.1%–0.5% increased risk of miscarriage [103,104]. **Invasive prenatal diagnosis** is indicated in cases of advanced maternal age, ultrasound suspicion of chromosomopathy, altered noninvasive prenatal testing, carriers of chromosomal rearrangements, oligoamnios-polyhydramnios, delayed intrauterine growth, and unique umbilical artery. Recently, Noninvasive Prenatal Testing (NIPT) for fetal aneuploidy has been introduced. NIPT allows detection of fetal chromosome abnormalities based on analysis of cell-free fetal DNA (cfDNA) present in maternal blood during pregnancy [105], reducing the need for invasive procedures and the number of couples that require amniocentesis or chorionic villi biopsy. However, invasive prenatal procedures are still required to confirm an abnormal NIPT result or when there is a suspicion of genetic abnormality not associated with abnormalities studied in NIPT.

References

[1] Hare WCD, Singh EL. Cytogenetics in animal reproduction. Slough: Commonwealth Agricultural Bureaux, UK; 1979.

[2] Caspersson T, Farber S, Foley GE, Kudynowski J, Modest EJ, Simonsson E, et al. Chemical differentiation along metaphase chromosomes. Exp Cell Res 1968;49(1):219–22.

[3] Caspersson T, Zech L, Modest EJ, Foley GE, Wagh U, Simonsson E. Chemical differentiation with fluorescent alkylating agents in Vicia faba metaphase chromosomes. Exp Cell Res 1969;58(1):128–40.

[4] Caspersson T, Zech L, Modest EJ, Foley GE, Wagh U, Simonsson E. DNA-binding fluorochromes for the study of the organization of the metaphase nucleus. Exp Cell Res 1969;58(1):141–52.

[5] Pardue ML, Gall JG. Chromosomal localization of mouse satellite DNA. Science 1970;168(3937):1356–8.

[6] Yunis JJ. High resolution of human chromosomes. Science 1976;191(4233):1268–70.

[7] McGowan-Jordan J., Simons A., Schmid M. ISCN 2016. An international system for human cytogenomic nomenclature basel. Karger; 2016.

[8] Shaffer LG, Bejjani BA. A cytogeneticist's perspective on genomic microarrays. Hum Reprod Update 2004;10 (3):221–6.

[9] ACC Professional Guidelines for Clinical Cytogenetics: General Best Practice v1.04, 2007.

[10] Hassold T, Hunt P. To err (meiotically) is human: the genesis of human aneuploidy. Nat Rev Genet 2001;2 (4):280–91.

[11] Simon C. Introduction: To transfer or not transfer... a mosaic embryo, that is the question. Fertil Steril 2017;107(5):1083–4.

[12] Martinez MC, Mendez C, Ferro J, Nicolas M, Serra V, Landeras J. Cytogenetic analysis of early nonviable pregnancies after assisted reproduction treatment. Fertil Steril 2010;93(1):289–92.

[13] Kolarski M, Ahmetovic B, Beres M, Topic R, Nikic V, Kavecan I, et al. Genetic Counseling and Prenatal Diagnosis of Triploidy During the Second Trimester of Pregnancy. Med Arch 2017;71(2):144–7.

[14] Gardner RJM, Sutherland GR, Schaffer LG. Chromosome abnormalities and genetic counseling. 4th ed. New York, NY: Oxford University Press; 2012.

[15] Huang T, Alberman E, Wald N, Summers AM. Triploidy identified through second-trimester serum screening. Prenat Diagn 2005;25(3):229–33.

[16] Jenderny J. Chromosome aberrations in a large series of spontaneous miscarriages in the German population and review of the literature. Mol Cytogenet 2014;7:38. Available from: https://doi.org/10.1186/1755-8166-7-38.eCollection2014.

[17] Schluth C, Doray B, Girard-Lemaire F, Favre R, Flori J, Gasser B, et al. Prenatal diagnosis of a true fetal tetraploidy in direct and cultured chorionic villi. Genet Couns. 2004;15:429–36.

[18] Fryns JP, Van Buggenhout G. Structural chromosome rearrangements in couples with recurrent fetal wastage. Eur J Obstet Gynecol Reprod Biol 1998;81(2):171–6.

[19] Therman E, Susman B, Denniston C. The nonrandom participation of human acrocentric chromosomes in Robertsonian translocations. Ann Hum Genet 1989;53 (1):49–65.

[20] Jacobs PA, Melville M, Ratcliffe S, Keay AJ, Syme J. A cytogenetic survey of 11,680 newborn infants. Ann Hum Genet 1974;37:359–76.

[21] Van Dyke DL, Weiss L, Roberson JR, Babu VR. The frequency and mutation rate of balanced autosomal rearrangements in man estimated from prenatal genetic studies for advanced maternal age. Am J Hum Genet 1983;35:301–8.

[22] Gardner RJM, Sutherland GR. Chromosome Abnormalities and Genetic Counseling. New York: Oxford University Press; 1996. p. 68–79.

[23] Fryns JP, Kleczkowska A, Kubien E, Petit P, Van den Berghe H. Cytogenetic survey in couples with recurrent fetal wastage. Hum Genet 1984;65:336–54.

[24] Worsham MJ, Miller DA, Devries JM, et al. A dicentric recombinant 9 derived from a paracentric inversion: phenotype, cytogenetics, and molecular analysis of centromeres. Am J Hum Genet 1989;44:115–23.

[25] HSU TC. Mammalian chromosomes in vitro. I. The karyotype of man. J Hered 1952;43:167–72.

[26] Hughes A. Some effects of abnormal tonicity on dividing cells in chick tissue cultures. Quart J Mirr Sci 1952;93:207–19.

[27] Balicek P. Pericentric inversion of human chromosomes and its risks. Cas Lek Cesk 2001;140(2):38–42.

[28] Bocian E, Suchenek K, Obersztyn E, Nowakowska B, Mazurczak T. Recombination aneusomy of subtelomeric regions of chromosome 5, resulting from a large familial pericentric inversion inv(5)(p15.33q35.3). J Appl Genet 2005;46(1):109–14.

[29] Saura R, Longy M, Sautarael M, Renouil M, Sandler B. Double trisomy and transmitted pericentric inversion (48, XXY, +21, inv(22)). Interchromosomal effect. Ann Genet 1983;26(3):180–2.

[30] Durkin SG, Glover TW. Chromosome fragile sites. Annu Rev Genet 2007;41:169–92.

[31] Berger R, Bloomfield CD, Sutherland GR. Report of the committee on chromosome rearrangements in neoplasia and on fragile sites. Cytogenet Cell Genet 1985;40(1–4):490–535.

[32] Sutherland GR, Jacky PB, Baker E, Manuel A. Heritable fragile sites on human chromosomes. X. New folate-sensitive fragile sites: 6p23, 9p21, 9q32, and 11q23. Am J Hum Genet 1983;35(3):432–7.

[33] Schmid M, Klett C, Niederhofer A. Demonstration of a heritable fragile site in human chromosome 16 with distamycin A. Cytogenet Cell Genet 1980;28 (1–2):87–94.

[34] Sutherland GR, Jacky PB, Baker EG. Heritable fragile sites on human chromosomes. XI. Factors affecting expression of fragile sites at 10q25, 16q22, and 17p12. Am J Hum Genet 1984;36(1):110–22.

[35] Scheres JM, Hustinx TW. Heritable fragile sites and lymphocyte culture medium containing BrdU. Am J Hum Genet 1980;32(4):628–9.

[36] Jacobs PA, Browne C, Gregson N, Joyce C, White H. Estimates of the frequency of chromosome abnormalities detectable in unselected newborns using moderate levels of banding. J Med Genet 1992;29(2):103–8.

[37] Wellesley D, Dolk H, Boyd PA, Greenlees R, Haeusler M, Nelen V, et al. Rare chromosome abnormalities, prevalence and prenatal diagnosis rates from population-based congenital anomaly registers in Europe. Eur J Hum Genet 2012;20(5):521–6.

[38] Kang SH, Shaw C, Ou Z, Eng PA, Cooper ML, Pursley AN, et al. Insertional translocation detected using FISH confirmation of array-comparative genomic hybridization (aCGH) results. Am J Med Genet A 2010;152A(5):1111–26.

[39] Neill NJ, Ballif BC, Lamb AN, Parikh S, Ravnan JB, Schultz RA, et al. Recurrence, submicroscopic complexity, and potential clinical relevance of copy gains detected by array CGH that are shown to be unbalanced insertions by FISH. Genome Res 2011;21 (4):535–44.

[40] Nowakowska BA, de Leeuw N, Ruivenkamp CA, Sikkema-Raddatz B, Crolla JA, Thoelen R, et al. Parental insertional balanced translocations are an important cause of apparently de novo CNVs in patients with developmental anomalies. Eur J Hum Genet 2012;20(2):166–70.

[41] Yip M-Y. Autosomal ring chromosomes in human genetic disorders. Transl Pediatr 2015;4:164–74.

[42] Guilherme RS, Meloni VF, Kim CA, Pellegrino R, Takeno SS, Spinner NB, et al. Mechanisms of ring chromosome formation, ring instability and clinical consequences. BMC Med Genet 2011;12:171–2350-12-171.

[43] Jacobs PA, Frackiewicz A, Law P, Hilditch CJ, Morton NE. The effect of structural aberrations of the chromosomes on reproductive fitness in man. II. Results. Clin Genet 1975;8(3):169–78.

[44] Lasan Trcić R, Hitrec V, Letica L, Cuk M, Begović D. Small supernumerary marker chromosome derived from proximal p-arm of chromosome 2: Identification

by fluorescent *in situ* hybridization. Croat Med J 2003;44:477–9.
[45] Woo HY, Cho HJ, Kong SY, Kim HJ, Jeon HB, Kim EC, et al. Marker chromosomes in Korean patients: Incidence, identification and diagnostic approach. J Korean Med Sci 2003;18:773–8.
[46] Jafari-Ghahfarokhi H, Moradi-Chaleshtori M, Liehr T, Hashemzadeh-Chaleshtori M, Teimori H, Ghasemi-Dehkordi P. Small supernumerary marker chromosomes and their correlation with specific syndromes. Adv Biomed Res 2015;4:140. Available from: https://doi.org/10.4103/2277-9175.161542.eCollection2015.
[47] Liehr T, Claussen U, Starke H. Small supernumerary marker chromosomes (sSMC) in humans. Cytogenet Genome Res 2004;107(1-2):55–67.
[48] Sahin FI, Yilmaz Z, Yuregir OO, Bulakbasi T, Ozer O, Zeyneloglu HB. Chromosome heteromorphisms: an impact on infertility. J Assist Reprod Genet 2008;25 (5):191–5.
[49] Madon PF, Athalye AS, Parikh FR. Polymorphic variants on chromosomes probably play a significant role in infertility. Reprod Biomed Online 2005;11 (6):726–32.
[50] Nakamura Y, Kitamura M, Nishimura K, Koga M, Kondoh N, Takeyama M, et al. Chromosomal variants among 1790 infertile men. Int J Urol 2001;8(2):49–52.
[51] Yakin K, Balaban B, Urman B. Is there a possible correlation between chromosomal variants and spermatogenesis? Int J Urol 2005;12(11):984–9.
[52] Morales R, Lledo B, Ortiz JA, Ten J, Llacer J, Bernabeu R. Chromosomal polymorphic variants increase aneuploidies in male gametes and embryos. Syst Biol Reprod Med 2016;62(5):317–24.
[53] Kaiser P. Pericentric inversions. Problems and significance for clinical genetics. Hum Genet 1984;68(1):1–47.
[54] Dana M, Stoian V. Association of pericentric inversion of chromosome 9 and infertility in romanian population. Maedica (Buchar) 2012;7(1):25–9.
[55] Zneimer SM. Cytogenetic abnormalities. Hoboken: John Wiley & Sons, Inc; 2014.
[56] Moorhead PS, Nowell PC, Mellman WJ, Battips DM, Hungerford DA. Chromosome preparations of leukocytes cultured from human peripheral blood. Exp Cell Res 1960;20:613–16.
[57] Howe B, Umrigar A, Tsien F. Chromosome preparation from cultured cells. J Vis Exp 2014;83:e50203.
[58] Nowell PC. Phytohemagglutinin: An initiator of mitosis in cultures of normal human leukocytes. Cancer Res 1960;20:462–6.
[59] Yunis JJ, Chandler ME. The chromosomes of man—clinical and biologic significance. A review. Am J Pathol 1977;88(2):466–96.
[60] Dutrillaux B, Lejeune J. Sur une nouvelle technique d'analyse du caryotype humain. Compt Rend Acad Sci Paris 1971;272:2638–40.
[61] Arrighi FE, Hsu TC. Localization of heterochromatin in human chromosomes. Cytogenetics 1971;10(2):81–6.
[62] Schreck RR, Disteche CM. Chromosome banding techniques. Curr Protoc Hum Genet 2001; Chapter 4: Unit 4.2.
[63] Rooney DE, editor. Human cytogenetics: constitutional analysis. 3rd edn Oxford: Oxford University Press; 2001.
[64] Swansbury J. Introduction to the analysis of the human G-banded karyotype. Methods Mol Biol 2003;220:259–69.
[65] Seabright M. A rapid banding technique for human chromosomes. (Letter.). Lancet 1971;2:971–2.
[66] Caspersson T, Zech L, Johansson C, Modest EJ. Identification of human chromosomes by DNA-binding fluorescent agents. Chromosoma 1970;30 215–27.
[67] Caspersson T, Lomakka G, Zech L. The 24 fluorescence patterns of the human metaphase chromosomes-distinguishing characters and variability. Hereditas (Lund.) 1971;67:89–102.
[68] Matsui S, Sasaki M. Differential staining of nucleolus organisers in mammalian chromosomes. Nature 1973;246(5429):148–50.
[69] Dutrillaux B. New system of chromosome banding: the T bands (author's transl). Chromosoma 1973;41 (4):395–402.
[70] Landegent JE, Jansen in de Wal N, Dirks RW, Baas F, van der Ploeg M. Use of the whole cosmid cloned genomic sequences for chromosomal localization by non-radioactive in situ hybridization. Hum Genet 1987;77:366–70.
[71] Pinkel D, et al. Fluorescence in situ hybridization with human chromosome specific libraries: detection of trisomy 21 and translocation of chromosome 4. Proc Natl Acad Sci USA 1988;85:9138–42.
[72] Cremer T, Lichter P, Borden J, Ward DC, Mannuelidis L. Detection of chromosome aberrations in metaphase and interphase tumor cells by in situ hybridization using chromosome-specific library probes. Hum Genet 1988;80:235–46.
[73] Shi Q, Martin RH. Aneuploidy in human sperm: a review of the frequency and distribution of aneuploidy, effects of donor age and lifestyle factors. Cytogenet Cell Genet 2000;90(3–4):219–26.
[74] Campana M, Serra A, Neri G. Role of chromosome aberrations in recurrent abortion: a study of 269 balanced translocations. Am J Med Genet 1986;24 (2):341–56.

[75] Chantot-Bastaraud S, Ravel C, Siffroi JP. Underlying karyotype abnormalities in IVF/ICSI patients. Reprod Biomed Online 2008;16:514–22.

[76] Dutta UR, Rajitha P, Pidugu VK, Dalal AB. Cytogenetic abnormalities in 1162 couples with recurrent miscarriages in southern region of India: report and review. J Assist Reprod Genet 2011;28(2):145–9.

[77] Frenny JS, Thomas L, Pritti K, Ralph A, Harsh JS, Jayesh JS. Chromosomal abnormalities in couples with repeated fetal loss: An Indian retrospective study. Indian J Hum Genet 2013;19(415):422.

[78] Elghezal H, Hidar S, Mougou S, Khairi H, Saad A. Prevalence of chromosomal abnormalities in couples with recurrent miscarriage. Fertil Steril 2007;88(3):721–3.

[79] Meza-Espinoza JP, Anguiano LO, Rivera H. Chromosomal abnormalities in couples with reproductive disorders. Gynecol Obstet Invest 2008;66(4):237–40.

[80] Regan L, BackosM, Rai R. Green-top Guideline No 17. The investigation and treatment of couples with recurrent first-trimester and second-trimester miscarriage. London: Royal College of Obstetricians and Gynaecologists (RCOG); 2011.

[81] Shekoohi S, Mojarrad M, Raoofian R, Ahmadzadeh S, Mirzaie S, Hassanzadeh-Nazarabadi M, et al. Chromosomal study of couples with the history of recurrent spontaneous abortions with diagnosed blightded ovum. Int J Mol Cell Med 2013;2:164–8.

[82] Hyde KJ, Schust DJ. Genetic considerations in recurrent pregnancy loss. Cold Spring Harb Perspect Med 2015;5:a023119.

[83] Sugiura-Ogasawara M, Ozaki Y, Katano K, Suzumori N, Kitaori T, Mizutani E. Abnormal embryonic karyotype is the most frequent cause of recurrent miscarriage. Hum Reprod 2012;27(8):2297–303.

[84] Carp H, Toder V, Aviram A, Daniely M, Mashiach S, Barkai G. Karyotype of the abortus in recurrent miscarriage. Fertil Steril 2001;75(4):678–82.

[85] Stephenson MD, Awartani KA, Robinson WP. Cytogenetic analysis of miscarriages from couples with recurrent miscarriage: a case-control study. Hum Reprod 2002;17(2):446–51.

[86] Stern JJ, Dorfmann AD, Gutierrez-Najar AJ, Cerrillo M, Coulam CB. Frequency of abnormal karyotypes among abortuses from women with and without a history of recurrent spontaneous abortion. Fertil Steril 1996;65(2):250–3.

[87] Sullivan AE, Silver RM, LaCoursiere DY, Porter TF, Branch DW. Recurrent fetal aneuploidy and recurrent miscarriage. Obstet Gynecol 2004;104(4):784–8.

[88] Ogasawara M, Aoki K, Okada S, Suzumori K. Embryonic karyotype of abortuses in relation to the number of previous miscarriages. Fertil Steril 2000;73(2):300–4.

[89] Mau-Holzmann UA. Somatic chromosomal abnormalities in infertile men and women. Cytogenet Genome Res 2005;111(3–4):317–36.

[90] Raziel A, Friedler S, Schachter M, Kasterstein E, Strassburger D, Ron-El R. Increased frequency of female partner chromosomal abnormalities in patients with high-order implantation failure after in vitro fertilization. Fertil Steril 2002;78(3):515–19.

[91] Stern C, Pertile M, Norris H, Hale L, Baker HW. Chromosome translocations in couples with in-vitro fertilization implantation failure. Hum Reprod 1999;14(8):2097–101.

[92] Garcia-Herrero S., Rodrigo L., Mateu E., et al. Medecine therapeutique/Medecine de la reproduction, gynecologie et endocrinologie. John Libbey Eurotext 2014;14(2):112–119.

[93] O'Flynn O'Brien KL, Varghese AC, Agarwal A. The genetic causes of male factor infertility: a review. Fertil Steril 2010;93(1):1–12.

[94] Ferlin A, Raicu F, Gatta V, Zuccarello D, Palka G, Foresta C. Male infertility: role of genetic background. Reprod Biomed Online 2007;14(6):734–45.

[95] Coates A, Hesla JS, Hurliman A, Coate B, Holmes E, Matthews R, et al. Use of suboptimal sperm increases the risk of aneuploidy of the sex chromosomes in preimplantation blastocyst embryos. Fertil Steril 2015;104(4):866–72.

[96] Elfateh F, Wang R, Zhang Z, Jiang Y, Chen S, Liu R. Influence of genetic abnormalities on semen quality and male fertility: a four-year prospective study. Iran J Reprod Med 2014;12(2):95–102.

[97] Kahraman S, Findikli N, Berkil H, Bakircioglu E, Donmez E, Sertyel S, Biricik A. Results of preimplantation genetic diagnosis in patients with Klinefelter's syndrome. Reprod Biomed Online 2003;73:346–52.

[98] Morales C, Sanchez A, Bruguera J, et al. Cytogenetic study of spontaneous abortions using semi-direct analysis of chorionic villi samples detects the broadest spectrum of chromosome abnormalities. Am J Med Genet 2008;146A(1):66–70.

[99] Guerneri S, Bettio D, Simoni G, Brambati B, Lanzani A, Fraccaro M. Prevalence and distribution of chromosome abnormalities in a sample of first trimester internal abortions. Hum Reprod 1987;2(8):735–9.

[100] Nagaishi M, Yamamoto T, Iinuma K, Shimomura K, Berend SA, Knops J. Chromosome abnormalities identified in 347 spontaneous abortions collected in Japan. J Obstet Gynaecol Res 2004;30(3):237–41.

[101] Yusuf RZ, Naeem R. Cytogenetic abnormalities in products of conception: a relationship revisited. Am J Reprod Immunol 2004;52(1):88–96.
[102] Campos-Galindo I, Garcia-Herrero S, Martinez-Conejero JA, Ferro J, Simon C, Rubio C. Molecular analysis of products of conception obtained by hysteroembryoscopy from infertile couples. J Assist Reprod Genet 2015;32(5):839–48.
[103] Akolekar R, Beta J, Picciarelli G, Ogilvie C, D'Antonio F. Procedure-related risk of miscarriage following amniocentesis and chorionic villus sampling: a systematic review and meta-analysis. Ultrasound Obstet Gynecol 2015;45(1):16–26.
[104] Simpson JL. Invasive procedures for prenatal diagnosis: any future left? Best Pract Res Clin Obstet Gynaecol 2012;26(5):625–38.
[105] Lo YM, Corbetta N, Chamberlain PF, Rai V, Sargent IL, Redman CW, et al. Presence of fetal DNA in maternal plasma and serum. Lancet 1997;350(9076):485–7.

CHAPTER

4

Molecular biology approaches utilized in preimplantation genetics: real-time PCR, microarrays, next-generation sequencing, karyomapping, and others

Almudena Devesa-Peiró[1,2], Josefa María Sánchez-Reyes[1,2] and Patricia Díaz-Gimeno[1,3]

[1]Department of Genomic & Systems Reproductive Medicine, IVI-RMA IVI Foundation, Valencia, Spain [2]Department of Pediatrics, Obstetrics and Gynaecology, School of Medicine, University of Valencia, Valencia, Spain [3]Biomedical Research Institute Hospital La Fe, Valencia, Spain

The success of assisted reproductive techniques relies on a synchronization between a genetically normal human embryo and a receptive endometrium to which it will attach. It has been reported that embryo abnormalities account for one third of implantation failures, while a defective endometrial stage is responsible for the other two thirds [1,2]. Consequently, the detection of these alterations and their correction have become a priority in assisted reproductive treatments (ARTs) to increase pregnancy rates and decrease recurrent miscarriages and implantation failures. While the embryo factor is typically assessed through preimplantation genetic testing (PGT) techniques, the endometrial factor is currently evaluated through gene expression-based diagnostic tools.

The embryo factor: preimplantation genetic testing techniques for embryo selection against chromosomal abnormalities and monogenic disorders

Although embryo morphological evaluation is currently the most clinically established method to assess embryo viability [3], it cannot evaluate chromosomal or gene abnormalities that may lead to miscarriages and implantation failures. PGT was first introduced in the late 1980s [4] to address this problem and offer an alternative to prenatal testing for couples at risk of having children affected with severe monogenic inherited diseases (PGT-M) and/or chromosome abnormalities, both numeric or aneuploidies (PGT-A) and structural (PGT-ST).

Human Reproductive Genetics
DOI: https://doi.org/10.1016/B978-0-12-816561-4.00004-1

PGT is indicated in the following situations: parent(s) that are carriers of a chromosomal or genetic disease, recurrent miscarriages, recurrent implantation failures, advanced maternal age, previous child with a chromosomal or genetic disease, and sex determination in the context of X-linked disease [5].

Overall, PGT techniques perform genetic testing on the DNA extracted typically from one or two cell biopsies of human embryos at a 6–10-cell stage on day 3 after in vitro fertilization (IVF) [6]. However, PGT is also applied to DNA obtained from polar bodies or one-cell zygotes just after IVF, or from 5 to 10 trophectoderm cells from a day 4–5 blastocyst [6]. Regardless of the source of DNA material, PGT techniques allow selection of those embryos without chromosomal or/and gene abnormalities before they are transferred to the uterus in an assisted reproduction treatment (ART). Genetic diagnosis may be achieved through different cytogenetic techniques, the most relevant being described in the following subsections.

Karyotyping

Karyotyping is a cytogenetic technique that was first introduced for prenatal genetic testing in 1966 and is aimed at pairing and ordering all the chromosomes of an organism using standardized staining procedures that reveal their characteristic structural and numerical features [7].

The scheme of the technique can be observed in Fig. 4.1. The process begins with the short-term culture of high-division cells (in this context: embryo-biopsied cells or/and progenitor's blood). After a period of cell growth and multiplication, dividing cells are arrested in metaphase or prometaphase by the addition of colchicine, which poisons the mitotic spindle. This is the cell cycle phase at which chromosomes assume their most condensed conformations. The cells are next treated with a hypotonic solution that causes their nuclei to swell and the cells to burst. After centrifugation, the nuclei are treated with a chemical fixative and various stains that reveal the structural features of the chromosomes when they are observed through a microscope [8,9].

The first karyotypes only detected changes in chromosome numbers or length at a low resolution. This changed with the development of different banding techniques, which are based on differential staining of chromosomal segments according to their enrichment in GC or AT nucleotides, thus enabling the detection of segmental chromosomal imbalances. In current clinical cytogenetics, G-banding and R-binding techniques are widely used. In G-banding, metaphase chromosome proteins are degraded with trypsin to relax the chromatin structure and facilitate Giemsa dye access to the DNA. Heterochromatic AT-enriched DNA segments incorporate more Giemsa and are visualized as dark segments. Alternatively, light segments represent euchromatic and GC-enriched DNA that is more transcriptionally active (Fig. 4.1). R-banding also involves Giemsa staining, but the procedure includes a heating step that melts AT-enriched DNA regions, leaving only the GC-enriched regions to take up the stain and thus generating the reverse pattern. In addition, there are other Giemsa-based banding techniques that are specialized in staining gene-rich telomeric (T-banding) and centromeric (C-banding) regions, which might be clinically useful for detecting abnormalities specifically targeting these structures [8,9].

Karyotyping is the gold standard in prenatal testing for the detection of genome-wide numerical and structural chromosomal aberrations since the first human prenatal testing took place in 1966 [10]. In the context of PGT, clinical cytogeneticists analyze human karyotypes to detect numeric chromosomal abnormalities associated with aneuploid conditions, such as trisomy 21 (Down syndrome), trisomy

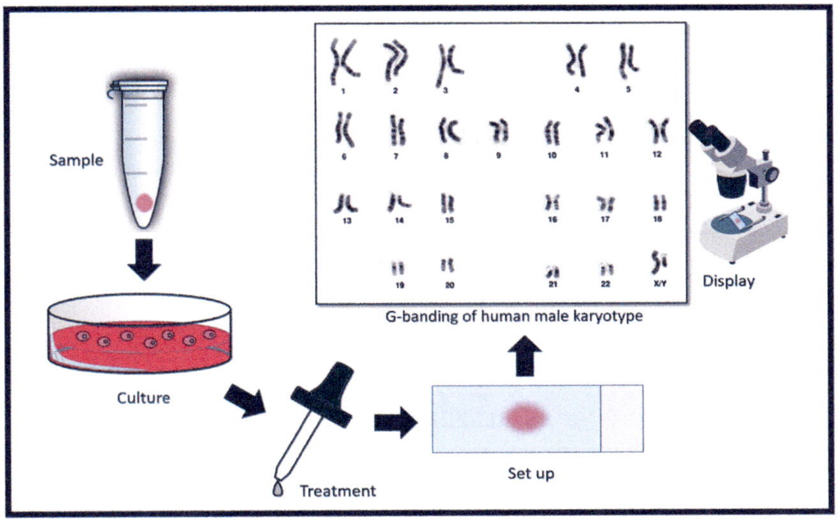

FIGURE 4.1 Scheme of different steps for karyotyping. Cell sample collection and short-term culture, treatments of cells for obtention of metaphase chromosomes, set up of banding chromosomes and display through the microscope. In this case, an example of G-banding of the human male karyotype is shown (*dark segments*: AT-enriched DNA; *light segments*: GC-enriched DNA).

18 (Edward syndrome), trisomy 13 (Patau syndrome), and X-linked chromosome alterations like Klinefelter syndrome (47, XXY) or Turner syndrome (45, X0). Karyotyping can also reveal chromosomal deletions, duplications, inversions, translocations or inversions related to other diseases as cri-du-chat syndrome (5p-) and Wolf-Hirschhorn (4p-) [11]. Karyotyping has several limitations, such as the need for cell cultures and visual screening (which requires skilled analysts and is time consuming), and a still low specific banding resolution, that have led to its replacement in PGT by the fluorescence in situ hybridization (FISH) technique [12].

Fluorescence in situ hybridization

Cytogenetics entered the molecular era in 1969 with the introduction of in situ hybridization (ISH), a procedure that locates the positions of specific DNA sequences on chromosomes with the aid of radioactive-labeled probes [13]. In 1986, radiation was replaced by fluorescence signals and FISH appeared [14,15]. FISH technology became the first cytogenetic technique that allowed aneuploidy detection in interphase nuclei (not only metaphase chromosomes), which eliminated the need to culture cells and provided results in a mere 2–3 days. This molecular cytogenetic technique was applied to PGT in 1992 [16] and ever since many variations of the procedure have been developed, and its sensitivity has increased enormously, becoming a very useful diagnosis tool.

The scheme of the technique can be observed in Fig. 4.2. After the DNA extraction (in this case from embryonic cells) and its fixation on a laboratory slide, the first step in the process is to develop the complementary probe that will be attached to the target DNA region of interest. FISH probes can be labeled either directly using fluorochrome-conjugated nucleotides (e.g., fluorescein-dUTP) or indirectly using reporter molecules (e.g., biotin-dUTP) by nick-translation, random priming, polymerase chain reaction (PCR), or various other molecular genetic techniques. Next, both the target and the probe sequences are denatured and mixed for hybridization based on

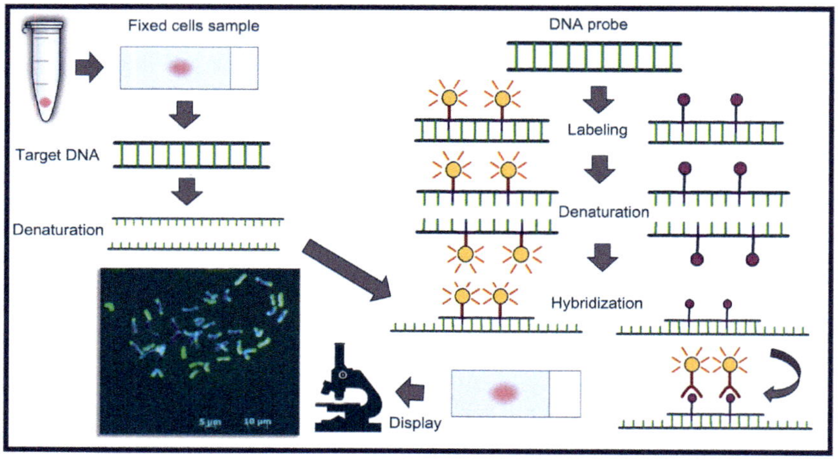

FIGURE 4.2 Scheme of steps for fluorescent in situ hybridization (FISH). On the left side, fixation of cell samples and denaturation of target DNA. On the right side, DNA probe preparation, two labeling types (direct on the left and indirect on the right), denaturation and hybridization with target DNA on a laboratory slide. Below, in the center, display through a fluorescence microscope.

target–probe complementarity, allowing the exploration of the target presence, number, and location on the chromosome. Fluorescent signals of bound probes are then inspected using a filter-equipped fluorescence microscope and computer software [12].

Nowadays, many different commercial and noncommercial probes are available for diagnostic purposes, including centromeric probes for chromosome enumeration and identification, and loci-specific probes and subtelomeric probes for detecting chromosomal rearrangements [12]. Cytogeneticists have also the option of using multifluor FISH, or spectral karyotyping [17], which paints each chromosome with a different color using a differentially labeled collection of hybridization probes scattered throughout each chromosome's whole length. This FISH variant, however, is only able to detect large chromosomal changes.

FISH applications in PGT allow the detection of numeric chromosomal abnormalities or aneuploidies (PGT-A), structural chromosomal alterations—deletions, duplications, inversions, and translocations—(preimplantation genetic testing for structural rearrangements) with higher resolution than karyotyping. Most laboratories use this technique to look for specific chromosomes including X, Y, 13, 16, 18, 21, and 22 as they are the most common aneuploidies seen in spontaneous miscarriages [18]. Nevertheless, FISH diagnosis is based on visual inspection and limited to the loci targeted by the probes used, and DNA-integrity and overlapping signals are a major problem [12].

Polymerase chain reaction

PCR was developed by Mullis et al. in 1983 [19] as a laboratory technique to amplify or make multiple copies of a specific segment of DNA. The scheme of this technique is shown in Fig. 4.3A. A basic PCR set up requires: a DNA template that contains the DNA target region to amplify (e.g., DNA of an embryonic cell); a DNA polymerase, enzyme that synthesizes new DNA strands from the DNA template (usually heat-resistant *Taq* polymerase); two DNA primers that are complementary to the 3′ ends of each of the sense and antisense strands of the DNA target and from which DNA polymerase can start to amplify; deoxynucleoside triphosphates that will be added by the DNA polymerase to the new DNA strand; and a buffer solution providing a suitable chemical environment for optimum activity and stability of the DNA polymerase,

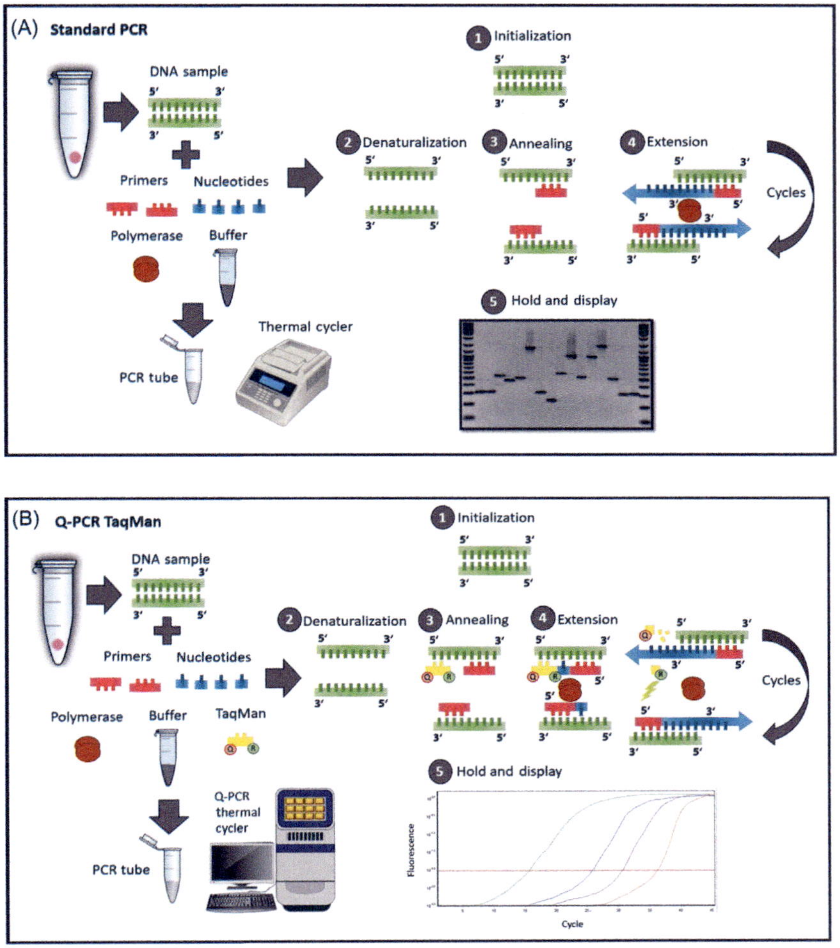

FIGURE 4.3 **General scheme of standard polymerase chain reaction (PCR) (A) and quantitative polymerase chain reaction (Q-PCR) based on TaqMan probes (B).** For each PCR technique, set up components are shown on the left, and the different steps of the PCR protocol (1–5) are schematized on the right. In comparison with the standard PCR protocol shown in (A), Q-PCR techniques (B) include the quantification of amplified DNA at real time thanks to the fluorescence emitted by the reporter of the TaqMan probe after its degradation by the DNA polymerase in the extension phase (4) in each cycle. The picture located next to the Hold and Display phase (5) represents the fluorescence signal emitted by the reporter of the TaqMan probes (y axis) in each Q-PCR cycle (x axis). *PCR*, Polymerase chain reaction; *Q*, quencher; *R*, reporter.

typically containing magnesium (Mg) and potassium (K) ions [20,21].

The whole amplification procedure takes place in a thermal cycler which increases and decreases the temperature in automatic, programmed steps. These steps are: initialization (94°C–96°C, 1–10 minutes) for DNA polymerase activation if necessary; denaturation (94°C–98°C, 20–30 seconds) for the separation of the double-stranded DNA (dsDNA) template into single strands; annealing (5°C below T_m or melting temperature of primers, usually 50°C–60°C, 20–40 seconds) allowing the annealing of the primers to each of the single-stranded DNA templates; extension (72°C, 20–40 seconds) for amplification by the DNA polymerase; optional elongation (72°C, 5–15 minutes) to ensure that any remaining single-stranded DNA is fully elongated; and final hold (4°C–15°C, indefinite time) for short-term storage of PCR products. Following synthesis and at the end of the first cycle, each dsDNA molecule consists of one new and one old DNA strand and will serve as templates in subsequent cycles (usually 25–35 cycles in total), which allow the DNA target to be exponentially amplified millions of times (2^n copies where n = the number of cycles). Finally, it is necessary to check whether the PCR successfully amplified the DNA target region, that is typically achieved by agarose gel electrophoresis that performs size separation of the PCR products and compares them to a reference DNA ladder [20,21].

This technique has been improved and several variants have been developed as real-time or quantitative fluorescence polymerase chain reaction (QF-PCR) that employs fluorescent dyes or probes to simultaneously amplify and quantify the DNA target [22]; reverse-transcription polymerase chain reaction (RT-PCR) for gene expression evaluation (see "The endometrial factor: gene expression diagnostic tools to assess endometrial receptivity" section); real-time or reverse-transcription quantitative polymerase chain reaction (RT-qPCR), a combination of the two former techniques [23]; and multiplex PCR methods that consist of the use of various sets of specific primers that simultaneously amplify different DNA regions [24].

In fact, quantitative polymerase chain reaction (Q-PCR) is a revolutionary tool for quantification of gene expression that is mostly employed in PGT to evaluate monogenic diseases. Overall, Q-PCR is based in monitoring the amplification of the targeted DNA molecule during each PCR cycle thanks to either (1) nonspecific fluorescent DNA-binding dyes (e.g., SYBR Green I) or (2) sequence-specific oligonucleotide probes labeled with a fluorescent reporter that gives signal only after hybridization of the probe with its complementary DNA sequence (e.g., TaqMan probes). Unlike conventional PCR methods, Q-PCR instruments have detectors that measure the fluorescence intensity after each PCR cycle. Here we describe the molecular procedures of the two most popular Q-PCR methods, which are based on SYBR Green I dyes and TaqMan probes [25].

SYBR Green I is a nonspecific dye that emits fluorescence when it binds to the minor groove of all dsDNA found in the PCR reaction tube. Therefore the increasing amount of dsDNA present in the reaction PCR tube after each cycle leads to a greater amount of bound dyes and thus an increasing fluorescent signal from SYBR Green I. This method is relatively cost efficient, and easy to use. However, these types of nonspecific dyes can potentially bind to all dsDNA PCR products, including primer dimers, that could interfere in the quantification of the targeted sequence [25]. This drawback is solved with sequence-specific probes such as TaqMan probes.

TaqMan probes are hydrolysis oligonucleotides consisting of a fluorophore (reporter), covalently attached to the 5′ end of the oligonucleotide probe, and a quencher attached at the 3′ end, that prevents the detection of the fluorescence emitted by the reporter when they are in proximity. These probes are designed to anneal within a specific DNA region amplified by a specific set of primers in the PCR. As the *Taq* polymerase extends the primer and synthesizes the nascent strand, the 5′ to 3′ exonuclease activity of this enzyme degrades the TaqMan probe that has annealed to the DNA template. This causes the separation of the reporter and the quencher, allowing the reporter's fluorescent signal to be liberated and detected by the Q-PCR instrument. A scheme of the Q-PCR technique using TaqMan probes is shown in Fig. 4.3B. The precision of this Q-PCR technique is equivalent to that of the SYBR Green I, but the specificity is higher, as TaqMan probes only detect targeted DNA sequences [25].

Since its first application in PGT [4] PCR-based methods have been important approaches in assisted reproduction clinics for a wide range of diagnostic applications. For instance, Q-PCR can use primers of informative polymorphic small tandem repeat markers to detect chromosomal aneuploidies in less than 24 hours [26], being an alternative method to FISH for prenatal testing and PGT-A [27]. In addition, Q-PCR is also used for the amplification and identification of single-nucleotide polymorphisms (SNPs) (see "High-resolution genome-wide approaches" section for more information on SNP genotyping) [28].

Nevertheless, the most widely used Q-PCR application in PGT is the detection of monogenic diseases (PGT-M) such as B-thalassemia or Becker and Duchenne muscular dystrophies [29]. In this sense, multiplex PCR methods have been applied together with Q-PCR based on TaqMan probes at a single-cell level to simultaneously diagnose several monogenic diseases and/or increase the reliability when only one disease is interrogated [30]. This is achieved by using different sets of primers that amplify distinct DNA regions (associated with the evaluation of the same or different monogenic diseases); and differentially labeled TaqMan probes that emit differentially colored fluorescent signals depending on the specific DNA region to which it binds.

Although PCR methods are very accurate and reproducible, the main limitation of these PCR technologies is their dependence on prior knowledge of the specific genomic loci to be amplified, which also limits the number of diseases that can be simultaneously evaluated [27].

High-resolution genome-wide approaches

The development of genome-wide approaches based on arrays and next-generation sequencing (NGS) has revolutionized the resolution of PGT, allowing cytogeneticists to interrogate the whole embryonic genome at a base-pair level. Since these genomic methods require hundreds of DNA nanograms and a single diploid human cell contains only about 7 picograms of DNA, the genome of the biopsied embryo cells must be amplified prior to the genetic analysis [6]. There are currently two major genome-wide amplification methods that are applied to single cells: multiple displacement amplification (MDA) and/or PCR amplification.

MDA is a non-PCR method that uses random primers and Φ29 DNA polymerase for faithful nucleotide amplification of the already-denatured single-cell DNA template [31]. In contrast, PCR methods can be based on linker adaptor PCR, primer extension preamplification-PCR [32], or degenerate oligonucleotide-primed-PCR [33]. Other WGA methods combine features of MDA- and PCR-based amplification. In general, the PCR-based WGA products deliver a more accurate copy-number profile [34] and can also be used for SNP genotyping and base-mutation detection [35]. However, MDA are still the preferred methods for these two latest purposes [34,36]. After DNA amplification, there are three main genome-wide approaches that can be applied for PGT: comparative genomic hybridization arrays (CGHa), SNP arrays, and NGS.

Comparative genomic hybridization arrays

In order to improve the resolution of the FISH technique and avoid using techniques of fixation of the cell onto a microscope slide, researchers developed comparative genomic hybridization (CGH) [37]. CGH was firstly applied for PGT in 1996 [38] and is a DNA-based method applicable to cells in any phase of the cell cycle.

This approach requires genomic DNA from both a reference subject (typically extracted from peripheral blood) and a test subject, which is extracted from the embryonic biopsied cells in the case of PGT. After a DNA amplification step, reference DNA fragments are labeled with red fluorescence and experimental DNA fragments with green fluorescence. Afterwards, both labeled DNA types are pooled together to be used in hybridization experiments [18,38].

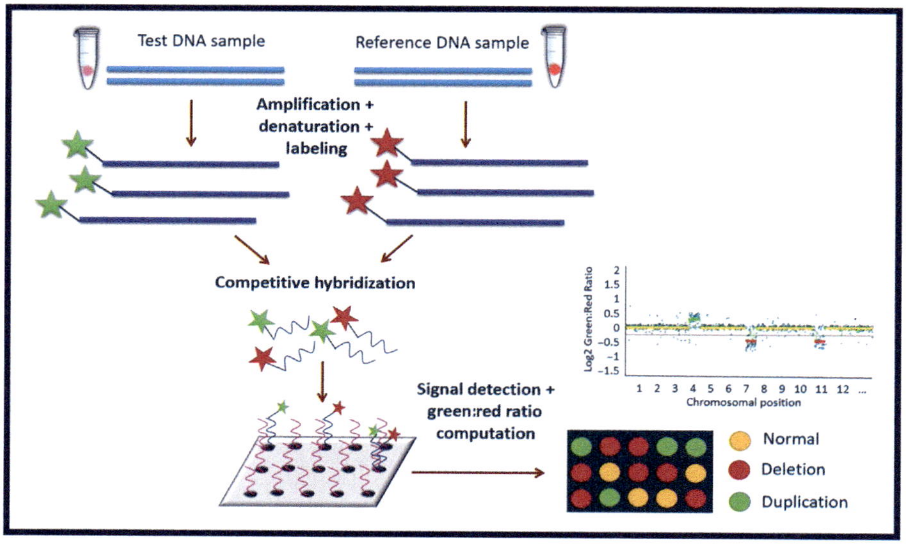

FIGURE 4.4 General scheme of comparative genomic hybridization array (CGHa). DNA previously extracted from the biopsied embryonic cells (test DNA) and reference sample is amplified, denatured, and differentially labeled with different fluorochromes. Afterwards, labeled test and reference DNA are pooled together and placed in the microarray for competitive hybridization with their complementary probes. Finally, fluorescent signals are scanned for each spot and the green:red ratio is computed for interpretation.

Conventional CGH employed this DNA pool as probes and hybridized them with normal metaphase chromosomes on a microscope slide for differentially painting them, a very labor-intensive methodology with limited resolution. With the advent of DNA microarrays [39] and its application to CGH, these limitations were overcome.

CGHa [40] uses for hybridization an array [39], that is, a solid surface containing thousands of DNA fragments (probes) located at specific positions, instead of metaphase chromosomes. Each of these probes corresponds to a known DNA sequence that is complementary of a human genome region of interest. The probes can be from oligonucleotides [25–85 base pairs (bp)] or chromosome-specific DNA, to genomic clones such as bacterial artificial chromosomes (80,000–200,000 bp). Because probes are several orders of magnitude smaller than metaphase chromosomes, the theoretical resolution of CGHa is proportionally higher than that of traditional CGH [3,18,40].

The experimental protocol of CGHa is schematized in Fig. 4.4. In the CGHa hybridization step, red (reference) and green (test) labeled DNA fragments compete to anneal to their complementary probes on the array. Next, digital imaging systems are used to capture and quantify the relative fluorescence intensities of the labeled DNA fragments that have hybridized to each probe. After that, the ratio of green:red fluorescence is computed to reveal the relative number of DNA copies for each region of interest in the test sample compared with the reference. For unaltered chromosomal regions, the green and red probes should bind equally, resulting in an orange/yellow color. However, if a chromosomal region was deleted in the test sample it will appear red and if it was amplified it will appear green, thus allowing detection of chromosomal abnormalities that can aid selection against chromosomally abnormal embryos before transfer [18,40].

In the context of PGT, CGHa has been successfully applied for the detection of aneuploidies (at the single chromosome level) and chromosome breakages and rearrangements (as translocations) in <48 hours or even <24 hours, involving many improvements with respect to FISH or conventional CGH. However, all these molecular cytogenetic techniques lack the capability to diagnose alterations at a gene level, such as those associated with monogenic diseases [3,18].

Single-nucleotide polymorphism array and karyomapping

Single-nucleotide polymorphism arrays (SNPa) were first introduced in 1998 to determine the linkage between a disease locus and a chromosomal region for genotype–phenotype association [41]. SNPs are single-nucleotide (A, T, C, and G) variations occurring approximately every 1200 bp of the DNA and present in <1% of the human population. Each of the bases that can occur at a single SNP is defined as an allele and, since SNPs are naturally biallelic and humans have two pairs of each chromosome, the genotype of each SNP can adopt three forms: homozygous for alleles A (AA) or B (BB), and heterozygous (AB).

Because specific groups of alleles belonging to different SNPs might be linked and inherited together as DNA blocks or haplotypes, SNP genotyping allows indirect diagnosis of monogenic disorders when the evaluated SNPs and the mutation locus belong to the same haplotype, which is an advantage over CGHa. Moreover, SNPa platforms contain probes designed for detection of copy-number variations—duplications, deletions, and insertions of >1 Kb—and indels—deletions and insertions of <1 Kb—at a gene resolution.

High-density SNPa can simultaneously genotype from tens of thousands up to millions of SNPs scattered through the whole genome, with two main SNPa chemistries (Fig. 4.5):

- Affymetrix SNPa [41,42] consist of 25-mer allele-specific oligonucleotide (ASO) probes that are synthesized in situ on a solid surface by photolithographic methods. For each interrogated SNP, ASO probes for its two possible alleles are in separate positions of the array. The overall strategy is based on the preferential hybridization of the previously amplified, fluorescently labeled and denatured DNA fragments with their perfect complementary ASO probes.
- Illumina Bead Chip SNPa [43,44] consist of 50-mer oligonucleotide probes that target one base upstream to the SNP rather than the SNP itself. These probes are attached to silica beads randomly distributed in array microwells and SNP alleles are distinguished by enzymatic single-base extension of the probe using the hybridized DNA target as a template and differentially fluorescent labeled nucleotides.

For both types of SNPa design, fluorescence signal intensities are detected and preprocessed, normalized, and summarized by probe replicates to compute pairs of allele measurements for each evaluated SNP, which are then used to address the embryo genotype and infer DNA abundance and SNP allele ratio [45]. Finally, these parameters are then compared with those of normal reference samples (usually a close relative) or the human HapMap reference genome to select nondefective embryos for transfer.

Karyomapping

One SNPa application that arose in 2010 to specifically select against embryos carrying monogenic inherited disorders was genome-wide haplotyping or karyomapping [46]. To build an embryo karyomap, DNA samples from the embryo and the peripheral blood of both progenitors and one or more relatives

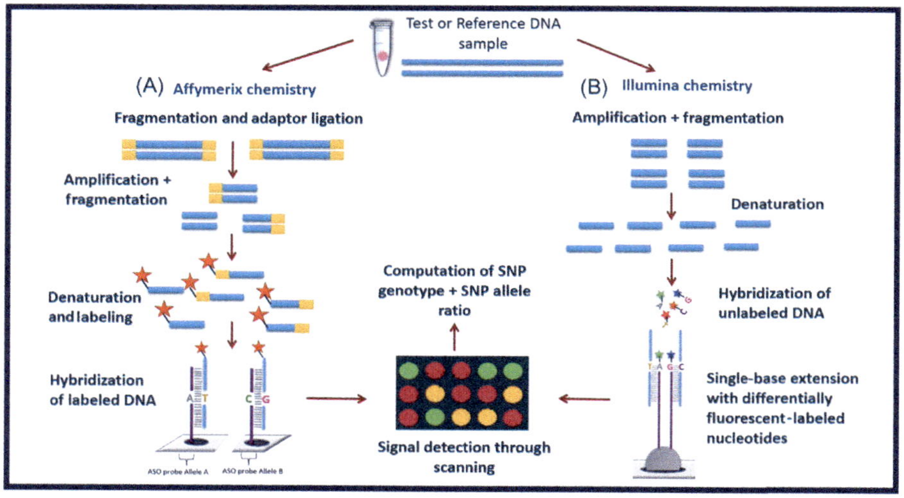

FIGURE 4.5 **General scheme of a single-nucleotide polymorphism array (SNPa).** Contrary to comparative genomic hybridization array (CGHa), in SNPa the DNA from tests and references is hybridized in separate microarrays. Once extracted, the DNA can follow two protocol chemistries. (A) The protocol followed by Affymetrix SNPa consists of DNA fragmentation and adapter ligation, followed by amplification, additional fragmentation, denaturalization, and fluorescence labeling and hybridization to ASO probes. (B) The protocol followed by Illumina SNPa includes a first amplification and fragmentation of the DNA, a denaturalization step, hybridization of nonlabeled DNA with probes that are complementary, and a single-base extension with nucleotides labeled with different fluorochromes. For both chemistries, after hybridization fluorescent signals are scanned and preprocessed for SNP genotyping and allele ratio computation. *ASO*, Allele-specific oligonucleotide; *SNP*, single-nucleotide polymorphism.

affected by (or carriers of) the genetic disorder are needed. These relatives would be established as the "references" and can be an already affected child and/or the parents of the progenitors [46]. These DNA samples are hybridized in separate SNPa that typically evaluate 300,000 informative SNPs designed to look for specific variations that are characteristic of a defective chromosome [47]. Genotypes from the parents are then compared to the reference to establish a DNA fingerprint for the chromosome that carries the defective haplotype. Finally, this DNA fingerprint is compared to that of the embryo to select for embryo transfer those that did not inherit the defective haplotype [48].

Karyomapping was first commercialized by Illumina in 2013 and is currently used in more than 1000 clinics worldwide as a routine option for parents that are known to be carriers of an inherited monogenic disease and want to avoid passing it to their offspring during an IVF treatment [47]. Advantages over other array-based methods include the simultaneous detection of monogenic and chromosomal disorders, the detection of loss of heterozygosity due to uniparental disomy or deletion, the identification of low levels of mosaicism or meiotic homologous recombination, the establishment of parental origin and follow up of genetic loci that can aid in future ARTs, and the selection of human leukocyte antigen-matching embryos to isolate cord blood stem cells at birth for transplantation to an existing child affected with a serious blood disorder [46,47,49,50].

Alternatively, the main limitations of these SNPa techniques are the need for reference samples, the fact that they do not genotype the mutation directly, and the impossibility of detecting de novo disease variants [46,51]. These drawbacks are being partially solved with the application of NGS techniques.

Next-generation sequencing

DNA sequencing techniques are aimed at determining the nucleotide order of a DNA fragment. The first sequencing method was proposed by Sanger [52], being successfully applied to human genome sequencing in 2001 [53]. However, this conventional method could only evaluate individual DNA fragments up to 1000 bp in length. NGS methods allowed fast, automatic, massive, and parallel sequencing of millions of DNA fragments in a single experiment, increasing the efficiency and accuracy and decreasing time and economic costs.

The molecular principles of NGS for PGT comprise several steps (Fig. 4.6). First, the embryo DNA sample is randomly fragmented, and adapters are added to both ends of each resulting molecule, which then undergo denaturalization and amplification by the previously described WGA PCR-based method. The amplified DNA fragments are then immobilized on a surface containing oligonucleotides that are complementary to the adapters. Afterwards, they are amplified to form small clonal clusters to be sequenced from one or both ends of the fragments—single-end or paired-end sequencing. There are several types of sequencing depending on the method used—fluorescence signals, pH changes—to identify the single nucleotides that are being incorporated to the DNA template during each cycle. Once the recorded signals are obtained for each DNA molecule, they are translated into sequence reads and mapped to the human reference genome for detecting genetic variants using different bioinformatic tools and databases.

One advantage of NGS-based PGT methods is that they interrogate almost every nucleotide

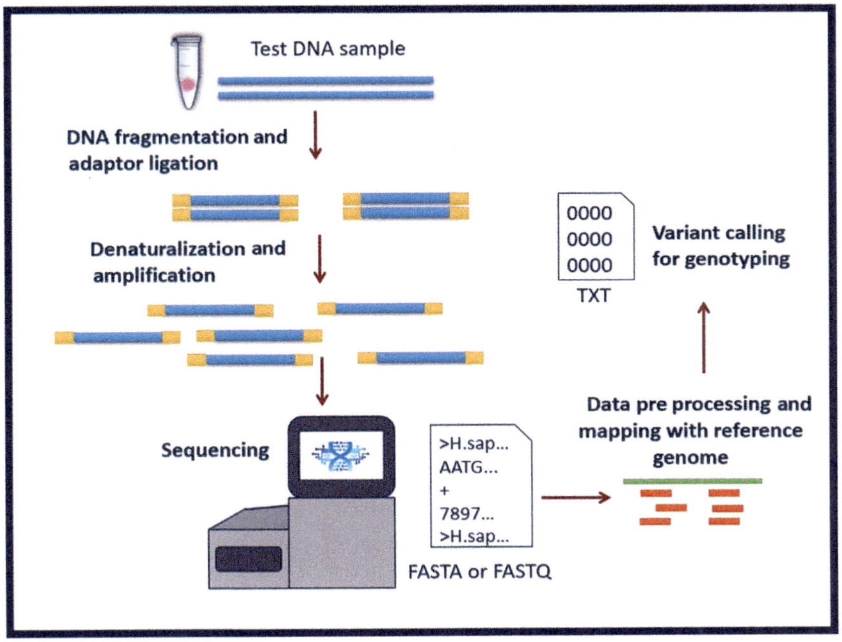

FIGURE 4.6 General scheme of the next-generation sequencing (NGS) technique. After extraction from the biopsied embryonic cells, DNA is fragmented, and adaptors are added to both ends. DNA fragments are then denaturalized and amplified for library preparation and sequencing. Reads are obtained in FASTA or FASTQ files and preprocessed for mapping with a reference genome. Finally, variant-calling bioinformatic tools are used for genotyping.

in the genome, allowing not only the detection of inherited abnormalities but also de novo discovery of disease-associated variants, copy-number aberrations, all types of structural variants, and mitochondrial DNA mutations [6].

In fact, there are several maternal inheritance diseases caused by mitochondrial DNA mutations [54]. A new technique to select embryos without this type of diseases has been recently applied. This approach is known as the "three-parent" technique and, in 2016, gave rise to a healthy baby from a mother who was carrier of Leigh syndrome [55]. The method approved in the United Kingdom is termed pronuclear transfer and involves fertilizing both the mother's egg and a donor egg with the father's sperm. Before the fertilized eggs start dividing into early-stage embryos, each nucleus is removed. The nucleus from the donor's fertilized egg is discarded and replaced by that from the mother's fertilized egg [56]. However, this technique was not appropriate for the couple that wanted to have a baby without Leigh syndrome because they were opposed to the destruction of two embryos. Therefore a different approach was taken, called spindle nuclear transfer. In this method, the nucleus is removed from one of the mother's eggs and inserted into a donor egg that had had its own nucleus removed. The resulting egg (with nuclear DNA from the mother and mitochondrial DNA from a donor) was then fertilized with the father's sperm. Five embryos were created, only one of which developed normally [55]. This embryo was transferred to mother's uterus and the healthy child was born 9 months later.

NGS technologies are more precise than microarray methods and can be applied to the whole genome, to only the exome or gene-coding regions, or to only a set of genes that are relevant for specific diseases [6]. This last approach is the most used in clinical practice due to its reduced costs. The main limitation of NGS techniques is the huge number of variants detected and the interpretation of those variants of uncertain significance [27].

The endometrial factor: gene expression diagnostic tools to assess endometrial receptivity

The endometrium is a highly complex and dynamic tissue that undergoes cyclic morphological and physiological changes regulated by hormones. This tissue becomes receptive to the embryo during a variable and limited period around 2–4 days within the mid-secretory phase, known as the window of implantation (WOI) [57]. Two thirds of implantation failures are associated with a nonreceptive or defective endometrium [1,2], and this percentage increases in ART as the embryo factor is ruled out with PGT before embryo transfer. Knowing the endometrial status would allow clinicians to personalize embryo transfer to the moment of receptiveness in ART, thus increasing implantation and pregnancy rates.

In the past few decades there have been huge efforts to develop diagnostic biomarkers of endometrial receptivity (ER) [2]. Conventional endometrial dating methods included luteinizing hormone urinary surge monitoring, ultrasound evaluation (including the widely investigated endometrial thickness) [2], and histological criteria [2,58]. However, these dating methods are currently being replaced by more precise techniques based on gene expression evaluation, such as RT-qPCR, DNA microarrays, or NGS transcriptomic technologies (RNA-Seq).

Since the molecular principles of PCR, DNA microarrays, and NGS have been described in the previous section for PGT of the embryo, here the focus is on their particularities and current clinical applications in assisted reproductive techniques for gene expression evaluation of the endometrial factor.

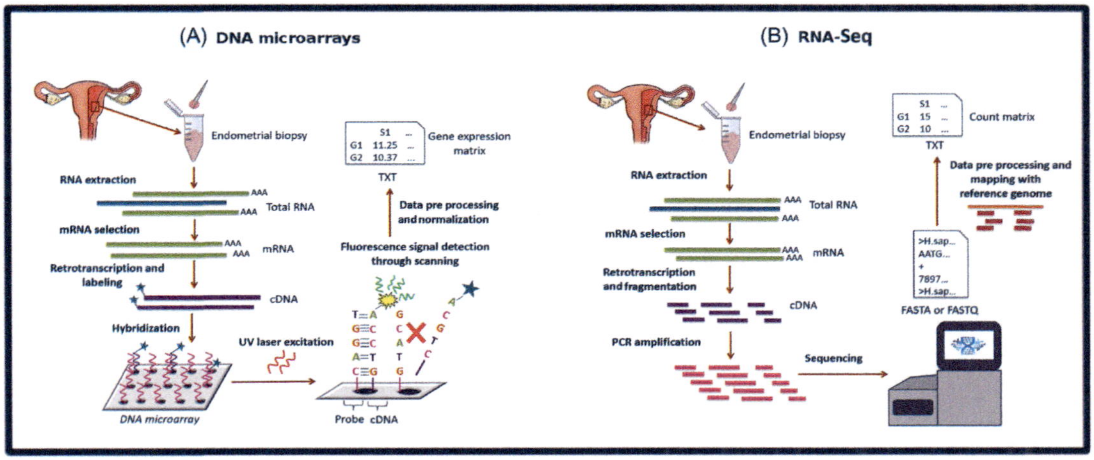

FIGURE 4.7 **General scheme of DNA microarrays (A) and RNA-Seq NGS technologies (B) for gene expression evaluation of the endometrial factor**. After total RNA extraction from the endometrial biopsy, mRNA transcripts are selected through their polyA tails, retrotranscribed and (A) fluorescently labeled and hybridized with complementary probes. Fluorescent signals are detected and preprocessed for gene expression measure; (B) PCR amplified and sequenced for read extraction, which are mapped against a reference genome and then preprocessed to generate a count matrix of gene expression values. *cDNA*, Complementary DNA; *mRNA*, messenger RNA; *PCR*, polymerase chain reaction.

For all three approaches, ER gene expression evaluation starts from an endometrial biopsy collected on the day in which the endometrium is expected to be receptive according to the assisted reproductive technique, and in the previous cycle of the transfer. Total ribonucleic acid (RNA) is extracted from the biopsy and then retrotranscribed to complementary DNA (cDNA). Most techniques include an additional step of isolation of messenger RNA (mRNA) through its poly A tails before the retrotranscription to select only protein-coding transcripts (Fig. 4.7). From this point, cDNA follows different preparations depending on whether gene expression is measured by RT-qPCR, DNA microarrays, or RNA-Seq.

Reverse-transcription real-time polymerase chain reaction

RT-qPCR [22,23] is a PCR-based method that quantifies gene expression at each amplification cycle thanks to the fluorescent labeling of the DNA strands that are being newly synthesized. The higher the expression of a gene is, the faster will be increase in the fluorescent signal after each cycle.

In 2013, the Window Implantation test (Win test) was commercialized to evaluate ER through quantification by RT-qPCR of the expression levels of 11 genes [59]. Five years later, a new endometrial receptivity test (ER Map/ER Grade) [60], also based on the RT-qPCR technique, was developed, evaluating the expression of 184 genes involved in endometrial proliferation and maternal immune response associated with embryonic implantation [2].

Despite RT-qPCR being successfully applied in the diagnostic field, its use as a diagnostic tool to assess ER is limited by the reduced number of biomarkers that can be analyzed. ER is a multifactorial and highly complex process that involves changes in the expression levels of a large number of genes. Consequently, the introduction of DNA microarrays and RNA-Seq panels has increased the diagnosis potential of ER, as these techniques are capable of simultaneously evaluating the expression of many genes. These high-throughput technologies have introduced the concept of transcriptomic profiles as the set of genes and their expression levels that are biomarkers of a given biological process or phenotype, such as a receptive endometrium [61,62].

DNA microarrays

When DNA microarrays are used to evaluate gene expression, the cDNA is labeled in the retrotranscription step and hybridized in the microarray with their respective complementary probes. The numeric values obtained from the fluorescence signals are then translated to expression levels of each evaluated gene through several bioinformatic steps, including background correction, normalization within and between arrays, and summarization from probe to gene, as a single gene may be represented by more than one probe in the array. This process is schematized in Fig. 4.7A.

In clinical practice, there are currently several commercialized arrays to assess ER, such as the endometrial receptivity analysis (ERA test), which evaluates the expression of 238 genes [61] that are predictive of ER. The ERA diagnostic tool allowed clinicians to personalize embryo transfer in the cycle following the endometrial evaluation, decreasing those cases of recurrent implantation failures that are due to displacement of the WOI, and thus increasing pregnancy rates [63]. Despite these promising results, a recent review pointed out that comparison between embryo transfer outcomes in receptive versus nonreceptive endometrial profiles assessed by the ERA test has yet to be evaluated, and that information about its clinical value is expected with the publication of an ongoing randomized controlled trial (ClinicalTrials.gov Identifier: NCT01954758) [2].

RNA-Seq

RNA-Seq uses NGS technologies to determine gene expression [64]. In contrast to DNA microarrays, cDNA is not labeled but fragmented and PCR amplified before being sequenced. The obtained sequences or reads are stored in a FASTA or FASTQ file and represent transcripts rather than genomic DNA. The number of reads generated is associated with the concepts of coverage and depth, which in RNA-Seq they are defined as the percentage of the sequenced transcriptome and the theoretical number of reads that could be mapped to the reference genome. Therefore a gene with high gene expression levels will have a high quantity of transcripts that will produce more reads after sequencing, which in turn will be translated into a deeper coverage in this region of the genome. After the preprocessing step, a gene expression matrix is generated by computing the number of reads associated with each gene. The whole process is illustrated in Fig. 4.7B.

Since NGS technologies have several advantages over DNA microarray technologies, including high resolution, accuracy, reliability, and the possibility of whole transcriptome evaluation without prior sequence knowledge, array-based commercialized ER tests are being gradually replaced by updated NGS versions or newly developed tests that use this technology. In fact, the ERA diagnostic tool is currently an ER predictive method based on an RNA-Seq panel that evaluates the expression of 236 genes, all of them included in the original 238 genes evaluated in the array version described in "DNA microarrays" section [65,66].

The use of DNA microarrays or RNA-Seq technologies, and the subsequent comparison through transcriptomic predictors between the obtained endometrial transcriptomic profiles at different times of the menstrual cycle, can then determine gene sets that are predictive of the receptive endometrial stage.

Transcriptomic predictors are generated computationally by machine learning algorithms applied to, for instance, microarray or RNA-Seq gene expression data of known samples (e.g., known menstrual cycle phase at time of endometrial biopsy) to make predictions for new unknown samples. To build a machine learning model, a set of samples, called a training set, is used as a reference. The learning process can occur from a labeled training set (supervised learning, e.g., transcriptomic predictors) or by using unlabeled transcriptomic information from the training set to structure data and define profiles (unsupervised learning, e.g., clustering methods) [67,68]. Based on Microarray Quality Control (MAQC) phase II and MAQC phase III consortia, the FDA has established guidelines for classification performance using transcriptomics for diagnosis in medicine. This type of models are performing a self-assessment in a process called cross-validation, where prediction performance for the model is estimated. The possibility of classifications using transcriptomic profile data is a powerful tool for clinical application and for personalizing reproductive medicine, especially in endometrial factors [67,68].

Further studies are needed to evaluate the clinical value of all these endometrial evaluation tests that are dating the endometrium, regardless of the technique used to measure gene expression [2]. Despite the acquired knowledge on the implantation process, little progress has been achieved regarding the development of diagnostic, prognostic, and treatment tests for suboptimal ER [2]. NGS and other "omics" techniques may offer an opportunity to discover new ER biomarkers able to address this highly complex and dynamic tissue. In addition, progress is being made on the discovery of ER biomarkers in endometrial fluid aspirate [2], as it is less invasive and may be performed without potentially affecting the pregnancy outcome [69].

Moreover, a new taxonomy of implantation failure has been published using transcriptomic predictors [70], indicating that patients who fail to implant due to the endometrial factor may have a displaced WOIWOI and/or a pathological WOI characterized by gene expression alterations. While a displaced WOI can be treated with personalized embryo transfer (pET), the establishment of a transcriptomic profile that is predictive of a pathological WOI is another issue. In addition, it has been reported that biomarker discovery associated with endometrial pathologies (e.g., recurrent implantation failure) is masked by the effect of the menstrual cycle and, consequently, this effect needs to be removed in advance to accurately identify those genes associated with a pathological WOI [70,71]. Future diagnostic tools aimed at evaluating the endometrial factor will need to consider these multiple causes of implantation failure to develop personalized treatments and to increase pregnancy rates.

General conclusion

The complementary clinical application in ARTs of PGT techniques (karyotyping, FISH, PCR, CGHa, SNPa, karyomapping, NGS) to select normal embryos, together with endometrial gene expression technologies (RT-qPCR, DNA microarrays, and RNA-Seq) to ensure an optimum endometrium, is a diagnostic procedure that will contribute to an increase in the reproductive success of ART patients. However, endometrial factor evaluation procedures and their clinical application should improve in the coming years. An integrative overview of all the molecular techniques described in this chapter for embryo and endometrial evaluation is shown in Fig. 4.8.

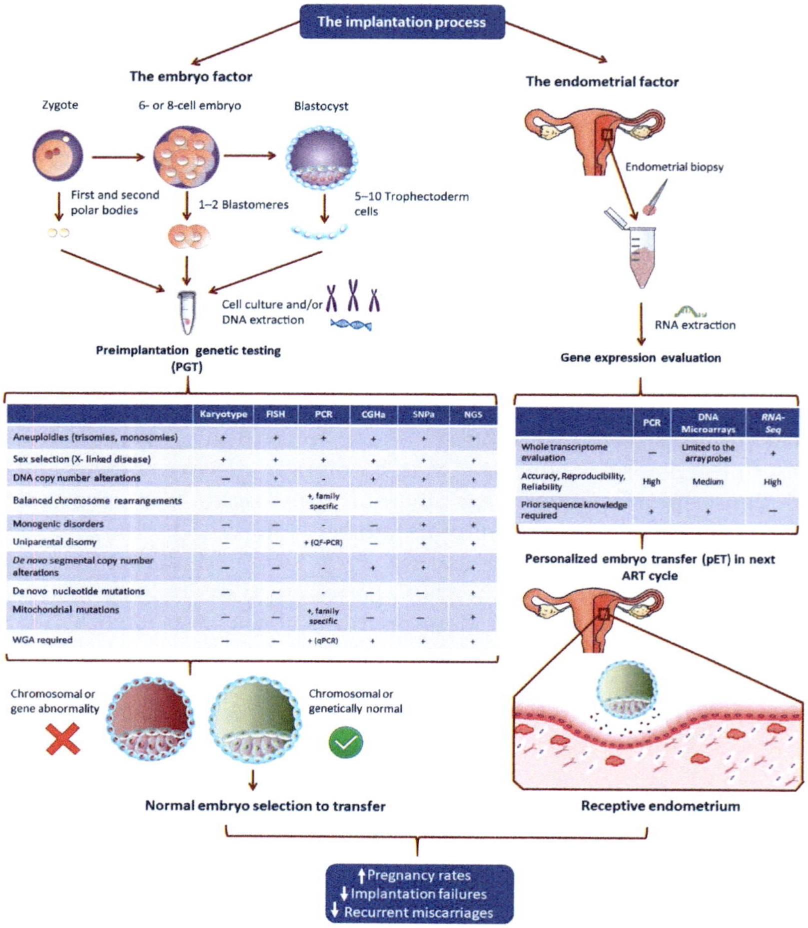

	Karyotype	FISH	PCR	CGHa	SNPa	NGS
Aneuploidies (trisomies, monosomies)	+	+	+	+	+	+
Sex selection (X- linked disease)	+	+	+	+	+	+
DNA copy number alterations	—	+	-	+	+	+
Balanced chromosome rearrangements	—	—	+, family specific	—	+	+
Monogenic disorders	—	—	-	—	+	+
Uniparental disomy	—	—	+ (QF-PCR)	—	+	+
De novo segmental copy number alterations	—	—	-	+	+	+
De novo nucleotide mutations	—	—	-	—	—	+
Mitochondrial mutations	—	—	+, family specific	—	—	+
WGA required	—	—	+ (qPCR)	+	+	+

	PCR	DNA Microarrays	*RNA-Seq*
Whole transcriptome evaluation	—	Limited to the array probes	+
Accuracy, Reproducibility, Reliability	High	Medium	High
Prior sequence knowledge required	+	+	—

FIGURE 4.8 **Integrative overview of molecular techniques currently used in preimplantation genetic testing (PGT) and in endometrial evaluation**. On the *left side*, the different embryonic sample sources and a comparison of the molecular techniques used for PGT evaluation of the embryo factor are shown. On the *right side*, the sampling procedure and a comparison between the different technologies for gene expression evaluation of endometrial receptivity (ER) are schematized. The transfer to a receptive endometrium of a genetically normal embryo contributes to increased reproductive success. *ART*, assisted reproductive treatment; *CGHa*, comparative genomic hybridization array; *FISH*, fluorescent in situ hybridization; *NGS*, next-generation sequencing; *pET*, personalized embryo transfer; *PGT*, preimplantation genetic testing; *QF-PCR*, quantitative fluorescence polymerase chain reaction; *qPCR*, quantitative polymerase chain reaction; *SNPa*, single-nucleotide polymorphism array.

References

[1] Edwards RG. Implantation, interception and contraception. Hum Reprod 1994;9:985–95.

[2] Craciunas L, Gallos I, Chu J, Bourne T, Quenby S, Brosens JJ, et al. Conventional and modern markers of endometrial receptivity: a systematic review and meta-analysis. Hum Reprod Update 2019;25:202–23.

[3] Wells D, Alfarawati S, Fragouli E. Use of comprehensive chromosomal screening for embryo assessment: microarrays and CGH. Mol Hum Reprod 2008;14:703–10.

[4] Handyside AH, Kontogianni EH, Hardy K, Winston RM. Pregnancies from biopsied human preimplantation embryos sexed by Y-specific DNA amplification. Nature 1990;344:768–70.

[5] Vaiarelli A, Cimadomo D, Capalbo A, Orlando G, Sapienza F, Colamaria S, et al. Pre-implantation genetic testing in ART: who will benefit and what is the evidence? J Assist Reprod Genet 2016;33:1273–8.

[6] Van der Aa N, Zamani Esteki M, Vermeesch JR, Voet T. Preimplantation genetic diagnosis guided by single-cell genomics. Genome Med 2013;5:71.

[7] Stebbins GL. Chapter XII: the karyotype. Variation and evolution in plants. Columbia University Press; 1950.

[8] Bates SE. Classical cytogenetics: karyotyping techniques. Methods Mol Biol 2011;177–90.

[9] Schreck RR, Distèche CM. Chromosome banding techniques. Curr Protoc Hum Genet. Hoboken, NJ: John Wiley & Sons, Inc; 2001.

[10] Steele MW, Breg WR. Chromosome analysis of human amniotic-fluid cells. Lancet 1966;1:383–5.

[11] Rooney DE, Czepulkowski B. Human cytogenetics: constitutional analysis: a practical approach. New York: Oxford University Press; 2001.
[12] Tönnies H. Modern molecular cytogenetic techniques in genetic diagnostics. Trends Mol Med 2002; 8:246–50.
[13] Pardue ML, Gall JG. Molecular hybridization of radioactive DNA to the DNA of cytological preparations. Proc Natl Acad Sci U S A 1969;64:600–4.
[14] Pinkel D, Straume T, Gray JW. Cytogenetic analysis using quantitative, high-sensitivity, fluorescence hybridization. Proc Natl Acad Sci U S A 1986;83:2934–8.
[15] Cremer T, Landegent J, Brückner A, Scholl HP, Schardin M, Hager HD, et al. Detection of chromosome aberrations in the human interphase nucleus by visualization of specific target DNAs with radioactive and non-radioactive in situ hybridization techniques: diagnosis of trisomy 18 with probe L1.84. Hum Genet 1986;74:346–52.
[16] Griffin DK, Wilton LJ, Handvside AH, Winston RML, Delhanty JDA. Dual fluorescent in situ hybridisation for simultaneous detection of X and Y chromosome-specific probes for the sexing of human preimplantation embryonic nuclei. Hum Genet 1992;89:18–22.
[17] Speicher MR, Gwyn Ballard S, Ward DC. Karyotyping human chromosomes by combinatorial multi-fluor FISH. Nat Genet 1996;12:368–75.
[18] Wilton L. Preimplantation genetic diagnosis and chromosome analysis of blastomeres using comparative genomic hybridization. Hum Reprod Update 2005; 11:33–41.
[19] Mullis KB, Erlich HA, Arnheim N, Horn GT, Saiki RK, Scharf SJ. Process for amplifying, detecting, and/or cloning nucleic acid sequences. Patent US 4800159A; 1989.
[20] Lorenz TC. Polymerase chain reaction: basic protocol plus troubleshooting and optimization strategies. J Vis Exp 2012;e3998.
[21] Waters DLE, Shapter FM. The polymerase chain reaction (PCR): general methods. Methods Mol Biol 2014;1099:65–75.
[22] Bustin SA, Benes V, Garson JA, Hellemans J, Huggett J, Kubista M, et al. The MIQE guidelines: minimum information for publication of quantitative real-time PCR experiments. Clin Chem 2009;55:611–22.
[23] Freeman WM, Walker SJ, Vrana KE. Quantitative RT-PCR: pitfalls and potential. Biotechniques 1999; 26:112–25.
[24] Chamberlain JS, Gibbs RA, Rainer JE, Nguyen PN, Thomas C. Deletion screening of the duchenne muscular dystrophy locus via multiplex DNA amplification. Nucleic Acids Res 1988;16:11141–56.
[25] Tajadini M, Panjehpour M, Javanmard SH. Comparison of SYBR Green and TaqMan methods in quantitative real-time polymerase chain reaction analysis of four adenosine receptor subtypes. Adv Biomed Res 2014;3:85.
[26] Vahab Saadi A, Kushtagi P, Gopinath P, Satyamoorthy K. Quantitative fluorescence polymerase chain reaction (QF-PCR) for prenatal diagnosis of chromosomal aneuploidies. Int J Hum Genet 2010;10:121–9.
[27] Vermeesch JR, Voet T, Devriendt K. Prenatal and pre--implantation genetic diagnosis. Nat Rev Genet 2016;17:643–56.
[28] Shen GQ, Abdullah KG, Wang QK. The TaqMan method for SNP genotyping. single nucleotide polymorfisms. Methods Mol Biol 2009;578:293–306.
[29] Traeger-Synodinos J. Real-time PCR for prenatal and preimplantation genetic diagnosis of monogenic diseases. Mol Aspects Med 2006;27:176–91.
[30] Lee VCY, Chow JFC, Yeung WSB, Ho PC. Preimplantation genetic diagnosis for monogenic diseases. Best Pract Res Clin Obstet Gynaecol 2017;44:69–75.
[31] Dean FB, Hosono S, Fang L, Wu X, Faruqi AF, Bray-Ward P, et al. Comprehensive human genome amplification using multiple displacement amplification. Proc Natl Acad Sci U S A 2002;99:5261–6.
[32] Zhang L, Cui X, Schmitt K, Hubert R, Navidi W, Arnheim N. Whole genome amplification from a single cell: implications for genetic analysis. Proc Natl Acad Sci U S A 1992;89:5847–51.
[33] Cheung VG, Nelson SF. Whole genome amplification using a degenerate oligonucleotide primer allows hundreds of genotypes to be performed on less than one nanogram of genomic DNA. Proc Natl Acad Sci U S A 1996;93:14676–9.
[34] Treff NR, Su J, Tao X, Northrop LE, Scott RT. Single-cell whole-genome amplification technique impacts the accuracy of SNP microarray-based genotyping and copy number analyses. Mol Hum Reprod 2011;17:335–43.
[35] Zong C, Lu S, Chapman AR, Xie XS. Genome-wide detection of single-nucleotide and copy-number variations of a single human cell. Science 2012;338:1622–6.
[36] Xu X, Hou Y, Yin X, Bao L, Tang A, Song L, et al. Single-cell exome sequencing reveals single-nucleotide mutation characteristics of a kidney tumor. Cell 2012;148:886–95.
[37] Kallioniemi A, Kallioniemi OP, Sudar D, Rutovitz D, Gray JW, Waldman F, et al. Comparative genomic hybridization for molecular cytogenetic analysis of solid tumors. Science 1992;258(80–):818–21.
[38] Wells D. Evaluating comparative genomic hybridization (CGH) as a strategy for preimplantation diagnosis of unbalanced chromosome complements. Eur J Hum Genet 1996;4:125.

[39] Schena M, Shalon D, Davis RW, Brown PO. Quantitative monitoring of gene expression patterns with a complementary DNA microarray. Science 1995;270:467–70.
[40] Pinkel D, Segraves R, Sudar D, Clark S, Poole I, Kowbel D, et al. High resolution analysis of DNA copy number variation using comparative genomic hybridization to microarrays. Nat Genet 1998; 20:207–11.
[41] Wang DG, Fan JB, Siao CJ, Berno A, Young P, Sapolsky R, et al. Large-scale identification, mapping, and genotyping of single-nucleotide polymorphisms in the human genome. Science 1998;280:1077–82.
[42] Matsuzaki H, Dong S, Loi H, Di X, Liu G, Hubbell E, et al. Genotyping over 100,000 SNPs on a pair of oligonucleotide arrays. Nat Methods 2004;1:109–11.
[43] Gunderson KL, Steemers FJ, Lee G, Mendoza LG, Chee MS. A genome-wide scalable SNP genotyping assay using microarray technology. Nat Genet 2005;37:549–54.
[44] Steemers FJ, Chang W, Lee G, Barker DL, Shen R, Gunderson KL. Whole-genome genotyping with the single-base extension assay. Nat Methods 2006;3:31–3.
[45] Lindgren D, Höglund M, Vallon-Christersson J. Genotyping techniques to address diversity in tumors. Adv Cancer Res 2011;112:151–82.
[46] Handyside AH, Harton GL, Mariani B, Thornhill AR, Affara N, Shaw M-A, et al. Karyomapping: a universal method for genome wide analysis of genetic disease based on mapping crossovers between parental haplotypes. J Med Genet 2010;47:651–8.
[47] Griffin DK, Gould RL. What is karyomapping and where does it fit in the world of preimplantation genetic diagnosis (PGD)? Med Res Arch 2017;5:1–18.
[48] Handyside AH. Live births following karyomapping—a "key" milestone in the development of preimplantation genetic diagnosis. Reprod Biomed Online 2015;31:307–8.
[49] Natesan SA, Bladon AJ, Coskun S, Qubbaj W, Prates R, Munne S, et al. Genome-wide karyomapping accurately identifies the inheritance of single-gene defects in human preimplantation embryos in vitro. Genet Med 2014;16:838–45.
[50] Van de Velde H, De Rycke M, De Man C, De Hauwere K, Fiorentino F, Kahraman S, et al. The experience of two European preimplantation genetic diagnosis centres on human leukocyte antigen typing. Hum Reprod 2009;24:732–40.
[51] Rechitsky S, Pomerantseva E, Pakhalchuk T, Pauling D, Verlinsky O, Kuliev A. First systematic experience of preimplantation genetic diagnosis for de-novo mutations. Reprod Biomed Online 2011;22:350–61.
[52] Sanger F, Nicklen S, Coulson AR. DNA sequencing with chain-terminating inhibitors. Proc Natl Acad Sci U S A 1977;74:5463–7.
[53] Venter JC, Adams MD, Myers EW, Li PW, Mural RJ, Sutton GG, et al. The sequence of the human genome. Science 2001;291:1304–51.
[54] Taylor RW, Turnbull DM. Mitochondrial DNA mutations in human disease. Nat Rev Genet 2005; 6:389–402.
[55] Zhang J, Liu H, Luo S, Chavez-Badiola A, Liu Z, Yang M, et al. First live birth using human oocytes reconstituted by spindle nuclear transfer for mitochondrial DNA mutation causing Leigh syndrome. Fertil Steril 2016;106:e375–6.
[56] Craven L, Tuppen HA, Greggains GD, Harbottle SJ, Murphy JL, Cree LM, et al. Pronuclear transfer in human embryos to prevent transmission of mitochondrial DNA disease. Nature 2010;465:82–5.
[57] Wilcox AJ, Baird DD, Weinberg CR. Time of implantation of the conceptus and loss of pregnancy. N Engl J Med 1999;340:1796–9.
[58] Noyes RW, Hertig AT, Rock J. Dating the endometrial biopsy. Am J Obstet Gynecol 1975;122:262–3.
[59] Hamamah S., Haouzi D., Methods for assessing endometrium receptivity of a patient. Win test. Patent Application Publication US 2013/0072748 A1, 2013; USA.
[60] Enciso M, Carrascosa JP, Sarasa J, Martínez-Ortiz PA, Munné S, Horcajadas JA, et al. Development of a new comprehensive and reliable endometrial receptivity map (ER Map/ER Grade) based on RT-qPCR gene expression analysis. Hum Reprod 2018;33:220–8.
[61] Díaz-Gimeno P, Horcajadas JA, Martínez-Conejero JA, Esteban FJ, Alamá P, Pellicer A, et al. A genomic diagnostic tool for human endometrial receptivity based on the transcriptomic signature. Fertil Steril 2011;95:50–60.e15.
[62] Shi L, Campbell G, Jones WD, Campagne F, Wen Z, Walker SJ, et al. The Microarray Quality Control (MAQC)-II study of common practices for the development and validation of microarray-based predictive models. Nat Biotechnol 2010;28:827–38.
[63] Ruiz-Alonso M, Blesa D, Díaz-Gimeno P, Gómez E, Fernández-Sánchez M, Carranza F, et al. The endometrial receptivity array for diagnosis and personalized embryo transfer as a treatment for patients with repeated implantation failure. Fertil Steril 2013;100:818–24.
[64] Wang Z, Gerstein M, Snyder M. RNA-Seq: a revolutionary tool for transcriptomics. Nat Rev Genet 2009;10:57–63.
[65] Igenomix. ERA® Endometrial Receptivity Analysis [Internet]. Spain: Igenomix; 2017. Available from: <https://www.igenomix.com/provider-tests/endometrial-receptivity-test-era>; 2017 [cited 16.07.19].

[66] Clemente-Císcar M, Ruiz-Alonso M, Blesa D, Jimenez-Almazan J, Bahceci M, Banker M, et al. Endometrial receptivity analysis (ERA) using a next generation sequencing (NGS) predictor improves reproductive outcome in recurrent implantation failure (RIF) patients when compared to ERA arrays. Abstracts of the 34th Annual Meeting of the European Society of Human Reproduction and Embryology. Human Reprod 2018;33(Suppl._1) Barcelona; Spain.

[67] Díaz-Gimeno P, Ruíz-Alonso M, Blesa D, Simón C. Transcriptomics of the human endometrium. Int J Dev Biol 2014;58:127–37.

[68] Diaz-Gimeno P, Ruiz-Alonso M, Sebastian-Leon P, Pellicer A, Valbuena D, Simon C. Window of implantation transcriptomic stratification reveals different endometrial subsignatures associated with live birth and biochemical pregnancy. Fertil Steril 2017;108:703–10.

[69] van der Gaast MH, Beier-Hellwig K, Fauser BCJM, Beier HM, Macklon NS. Endometrial secretion aspiration prior to embryo transfer does not reduce implantation rates. Reprod Biomed Online 2003;7:105–9.

[70] Sebastian-Leon P, Garrido N, Remohí J, Pellicer A, Diaz-Gimeno P. Asynchronous and pathological windows of implantation: two causes of recurrent implantation failure. Hum Reprod 2018;33(4):626–35.

[71] Devesa-Peiro A, Sebastian-Leon P, Pellicer A, Diaz-Gimeno P. Biomarker discovery associated with endometrial-related conditions is biased by the menstrual cycle effect in the transcriptomic analysis. Abstracts of the 35th Annual Meeting of the European Society of Human Reproduction and Embryology. Human Reprod 2019;34(Suppl. 1) Vienna; Austria.

Further reading

Su Z, Łabaj PP, Li S, Thierry-Mieg J, Thierry-Mieg D, Shi W, et al. A comprehensive assessment of RNA-seq accuracy, reproducibility and information content by the Sequencing Quality Control Consortium. Nat Biotechnol 2014;32:903–14.

CHAPTER

5

Epigenetics and imprinting in assisted reproduction

Diego Marin[1,2] *and Emre Seli*[1,3]

[1]IVIRMA New Jersey, Basking Ridge, NJ, United States [2]Thomas Jefferson University, Philadelphia, PA, United States [3]Yale School of Medicine, New Haven, CT, United States

Introduction

In the winter of 1944, German troops occupied most parts of Europe, including the Netherlands. Because of the usual shortages of that time and a railway strike, German authorities implemented a policy that limited food rations allocated to the population of the Western region of the Netherlands. This episode in history is known as the Dutch famine. And as brutal and tragic as it was, this event ended up helping us better understand how the environment plays a crucial role in human development [1]. It turns out that the Dutch population in question included pregnant women, meaning that individuals who had an in utero exposure to the famine were born and were followed up. The level of detail in which demographic and medical records were kept in the Netherlands allowed for the design of elegant human studies to evaluate the health consequences of intrauterine food deprivation [2]. Most of these studies concluded that the environment did have an effect on the fetuses in utero, and that changes caused by food deprivation, such as higher adiposity and increased risk for disease, persisted through adulthood [2,3].

Given that the undernutrition period was transitory, one might ask, how was it possible to observe health effects 70 years later? In fact, there is evidence of transgenerational effects such as increased adiposity and morbidity due to prenatal exposure to those harsh conditions in utero [4,5]. Can the accessibility of our DNAs be modified by the environment? Are those modifications heritable? Does DNA have memory for these modifications? All these are examples of changes attributed to epigenetics. Although our DNA sequence is relatively stable (apart from de novo mutations and chromosome rearrangements), it turns out that the way it is packed and how its transcription is regulated can indeed be modified. In addition, although those modifications are also stable through time, they are prone to changes

Human Reproductive Genetics
DOI: https://doi.org/10.1016/B978-0-12-816561-4.00005-3

induced by environmental factors. Therefore we can define epigenetics as another level of organization of our DNA that regulates how and when genes are expressed.

All cells in our body have the same genetic constitution in terms of DNA sequence (except for gametes produced in our gonads), yet a neuron has completely different structure and function than an epithelial cell, or a Sertoli cell. How does this programming originate? This is another phenomenon, that is, largely attributed to epigenetics. Although the DNA backbone is the same for all cells, the way it is organized and how some parts of that sequence get transcribed and expressed while others are silenced is regulated by several chemical and physical modifications. It has been suggested that epigenetics is the bridge between genotype and phenotype, given that the phenotype is the direct consequence of how the genome is expressed and not what it codes for [6].

This chapter will focus on describing the major levels of epigenetic regulation in mammals, as well as its implications in other known phenomena such as aging and imprinting. In addition, special emphasis will be placed on the relationship between assisted reproductive treatment (ART) and epigenetic regulation. This is because, as we will discuss shortly, some of the most critical moments of epigenetic programming occur during preimplantation development, a time when ART may impose different types of stress upon the early embryo compared to natural conception.

Molecular mechanisms of epigenetic regulation

As stated above, several chemical modifications and physical interactions with other molecules are pivotal in determining which sections of the DNA will be expressed. These determine when and where genes are turned on and off. These modifications can be categorized into three main levels of epigenetic regulation: DNA methylation, histone modifications, and noncoding RNA regulation. The main features of each of these mechanisms and the most feasible methods to analyze them are described below.

DNA methylation

Methylation refers to the addition of a methyl group (−CH3) to a molecule. As simple as it may sound, this molecular change can determine how the corresponding region of the DNA molecule is interpreted by the cell, and therefore how its genes are either silenced or highly expressed. Usually, the addition of methyl groups occurs on the nucleotide cytosine, changing its nomenclature to 5-methylcytosine, and almost exclusively when it is followed by a guanine, thus forming a methylated CpG dinucleotide (where "p" simply indicates that "C" and "G" are connected by a phosphodiester bond). Methylation is made possible by the enzymes called DNA methyltransferases, which not only mediate de novo DNA methylation (such as the one observed during development and differentiation), but also help maintain DNA methylation status from one division to another [7,8] (because epigenetic markers have a mitotic inheritance, meaning that all cells stemming from a tissue or exerting the same function will have a similar epigenetic arrangement, i.e., established immediately upon cell division). Importantly, CpG dinucleotides tend to be clustered in what is called a CpG island [9], or regions of the genome of around 200 bases with a C + G content of around 50% and a ratio of observed versus expected CpG frequency of at least 0.6 [10]. CpG islands are generally associated with gene promoter regions [11], where, when methylated, they result in gene silencing. Although other nucleotides can become methylated, in mammals DNA methylation occurs almost exclusively in CpG dinucleotides, and that is why the chemistry of methods to detect and analyze this phenomenon focus entirely on cytosine methylation.

Several methods are currently available to quantify DNA methylation, each with advantages and limitations. When the main goal is to profile global methylation of the genome, it is not critical to determine methylation levels for specific loci. Instead, an overall picture of the methylation level of a genome in question is obtained. Although these measurements may seem somewhat uninformative, altered global DNA methylation occurs in various diseases and has also been associated with tumors [12,13] and aging [14,15]. In addition, whole-genome methylation may also be used as an indirect measure of the methylation machinery function that operates in a cell [16,17].

If measuring overall DNA methylation is the ultimate goal, then the method considered as gold standard is high-performance liquid chromatography or its variants [18–20]. Briefly, the DNA input is digested so that all nucleotides are hydrolyzed from the main DNA and separated by chromatographic approaches. Since methylated and unmethylated cytosines have different molecular weights, they can be separated and quantified [18]. A ratio of the measurements obtained for methylated and unmethylated cytosines serves as an indicator of global methylation that can be useful when comparing different tissues or experimental treatments. However, this technique requires large amounts of DNA ($>3\ \mu g$), not to mention highly complex instruments. As a result, other methods to quantify global methylation have been developed. Some rely on enzymatic digestion, meaning that the DNA input is treated with enzymes that cut the DNA in specific sites where there are CpG dinucleotides. Likewise, some enzymes will only cut if there is no methyl group that can hinder enzyme–DNA binding. Therefore by detecting and quantifying DNA fragments after enzymatic digestion an overall estimate of CpG methylation becomes available for that sample [21–25].

Before describing the methods for locus-specific methylation, it is important to mention that several techniques that measure both global and locus-specific methylation are based on a chemical reaction called bisulfite conversion (Fig. 5.1). This method consists of inducing deamination (removal of the amine group –NH3) of the nucleotide cytosine using bisulfite (HSO_3^-), which changes the cytosine into uracil. This conversion is often followed by polymerase chain reaction (PCR) to amplify the bisulfite-treated templates. Since cytosine methylation blocks the bisulfite conversion, those unmethylated cytosines will appear as thymines in the new PCR products, while the methylated ones will continue to be sequenced as cytosines [26–29].

Whole-genome bisulfate sequencing (WGBS) is a widespread assay that merges bisulfate conversion with next-generation sequencing. After DNA is fragmented, treated with bisulfite and sequenced, overall estimations of cytosine methylation can be performed. Nevertheless, coverage of the genome is not optimal in many cases, and may therefore require more sequencing at higher costs if an acceptable representation of genomic CpGs is desired [30,31].

Additional methods relying on bisulfite conversion chemistry are available to determine the methylation status of specific loci in the genome. A common assay similar to WGBS is reduced representation bisulfite sequencing [32]. In this case, only a fraction of the genome enriched in CpG dinucleotides is sequenced. After DNA enzymatic digestion, this technique can provide information for around 85% of all CpG island sites [33]. In addition, commercial arrays are available that do not involve sequencing, but have probes that bind to either uracil or cytosine after bisulfite conversion. By following this method, not only are experiment costs dramatically decreased, but specific loci can be tested for methylation, depending on how primers are designed [34,35].

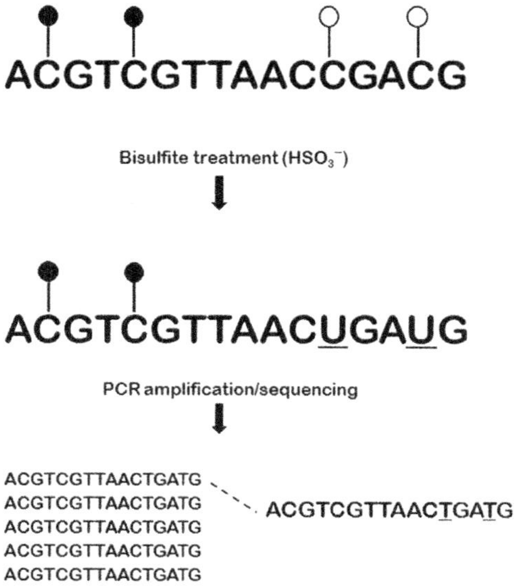

FIGURE 5.1 Bisulfite conversion. An example of a DNA sequence with both methylated and unmethylated cytosines is depicted in this figure. When the DNA sample is treated with the ion bisulfite (HSO_3^-), cytosines that are not methylated lose their amine group (−NH3) in a reaction called deamination, resulting in the nucleotide uracil (*underlined*). On the other hand, methylated cytosines remain intact after bisulfite treatment and therefore persist as cytosines. This DNA product is further amplified by polymerase chain reaction (PCR), where the nucleotide thymine is incorporated instead of uracil (*underlined*) in subsequent rounds of DNA amplification. The final amplified DNA can undergo sequencing or hybridization to customized arrays where information regarding methylation sites can be retrieved. If a cytosine residue remains as a cytosine after bisulfite conversion and sequence amplification, this finding indicates that it was originally methylated. Conversely, if a cytosine residue is changed to a thymine, this suggests that it was not methylated.

Histone modifications

Histones are the proteins with which the DNA is packed and organized in most cells. A DNA double strand coiled around a core of histones constitutes a structural unit called the nucleosome (Fig. 5.2) [36,37]. A major determinant of whether a gene is expressed or not is its accessibility. Indeed, while transcription factors might be available and the cell's transcriptional machinery active, the DNA region coding for that gene should be accessible for effective generation of messenger ribonucleic acid (mRNA). Histones play a major role in the regulation of chromatin accessibility due to the fact that these proteins may undergo more than 100 types of posttranscriptional modifications that will either loosen the DNA packaging, thus making it available for transcription or replication, or that will tightly pack the nucleosome so that access to the DNA is limited. In addition, modified histones can either promote or impede protein recruitment [38,39]. The transcription process has several steps with various proteins being indispensable, therefore modifying protein recruitment directly alters whether DNA is transcribed or not. As a result, genes can be turned on and off by modifying how DNA is packed and which proteins are allowed to interact with it [40,41].

Histone modification is defined as any covalent addition of a chemical group (acetylation, methylation, ubiquitination, phosphorylation, etc.) that occurs posttranscriptionally. These chemical changes can affect internucleosome interactions, and also protein recruitment as

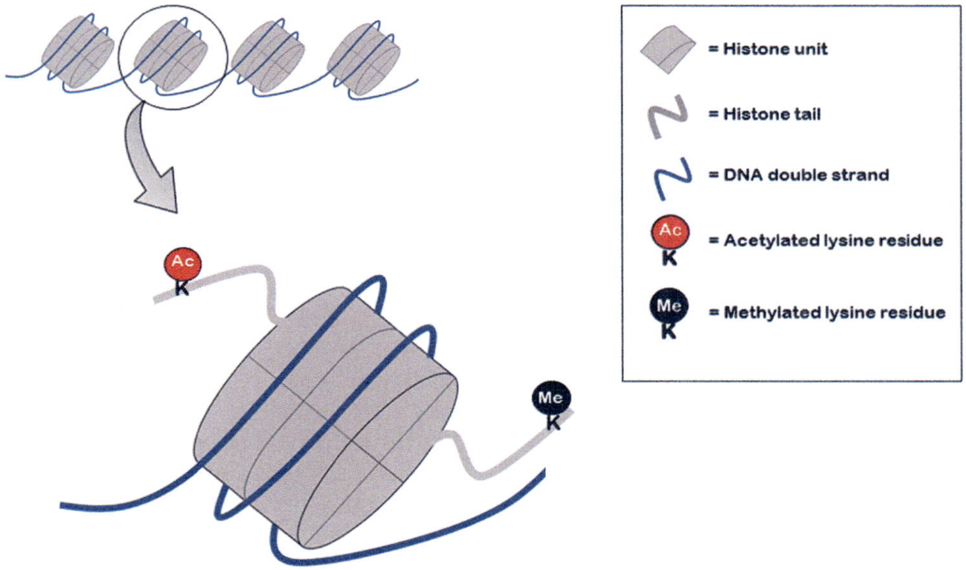

FIGURE 5.2 The nucleosome. A nucleosome is the structural unit in which DNA is packed and organized in the cell nucleus. The DNA double strand is coiled around a core of proteins called histones. Nucleosome structures are dynamic and are major regulators of chromatin accessibility and therefore gene expression. Protrusions of histone proteins from the nucleosome proteic core are known as histone tails. Most histone modifications occur in these tails. Examples of acetylated and methylated lysine residues are shown in this figure. These are moieties covalently linked to histones that exert a regulatory function in chromatin structure and accessibility.

stated above [40]. Among the different types of histone modification, acetylation was one of the first to be characterized [42,43]. It was observed that when a lysine residue of the N-terminal tail of the histone is acetylated, transcriptional activity and chromatin accessibility are enhanced. On the other hand, if the modification is the addition of a methyl group, an opposite effect occurs [44]. Importantly, the type of histone modification (whether it is an acetylation, methylation, or the addition of a phosphate group) is not as important as the target, since depending on which histone residue is modified, the result can be either silencing or increased expression of the gene of interest [45].

Due to the effects of histone modifications on chromatin accessibility by transcription factors and other proteins, quantifying the extent to which DNA is accessible provides a useful measure of the epigenetic regulation exerted by histones. This is accomplished mostly by determining how susceptible a DNA sequence is to cleavage or other enzymatic modifications [46]. For example, one of the first methods that coupled DNA susceptibility to cleavage and PCR amplification, treated DNA samples with DNase I, an enzyme that cleaves DNA. Under the principle that inaccessible DNA is protected from enzymatic action, PCR and further array hybridization or sequencing technologies enable the researcher to interrogate to what extent chromatin is accessible by quantifying lengths of fragments and where DNase cleavages take place more often [47–50]. Likewise, the method micrococcal nuclease sequencing (MNase-seq) also performs DNA digestion, but in this case the intact DNA that remains bound to a nucleosome is isolated and sequenced, and thus regions of restricted accessibility are unveiled [51,52].

Furthermore, chromatin immunoprecipitation (ChIP) assays have also been exploited to interrogate what segments of the DNA sequence are more tightly associated with the proteic core of the nucleosome. In a ChIP assay, DNA is cross-linked to proteins that interact with that specific sequence at a specific moment or developmental stage. Next, chromatin undergoes fragmentation and any protein–DNA complex is captured by an antibody specific for the protein in question. Antibodies for histones and even specific histone modifications would shed light on what regions of chromatin are associated with them. Finally, DNA is dissociated from the precipitated proteins and is subjected to either hybridization to an array with selected probes or sequencing [53]. The latter is known as ChIP-seq, which has gradually replaced its array counterpart since it allows to analyze a much larger portion of the genome at lower costs. Nonetheless, a high-quality DNA input is vital in this assay to achieve adequate sequencing depth for data analysis [54].

Another method that has recently gained popularity for these measurements is the assay for transposase-accessible chromatin using sequencing. For this technique, DNA sequences that work as adapters for downstream sequencing are inserted into open and accessible chromatin regions. By following this protocol, very proximal DNA fragments with adapters indicate that chromatin was easily accessible. On the other hand, DNA regions with limited accessibility are not sequenced and silenced gene activity can be inferred [55,56].

Finally, an additional method to assess chromatin accessibility is based on DNA methylation and the bisulfite conversion chemistry mentioned above. In this case, methylation of DNA is an indirect indicator of open and accessible chromatin, since only these regions are accessible by methyltransferases. As a result, and after bisulfite treatment and sequencing, CpG methylation indicates open chromatin regions versus the unmethylated ones, which are most likely regions tightly packed and with absent transcriptional activity. This method is known as nucleosome occupancy and methylome sequencing [57,58].

Noncoding RNAs

As mentioned above, DNA methylation and histone modification are the two major mechanisms of epigenetic regulation in mammals. Nevertheless, recent findings suggest that the definition of epigenetic regulation goes beyond these two processes. Noncoding RNAs have been proposed as a third level of epigenetic regulation because they play pivotal roles in regulating gene expression without causing a change in the DNA sequence, which is the basic definition of epigenetics.

Only around 2% of the human genome is estimated to be transcribed and translated into protein, while the vast majority of the genome is transcribed but not translated [59]. Several of the untranslated RNA species have been found to interact with both the DNA and it binding protein complexes, resulting in either enhancement or suppression of gene expression. These RNA species can be divided into two major groups based on their length: long noncoding RNAs (lncRNA) are longer than 200 base pairs (bp) and may originate from transcribed introns or other coding sequences. Short noncoding RNAs have less than 200 bp and their mechanism of function, cell origin, and role in disease and diagnostics have been hitherto extensively studied, most importantly due to their high stability in contrast to other RNA species [60,61].

How these noncoding RNAs actually exert epigenetic regulation depends on numerous mechanisms and pathways, but a common denominator is protein recruitment. In the case of lncRNAs, protein complexes such as the polycomb group (PcG) are recruited once an lncRNA finds complementarity to a certain DNA sequence, and start the formation of heterochromatin (tightly packed and inaccessible chromatin), as is the case of chromosome X inactivation, where gene expression is totally silenced [62–64]. Among the short noncoding RNAs, micro-RNAs (miRNAs) have been extensively characterized. Not only do miRNAs recruit protein complexes that silence and/or degrade mature mRNAs [65,66], they also regulate the expression of proteins that have direct epigenetic functions such as the PcG, methyltransferases, and deacetylases [67–69].

Epigenetics of aging

The phenomenon of aging is a highly complex process that involves a myriad of biological changes in cell function caused by numerous biochemical events. This process can be understood as a gradual loss of functionality (either at a cell or organism level) that results in increased risk of disease, and eventually death [70–72].

Since aging involves major changes in cell function and since the epigenome plays a crucial role in the regulation of gene expression and cell fate decisions, aging research has recently focused on the epigenetic mechanisms as a potential master-regulator of this process. The fact that two organisms that share the same genetic background can age differently and present diverse lifespans is another argument in favor of how environmental changes affect the aging process [73]. In fact, epigenetic studies have provided evidence that most environmentally induced modifications in cellular function are mediated by epigenetic changes such as histone modifications, alterations in DNA methylation, and even expression of noncoding RNAs, all described above.

Histone modifications and aging

One important event linking epigenetics and aging is loss of histones. In many organisms, including invertebrate animal models and mammals, global loss of histones has been reported in aged organisms compared to younger populations [74,75]. As stated above, histones are the core component of nucleosomes and are highly responsible for regulating chromatin organization and accessibility. Consequently, depletion of histones results in loss of nucleosomal structures, which translates into open and accessible chromatin. Indeed, a well-characterized phenomenon associated with aging cells is loss of heterochromatin (regions of tightly packed DNA, i.e., transcriptionally silent) [76], with significant potential repercussions, two of which have been proposed as pivotal in the aging process: gene expression deregulation and genome instability.

Transcriptional deregulation has been evidenced in aged cells due to excessive open chromatin. Transcriptional deregulation can result in increased global transcriptional amplification, meaning that genes start to be expressed uncontrollably, culminating in unendurable cell instability and eventually loss of function. Similarly, genes that are supposed to be silent may become accessible by the transcriptional machinery and upregulated, inducing cellular chaos and suboptimal functionality [77]. In addition, noncoding genomic regions that are normally silent and packed in heterochromatin domains may become accessible and transcribed once the nucleosomes cease to exist. Some of the resulting transcripts originate from retrotransposable elements, which are genomic regions that can move and become inserted into other genomic positions causing insertional mutations, copy number variations, and even gene conversions [78]. This genomic instability is typical of aging cells and happens because those unwanted transcripts may undergo reverse transcription, resulting in the formation of complementary DNA copies that may subsequently be inserted into the genome [79,80].

Although loss of histones primarily results in loss of heterochromatin and increased chromatin accessibility, heterochromatization in otherwise normally open chromatin has also been reported in aging models. In fact, this is a feature of senescent cells [81,82]. Senescence refers to the process where cells undergo programmed growth arrest due to various cues. While cell senescence often occurs in the context of aging, these are two distinct processes, since senescence has also been observed in embryonic stages as a mechanism to orchestrate cell fate [83,84]. Heterochromatization during aging is mainly due to altered histone modifications, potentially caused by defective enzymatic activity on histone residues. For instance, both methylation and demethylation of histones have been associated with restructuring of the nucleosome and increased heterochromatin [85,86]. Conversely, increased histone acetylation has been observed in human aged cell lines, resulting in increased chromatin accessibility and expression of genes important for autophagy and stress response [87].

Therefore both loss and gain of heterochromatin (the latter mostly associated with senescence [88]) are observed in aging organisms, depending on specific epigenetic cues. As a result, the term heterochromatin redistribution has been proposed as a significant process mediating cellular aging, highlighting the importance of the epigenome [89].

DNA methylation and aging

DNA methylation is also a major player in linking epigenetics and aging. As mentioned above, CpG methylation in mammals is mostly associated with repression of gene expression. In aged organisms, however, the observed pattern is gradual loss of DNA methylation [90–92]. The consequences of this are somewhat similar to those described for chromatin reorganization resulting from loss of histones, where genomic regions that used to be transcriptionally silent become accessible, resulting in transcriptional deregulation and genome instability. DNA methyltransferases play a key role in maintaining methylation, which is why depletion of these enzymes is usually implicated in the process of aging [93,94]. However, similar to the paradox of heterochromatin in aging, locus-specific DNA hypermethylation has also been reported in aged individuals [95].

Furthermore, age-associated changes in methylation of specific loci seem to be surprisingly predictable in somatic cells and form the basis of the "epigenetic clock" concept. Indeed, Steve Horvath developed a model based on DNA methylation status of 353 specific CpG sites, which proved to be highly predictive of chronological age in a study with unprecedented sample size and quality [96], a finding that was reproduced with a smaller set of CpG sites (71 CpGs) by Hannum et al. [97]. In both models, only the CpG sites most strongly associated with the subjects' chronological age were included. Moreover, in the same study it was also observed that some subjects were predicted as older than their chronological age by the epigenetic aging model, a circumstance also known as epigenetic age acceleration. This age acceleration was notably evidenced in cancer tissues and those harboring mutations on tumor suppressor genes [96], which suggests that the epigenetic clock could provide additional information regarding biological aging. This last term refers to an organism's functional decline strongly associated with morbidity and mortality. For instance, two individuals of the same chronological age could differ greatly in their biological age [98].

In fact, since these epigenetic aging models were designed based solely on the high predictability of an individual's chronological age, some have questioned their applicability to predict risk of disease or other aspects of clinical relevance [98]. Nevertheless, using the epigenetic aging model proposed by Horvath [96] in a cohort of semisupercentenarians (individuals reaching ages of 105–109 years) it was found not only that centenarian subjects were predicted younger by the epigenetic clock, but also that their offspring were predicted younger than age-matched controls [99], suggesting that these epigenetic predictions are also indicative of biological age. Likewise, the same group developed another similar epigenetic aging model that included phenotypic traits of the study subjects and that set prediction of phenotypic age rather than chronological as the primary endpoint. This novel model proved to be superior to the previous ones in terms of prediction of all-cause mortality, cancers, and healthspan [100,101], which in turn highlights its clinical applicability. In sum, this innovative concept of the "epigenetic clock" provides further and strong evidence that epigenetics and aging are inextricably linked phenomena [102].

Epigenetics and reproductive aging

Given the clear association between the epigenome and the aging process described so far, it is expected that epigenetic regulation is also vital in reproductive aging, especially as it is well established that fertility declines with increased age in most organisms [103]. With respect to female reproductive aging, ovarian aging seems to be the primary focus, and it refers to the declining capability of ovaries to generate oocytes of good quality and in good number after controlled ovarian stimulation [104]. In fact, it has been shown that gene expression in oocytes of women of advanced maternal age is altered compared to younger women [105]. These age-dependent changes to the oocyte transcriptome can be explained by altered epigenetic cues and regulators. Expression of DNA methyltransferases, the enzymes responsible for DNA methylation, has been reported to differ between oocytes from young and old mice [106], and can therefore be the cause of the global transcriptional changes observed during ovarian aging. In addition, other key epigenetic regulators such as histone modifications are altered in aged oocytes. For instance, histone methylation patterns in immature oocytes from mice are significantly different between young and older females [107]. Likewise, maternal age has also been linked to decreased histone deacetylation in human oocytes [108].

As mentioned above, DNA methylation patterns of selected loci in the genome proved to be predictive of an individual's age and were therefore referred as the "epigenetic clock" described by Horvath [96,102]. Following a similar hypothesis, a recent study posed the question of whether the somatic methylome measured in cumulus cells using the Horvath model (based on 353 CpG sites) predicted age or ovarian response to stimulation in women undergoing in vitro fertilization (IVF). Four groups were compared: younger women (<35 years old) with normal response, younger women with poor response, older women (>40 years old) with expected response, and older women (>40 years old) with high response. Interestingly, the age predicted in cumulus cells was much younger then chronological age (approximately 10 years old), and did not differ between younger and older reproductive-age women or between those with normal or poor response [109]. The findings of this study suggest that the mechanisms of epigenetic regulation in reproductive tissues might be different than in nonreproductive somatic tissues.

Paternal age has been shown to negatively impact fertility in various ways such as increased time to pregnancy, altered sperm epigenome, and disease susceptibility in the offspring [110]. The most studied epigenetic mark in sperm is DNA methylation. In sperm from older rats, for instance, a global hypermethylation was observed, while loci-specific demethylation was also reported [111]. This is in contrast to most somatic tissues which show the opposite methylation patterns [6]. An elegant study that compared sperm methylation patterns of samples collected from the same men 10–20 years apart identified specific loci that undergo predictable changes in DNA methylation [112]. Moreover, the same group found that loci that undergo age-related methylation changes in sperm retain those changes after fertilization and can potentially transmit to their offspring, a phenomenon already described in mice [113]. In addition, the theory of the "epigenetic clock" described above was also tested with sperm samples [96]. The study identified 51 CpG sites that predict a man's age with an accuracy of 94% [114].

A special aspect of epigenetics: imprinting

It is well established that abnormal fertilization can result in embryonic arrest, improper preimplantation development, and in some cases aberrant phenotypes in implanted embryos. Studies in mice have reported that when the male pronucleus is replaced by a second female pronucleus in a fertilized oocyte, the resulting monoparental embryo does not develop normally and becomes a teratoma [115]. Similarly, when an embryo has only paternal genomes, for example, by fertilization of a genetically void oocyte by two sperms, the resulting embryo undergoes excessive trophoblast proliferation and forms a hydatidiform mole [116,117]. These two phenomena indicate that in addition to having the correct DNA copy number, normal embryonic development requires parental genomes of both sexes to be present. This requisite for normal development is explained by the fact that some loci in our genome are expressed in a parent-of-origin specific manner. This phenomenon is known as genomic imprinting [118]. Unlike the vast majority of our genes, which are expressed equally irrespective of whether they are inherited from our father or mother, approximately 100 imprinted genes are expressed or silenced based on the parental origin of the chromosome in which they are located [119–121]. When the required paternal or maternal genome is absent for imprinted genes, transcriptional imbalances occur and lead to abnormal development and clinical syndromes.

Before the molecular basis of imprinting is described, it is paramount to first understand how epigenetic marks are reprogrammed during development and how imprinted regions slightly differ from the global genome in the way they are reprogrammed. The importance of DNA methylation as an epigenetic regulator was described in detail above. DNA methylation is also a major regulator of genome-wide reprogramming during germ cell and embryo development. All cells in our body possess different methylation patterns since they vary in function and therefore in transcriptional programs. During embryonic development, those cells that will give rise to gametes undergo global demethylation, losing all epigenetic marks that other somatic tissues retain for normal function [122–124]. These cells are called primordial germ cells (PGC) and their reprogramming is indispensable for continuing differentiation into gamete precursors and eventually oocytes or sperm. In mammals, this reprogramming phase occurs before and during PGCs' migration to the genital ridge [125]. This global methylation is then followed by a round of remethylation, which introduces parental specific epigenetic signatures to germ cells. For example, in males, the de novo methylation finalizes before birth and is maintained by spermatogonial stem cells and the meiotically produced spermatozoa. In contrast, de novo methylation in females starts before birth in meiotically arrested oocytes and culminates at the germinal vesicle stage [123,126]. These DNA methylation dynamics result in mature gametes with distinct methylation patterns reflecting their parental origin.

Furthermore, once the oocyte is fertilized, a second round of demethylation or reprogramming occurs again with differential parental origin dynamics. DNA in the male pronucleus undergoes rapid demethylation, whereas in the female genome the reprogramming is more gradual [127,128]. However, the important aspect to note in this second reprogramming event during preimplantation development is that the demethylation is not 100% complete, because some loci retain their parental methylation patterns; these are the so-called imprinted regions. Finally, tissue-specific methylation patterns start being set during the blastocyst stage and in the postimplantation embryo establishing cell lineages, while simultaneously maintaining the imprinted marks that resisted the previous global reprogramming [129,130].

When imprinting goes bad

Having established the dynamics of epigenetic reprogramming and how imprinted marks are retained after fertilization, it should be mentioned that this is an error-prone biological process that may have significant consequences. First, imprinted marks are generally cytosine methylations that mostly are not located in the coding DNA sequence, but rather in regulatory sequences. These regulatory imprinted regions are known as imprinted centers containing differentially methylated regions [131], which, depending on their methylation levels, can enhance or block transcription by orchestrating protein recruitment or inducing chromatin changes. Therefore an error in DNA methylation or failure to maintain imprinted marks in these locations will result in abnormal gene expression.

For example, epimutations are changes in the epigenetic marks of those regulatory regions or other chromatin modifications caused stochastically or by environmental stressors without modifying the DNA sequence [132–135]. If erasure of the maternal imprint is suboptimal during PGC reprogramming in a male, the produced sperm would retain its maternal imprints, thus resulting in an epigenetic imbalance once an oocyte is fertilized with that sperm. In addition, failure of maintenance of imprinted loci during the remethylation wave that occurs in the peri- and postimplantation stages of embryo development could result in some cells presenting hypermethylated imprinted loci, giving rise to epigenetic mosaicism since the epimutation happens postzygotically [135]. Imprinting disorders such as the Prader–Willi syndrome (PWS), Angelman syndrome (AS), and Beckwith–Wiedemann syndrome (BWS) are caused by these phenomena [131,134].

Assisted reproductive treatment and the epigenome

Assisted reproductive technology is defined as "all interventions that include in vitro handling of both human oocytes and sperm or of embryos for the purpose of reproduction" [136]. As a result, it is more than legitimate to hypothesize that ART can potentially affect the epigenetics of future babies since most of the major events of establishment of epigenetic marks and maintenance of imprinted regions occur in gametes and the preimplantation embryos, which are manipulated in vitro in IVF laboratories. Likewise, the epigenome seems to be the most plausible molecular mechanism in which environmental changes can permanently affect an organism through its lifespan [137]. In fact, the potential effects of ART on the epigenome have been investigated and reviewed exhaustively [138–142].

For instance, it was reported by several studies that children born through ART are more susceptible to suffer imprinting disorders such as AS and BWS [139], although the absolute risk remains minimal. Moreover, studies in animal models have postulated that in vitro culture of mammalian embryos affects not only gene expression patterns [143], but also DNA methylation at imprinted loci [144–146]. Despite the ease with which in vitro and animal models can study causation, establishing a causal relationship between an intervention (or an insult) and a clinical outcome in the newborn within the context of ART remains a challenge due to the relatively unknown impact of parental infertility [147]. Therefore it is possible that many of the so far reported associations between ART and imprinting disorders are caused by infertility, rather than the ART treatment. Indeed, a Dutch study revealed that after correcting for parental infertility factors, there was no apparent association between ART and AS, PWS, or BWS [148].

Although it is clear that ART imposes nonphysiological and many times invasive manipulations on gametes and embryos, and investigation of possible detrimental effects of ART in children is more than encouraged, it is also of the utmost importance to investigate epigenetics as a tool that could potentially improve culture conditions, micromanipulation techniques, and ultimately clinical outcomes. Moreover, our recently deeper understanding of epigenetics has allowed reproductive research to focus on the epigenome as a potential source of biomarkers for reproductive competence, as described below.

The epigenome as a tool to improve assisted reproductive treatment

The implementation of preimplantation genetic testing for aneuploidies in in vitro generated embryos has provided the field of ART with substantial benefits, such as higher implantation rates per transfer, reduced miscarriage rates, and shorter time to achieve pregnancy. However, roughly one third of chromosomally normal embryos fail to implant, stressing the need for additional biomarkers for reproductive fitness [149]. A recent study assessed the global DNA methylation levels by means of WGBS of trophoectoderm biopsies from IVF-generated human embryos donated for research in order to establish the grounds for investigating global methylation as a potential biomarker in human blastocysts. The authors found that global methylation was significantly higher in aneuploid embryos compared to euploid embryos and that embryos from older patients also presented overall higher DNA methylation levels [150].

Not only was this study motivated by the urge of finding potential biomarkers of embryo viability in the epigenome, but it also highlighted the challenges of epigenetic assessments. For example, although data in animal models have provided some hints about DNA methylation in preimplantation embryos, it is imperative to first establish what would be considered normal values in human embryos before identifying abnormal deviations that could become potential biomarkers of embryonic competence; a step that would require a large sample size. In addition, it is highly likely that once the method for DNA methylation quantification is well validated and embryos with diverse outcomes are analyzed, the differences between embryos that implant and those that do not might be so small that the implemented method may not be sensitive enough to detect them.

Summary and conclusions

Epigenetic marks are pivotal determinants of how cellular identity and lineages are established during development. As stated above and proposed elsewhere, the epigenome is the bridge between the genotype and the phenotype. DNA methylation, histone modifications, and noncoding RNAs are the three major levels of epigenetic regulation in mammals. Currently, several methodologies are available to study these epigenetic marks, shedding light on the dynamics of epigenetic regulation and how aberrations in chromatin accessibility may result in disease and aging. Both male and female reproductive aging are associated with epigenetic changes, where the role of DNA methylation has been widely studied. Furthermore, genomic imprinting mandates that both the maternal and paternal genomes are present in cells for normal development, due to the parent-of-origin differential gene expression seen for some genes in mammals.

The overlap that exists between the most remarkable events of epigenetic reprogramming that occur during preimplantation development and the developmental stages at which gametes and embryos are manipulated in ART raises concerns regarding potential untoward effects on the epigenetic landscape of ART-born children. Nevertheless, clear evidence for causation between ART and imprinting or epigenetic disorders in humans is still lacking. Finally, a better understanding of epigenetics and how it regulates early mammalian development has encouraged recent research to address the epigenome as a tool for improvements in ART.

References

[1] Schulz LC. The Dutch Hunger Winter and the developmental origins of health and disease. Proc Natl Acad Sci U S A 2010;107(39):16757–8.

[2] Heijmans BT, Tobi EW, Stein AD, Putter H, Blauw GJ, Susser ES, et al. Persistent epigenetic differences associated with prenatal exposure to famine in humans. Proc Natl Acad Sci U S A 2008;105(44):17046–9.

[3] Roseboom T, de Rooij S, Painter R. The Dutch famine and its long-term consequences for adult health. Early Hum Dev 2006;82(8):485–91.

[4] Veenendaal MV, Painter RC, de Rooij SR, Bossuyt PM, van der Post JA, Gluckman PD, et al. Transgenerational effects of prenatal exposure to the 1944-45 Dutch famine. BJOG Int J Obstet Gynaecol 2013;120(5):548–53.

[5] Painter RC, Osmond C, Gluckman P, Hanson M, Phillips DI, Roseboom TJ. Transgenerational effects of prenatal exposure to the Dutch famine on neonatal adiposity and health in later life. BJOG Int J Obstet Gynaecol 2008;115(10):1243–9.

[6] Pal S, Tyler JK. Epigenetics and aging. Sci Adv 2016;2(7):e1600584.

[7] Bird A. DNA methylation patterns and epigenetic memory. Genes Dev 2002;16(1):6–21.

[8] Goll MG, Bestor TH. Eukaryotic cytosine methyltransferases. Annu Rev Biochem 2005;74:481–514.

[9] Takai D, Jones PA. Comprehensive analysis of CpG islands in human chromosomes 21 and 22. Proc Natl Acad Sci U S A 2002;99(6):3740–5.

[10] Gardiner-Garden M, Frommer M. CpG islands in vertebrate genomes. J Mol Biol 1987;196(2):261–82.

[11] Wang Y, Leung FC. An evaluation of new criteria for CpG islands in the human genome as gene markers. Bioinformatics (Oxford, Engl) 2004;20(7):1170–7.

[12] Bujko M, Musialik E, Olbromski R, Przestrzelska M, Libura M, Pastwinska A, et al. Repetitive genomic elements and overall DNA methylation changes in acute myeloid and childhood B-cell lymphoblastic leukemia patients. Int J Hematol 2014;100(1):79–87.

[13] Calvo X, Nomdedeu M, Navarro A, Tejero R, Costa D, Munoz C, et al. High levels of global DNA methylation are an independent adverse prognostic factor in a series of 90 patients with de novo myelodysplastic syndrome. Leukemia Res 2014;38(8):874–81.

[14] Bellizzi D, D'Aquila P, Montesanto A, Corsonello A, Mari V, Mazzei B, et al. Global DNA methylation in old subjects is correlated with frailty. Age (Dordrecht, Neth) 2012;34(1):169–79.

[15] Thompson RF, Atzmon G, Gheorghe C, Liang HQ, Lowes C, Greally JM, et al. Tissue-specific dysregulation of DNA methylation in aging. Aging Cell 2010;9(4):506–18.

[16] Arakawa Y, Watanabe M, Inoue N, Sarumaru M, Hidaka Y, Iwatani Y. Association of polymorphisms in DNMT1, DNMT3A, DNMT3B, MTHFR and MTRR genes with global DNA methylation levels and prognosis of autoimmune thyroid disease. Clin Exp Immunol 2012;170(2):194–201.

[17] Conti A, Kobets T, Escudero-Lourdes C, Montgomery B, Tryndyak V, Beland FA, et al. Dose- and time-dependent epigenetic changes in the livers of Fisher 344 rats exposed to furan. Toxicol Sci Off J Soc Toxicol 2014;139(2):371–80.

[18] Kuo KC, McCune RA, Gehrke CW, Midgett R, Ehrlich M. Quantitative reversed-phase high performance liquid chromatographic determination of major and modified deoxyribonucleosides in DNA. Nucleic Acids Res 1980;8(20):4763–76.

[19] Fraga MF, Uriol E, Borja Diego L, Berdasco M, Esteller M, Canal MJ, et al. High-performance capillary electrophoretic method for the quantification of 5-methyl 2′-deoxycytidine in genomic DNA: application to plant, animal and human cancer tissues. Electrophoresis 2002;23(11):1677–81.

[20] Wilson VL, Smith RA, Autrup H, Krokan H, Musci DE, Le NN, et al. Genomic 5-methylcytosine determination by 32P-postlabeling analysis. Anal Biochem 1986;152(2):275–84.

[21] Aung HT, Harrison DK, Findlay I, Mattick JS, Martin NG, Carroll BJ. Stringent programming of DNA methylation in humans. Twin Res Hum Genet Off J Int Soc Twin Stud 2010;13(5):405–11.

[22] Jaligot E, Beule T, Rival A. Methylation-sensitive RFLPs: characterisation of two oil palm markers showing somaclonal variation-associated polymorphism. Theor Appl Genet (TAG) 2002;104(8):1263–9.

[23] Jorda M, Rodriguez J, Frigola J, Peinado MA. Analysis of DNA methylation by amplification of intermethylated sites (AIMS). Methods Mol Biol (Clifton, NJ) 2009;507:107–16.

[24] Karimi M, Johansson S, Ekstrom TJ. Using LUMA: a Luminometric-based assay for global DNA-methylation. Epigenetics 2006;1(1):45–8.

[25] Karimi M, Johansson S, Stach D, Corcoran M, Grander D, Schalling M, et al. LUMA (LUminometric Methylation Assay)—a high throughput method to the analysis of genomic DNA methylation. Exp Cell Res 2006;312(11):1989–95.

[26] Wang RY, Gehrke CW, Ehrlich M. Comparison of bisulfite modification of 5-methyldeoxycytidine and deoxycytidine residues. Nucleic Acids Res 1980;8(20):4777–90.

[27] Frommer M, McDonald LE, Millar DS, Collis CM, Watt F, Grigg GW, et al. A genomic sequencing protocol that yields a positive display of 5-methylcytosine residues in individual DNA strands. Proc Natl Acad Sci U S A 1992;89(5):1827–31.

[28] Grunau C, Clark SJ, Rosenthal A. Bisulfite genomic sequencing: systematic investigation of critical experimental parameters. Nucleic Acids Res 2001;29(13) E65.

[29] Clark SJ, Harrison J, Paul CL, Frommer M. High sensitivity mapping of methylated cytosines. Nucleic Acids Res 1994;22(15):2990–7.

[30] Ziller MJ, Hansen KD, Meissner A, Aryee MJ. Coverage recommendations for methylation analysis by whole-genome bisulfite sequencing. Nat Methods 2015;12(3):230–2.

[31] Suzuki M, Liao W, Wos F, Johnston AD, DeGrazia J, Ishii J, et al. Whole-genome bisulfite sequencing with improved accuracy and cost. Genome Res 2018;28(9):1364–71.

[32] Meissner A, Gnirke A, Bell GW, Ramsahoye B, Lander ES, Jaenisch R. Reduced representation bisulfite sequencing for comparative high-resolution DNA methylation analysis. Nucleic Acids Res 2005;33(18):5868–77.

[33] Chatterjee A, Rodger EJ, Stockwell PA, Weeks RJ, Morison IM. Technical considerations for reduced representation bisulfite sequencing with multiplexed libraries. J Biomed Biotechnol 2012;2012:741542.

[34] Estecio MR, Yan PS, Ibrahim AE, Tellez CS, Shen L, Huang TH, et al. High-throughput methylation profiling by MCA coupled to CpG island microarray. Genome Res 2007;17(10):1529–36.

[35] Wilhelm-Benartzi CS, Koestler DC, Karagas MR, Flanagan JM, Christensen BC, Kelsey KT, et al. Review of processing and analysis methods for DNA methylation array data. Br J Cancer 2013;109(6):1394–402.

[36] Luger K, Mader AW, Richmond RK, Sargent DF, Richmond TJ. Crystal structure of the nucleosome core particle at 2.8 A resolution. Nature 1997;389(6648):251–60.

[37] Olins DE, Olins AL. Chromatin history: our view from the bridge. Nat Rev Mol Cell Biol 2003;4(10):809–14.

[38] Dann GP, Liszczak GP, Bagert JD, Müller MM, Nguyen UTT, Wojcik F, et al. ISWI chromatin remodellers sense nucleosome modifications to determine substrate preference. Nature 2017;548:607.

[39] Allis CD, Jenuwein T. The molecular hallmarks of epigenetic control. Nat Rev Genet 2016;17(8):487–500.

[40] Kouzarides T. Chromatin modifications and their function. Cell 2007;128(4):693–705.

[41] Bannister AJ, Kouzarides T. Regulation of chromatin by histone modifications. Cell Res 2011;21(3):381–95.

[42] Allfrey VG, Faulkner R, Mirsky AE. Acetylation and methylation of histones and their possible role in the regulation of RNA synthesis. Proc Natl Acad Sci U S A 1964;51(5):786–94.

[43] Verdin E, Ott M. 50 years of protein acetylation: from gene regulation to epigenetics, metabolism and beyond. Nat Rev Mol Cell Biol 2015;16(4):258–64.

[44] Kayne PS, Kim UJ, Han M, Mullen JR, Yoshizaki F, Grunstein M. Extremely conserved histone H4 N terminus is dispensable for growth but essential for repressing the silent mating loci in yeast. Cell. 1988;55 (1):27–39.
[45] Megee PC, Morgan BA, Mittman BA, Smith MM. Genetic analysis of histone H4: essential role of lysines subject to reversible acetylation. Science 1990;247 (4944):841.
[46] Klemm SL, Shipony Z, Greenleaf WJ. Chromatin accessibility and the regulatory epigenome. Nat Rev Genet 2019;20(4):207–20.
[47] Crawford GE, Davis S, Scacheri PC, Renaud G, Halawi MJ, Erdos MR, et al. DNase-chip: a high-resolution method to identify DNase I hypersensitive sites using tiled microarrays. Nat Methods 2006;3 (7):503–9.
[48] Rao S, Procko E, Shannon MF. Chromatin remodeling, measured by a novel real-time polymerase chain reaction assay, across the proximal promoter region of the IL-2 gene. J Immunol (Baltimore, MD: 1950) 2001;167 (8):4494–503.
[49] Sabo PJ, Kuehn MS, Thurman R, Johnson BE, Johnson EM, Cao H, et al. Genome-scale mapping of DNase I sensitivity in vivo using tiling DNA microarrays. Nat Methods 2006;3(7):511–18.
[50] Boyle AP, Davis S, Shulha HP, Meltzer P, Margulies EH, Weng Z, et al. High-resolution mapping and characterization of open chromatin across the genome. Cell 2008;132(2):311–22.
[51] Mueller B, Mieczkowski J, Kundu S, Wang P, Sadreyev R, Tolstorukov MY, et al. Widespread changes in nucleosome accessibility without changes in nucleosome occupancy during a rapid transcriptional induction. Genes Dev 2017;31(5):451–62.
[52] Mieczkowski J, Cook A, Bowman SK, Mueller B, Alver BH, Kundu S, et al. MNase titration reveals differences between nucleosome occupancy and chromatin accessibility. Nat Commun 2016;7:11485.
[53] O'Geen H, Echipare L, Farnham PJ. Using ChIP-seq technology to generate high-resolution profiles of histone modifications. Methods Mol Biol (Clifton, NJ) 2011;791:265–86.
[54] Ho JW, Bishop E, Karchenko PV, Negre N, White KP, Park PJ. ChIP-chip versus ChIP-seq: lessons for experimental design and data analysis. BMC Genomics 2011;12:134.
[55] Corces MR, Trevino AE, Hamilton EG, Greenside PG, Sinnott-Armstrong NA, Vesuna S, et al. An improved ATAC-seq protocol reduces background and enables interrogation of frozen tissues. Nat Methods 2017;14:959.
[56] Buenrostro JD, Giresi PG, Zaba LC, Chang HY, Greenleaf WJ. Transposition of native chromatin for fast and sensitive epigenomic profiling of open chromatin, DNA-binding proteins and nucleosome position. Nat Methods 2013;10:1213.
[57] Lay FD, Kelly TK, Jones PA. Nucleosome Occupancy and Methylome Sequencing (NOMe-seq). Methods Mol Biol (Clifton, NJ) 2018;1708:267–84.
[58] Krebs AR, Imanci D, Hoerner L, Gaidatzis D, Burger L, Schübeler D. Genome-wide single-molecule footprinting reveals high RNA polymerase II turnover at paused promoters. Mol Cell 2017;67(3):411–422e.4.
[59] The EPC, Dunham I, Kundaje A, Aldred SF, Collins PJ, Davis CA, et al. An integrated encyclopedia of DNA elements in the human genome. Nature 2012;489:57.
[60] Peschansky VJ, Wahlestedt C. Non-coding RNAs as direct and indirect modulators of epigenetic regulation. Epigenetics 2014;9(1):3–12.
[61] Frias-Lasserre D, Villagra CA. The importance of ncRNAs as epigenetic mechanisms in phenotypic variation and organic evolution. Front Microbiol 2017;8:2483.
[62] Brown CJ, Hendrich BD, Rupert JL, Lafreniere RG, Xing Y, Lawrence J, et al. The human XIST gene: analysis of a 17 kb inactive X-specific RNA that contains conserved repeats and is highly localized within the nucleus. Cell 1992;71(3):527–42.
[63] Lee JT, Davidow LS, Warshawsky D. Tsix, a gene antisense to Xist at the X-inactivation centre. Nat Genet 1999;21(4):400–4.
[64] Mak W, Baxter J, Silva J, Newall AE, Otte AP, Brockdorff N. Mitotically stable association of polycomb group proteins eed and enx1 with the inactive x chromosome in trophoblast stem cells. Curr Biology (CB) 2002;12(12):1016–20.
[65] Bartel DP. MicroRNAs: target recognition and regulatory functions. Cell 2009;136(2):215–33.
[66] Fabian MR, Sonenberg N. The mechanics of miRNA-mediated gene silencing: a look under the hood of miRISC. Nat Struct Mol Biol 2012;19(6):586–93.
[67] Wellner U, Schubert J, Burk UC, Schmalhofer O, Zhu F, Sonntag A, et al. The EMT-activator ZEB1 promotes tumorigenicity by repressing stemness-inhibiting microRNAs. Nat Cell Biol 2009;11(12):1487–95.
[68] Sander S, Bullinger L, Klapproth K, Fiedler K, Kestler HA, Barth TF, et al. MYC stimulates EZH2 expression by repression of its negative regulator miR-26a. Blood 2008;112(10):4202–12.
[69] Kanhere A, Viiri K, Araujo CC, Rasaiyaah J, Bouwman RD, Whyte WA, et al. Short RNAs are transcribed from repressed polycomb target genes and interact with polycomb repressive complex-2. Mol Cell 2010;38 (5):675–88.

[70] Sen P, Shah PP, Nativio R, Berger SL. Epigenetic mechanisms of longevity and aging. Cell 2016;166 (4):822–39.
[71] Kennedy BK, Berger SL, Brunet A, Campisi J, Cuervo AM, Epel ES, et al. Geroscience: linking aging to chronic disease. Cell 2014;159(4):709–13.
[72] Brunet A, Berger SL. Epigenetics of aging and aging-related disease. J Gerontol Ser A Biol Sci Med Sci 2014;69(Suppl. 1):S17–20.
[73] Fraga MF, Ballestar E, Paz MF, Ropero S, Setien F, Ballestar ML, et al. Epigenetic differences arise during the lifetime of monozygotic twins. Proc Natl Acad Sci U S A 2005;102(30):10604–9.
[74] Ivanov A, Pawlikowski J, Manoharan I, van Tuyn J, Nelson DM, Rai TS, et al. Lysosome-mediated processing of chromatin in senescence. J Cell Biol 2013;202 (1):129–43.
[75] O'Sullivan RJ, Kubicek S, Schreiber SL, Karlseder J. Reduced histone biosynthesis and chromatin changes arising from a damage signal at telomeres. Nat Struct Mol Biol 2010;17(10):1218–25.
[76] Villeponteau B. The heterochromatin loss model of aging. Exp Gerontol 1997;32(4-5):383–94.
[77] Hu Z, Chen K, Xia Z, Chavez M, Pal S, Seol JH, et al. Nucleosome loss leads to global transcriptional up-regulation and genomic instability during yeast aging. Genes Dev 2014;28(4):396–408.
[78] Callinan PA, Batzer MA. Retrotransposable elements and human disease. Genome Dyn 2006;1:104–15.
[79] Wood JG, Helfand SL. Chromatin structure and transposable elements in organismal aging. Front Genet 2013;4:274.
[80] Sedivy JM, Kreiling JA, Neretti N, De Cecco M, Criscione SW, Hofmann JW, et al. Death by transposition—the enemy within? BioEssays 2013;35 (12):1035–43.
[81] van Deursen JM. The role of senescent cells in ageing. Nature 2014;509:439.
[82] Chandra T, Kirschner K, Thuret J-Y, Pope Benjamin D, Ryba T, Newman S, et al. Independence of repressive histone marks and chromatin compaction during senescent heterochromatic layer formation. Mol Cell 2012;47(2):203–14.
[83] Munoz-Espin D, Canamero M, Maraver A, Gomez-Lopez G, Contreras J, Murillo-Cuesta S, et al. Programmed cell senescence during mammalian embryonic development. Cell 2013;155(5):1104–18.
[84] Storer M, Mas A, Robert-Moreno A, Pecoraro M, Ortells MC, Di Giacomo V, et al. Senescence is a developmental mechanism that contributes to embryonic growth and patterning. Cell 2013;155(5):1119–30.
[85] Greer EL, Maures TJ, Hauswirth AG, Green EM, Leeman DS, Maro GS, et al. Members of the H3K4 trimethylation complex regulate lifespan in a germline-dependent manner in *C. elegans*. Nature 2010;466:383.
[86] Shah PP, Donahue G, Otte GL, Capell BC, Nelson DM, Cao K, et al. Lamin B1 depletion in senescent cells triggers large-scale changes in gene expression and the chromatin landscape. Genes Dev 2013;27 (16):1787–99.
[87] Eisenberg T, Knauer H, Schauer A, Büttner S, Ruckenstuhl C, Carmona-Gutierrez D, et al. Induction of autophagy by spermidine promotes longevity. Nat Cell Biol 2009;11:1305.
[88] Narita M, Nunez S, Heard E, Narita M, Lin AW, Hearn SA, et al. Rb-mediated heterochromatin formation and silencing of E2F target genes during cellular senescence. Cell. 2003;113(6):703–16.
[89] Sedivy JM, Banumathy G, Adams PD. Aging by epigenetics—a consequence of chromatin damage? Exp Cell Res 2008;314(9):1909–17.
[90] Bjornsson HT, Sigurdsson MI, Fallin MD, Irizarry RA, Aspelund T, Cui H, et al. Intra-individual change over time in DNA methylation with familial clustering. JAMA 2008;299(24):2877–83.
[91] Bollati V, Schwartz J, Wright R, Litonjua A, Tarantini L, Suh H, et al. Decline in genomic DNA methylation through aging in a cohort of elderly subjects. Mech Ageing Dev 2009;130(4):234–9.
[92] Bormann F, Rodriguez-Paredes M, Hagemann S, Manchanda H, Kristof B, Gutekunst J, et al. Reduced DNA methylation patterning and transcriptional connectivity define human skin aging. Aging Cell 2016;15 (3):563–71.
[93] Liu L, van Groen T, Kadish I, Li Y, Wang D, James SR, et al. Insufficient DNA methylation affects healthy aging and promotes age-related health problems. Clin Epigenetics 2011;2(2):349–60.
[94] Jung M, Pfeifer GP. Aging and DNA methylation. BMC Biol 2015;13:7.
[95] Christensen BC, Houseman EA, Marsit CJ, Zheng S, Wrensch MR, Wiemels JL, et al. Aging and environmental exposures alter tissue-specific DNA methylation dependent upon CpG island context. PLoS Genet 2009;5(8):e1000602.
[96] Horvath S. DNA methylation age of human tissues and cell types. Genome Biol 2013;14(10):R115.
[97] Hannum G, Guinney J, Zhao L, Zhang L, Hughes G, Sadda S, et al. Genome-wide methylation profiles reveal quantitative views of human aging rates. Mol Cell 2013;49(2):359–67.
[98] Field AE, Robertson NA, Wang T, Havas A, Ideker T, Adams PD. DNA methylation clocks in aging: categories, causes, and consequences. Mol Cell 2018;71 (6):882–95.

[99] Horvath S, Pirazzini C, Bacalini MG, Gentilini D, Di Blasio AM, Delledonne M, et al. Decreased epigenetic age of PBMCs from Italian semi-supercentenarians and their offspring. Aging 2015;7(12):1159–70.
[100] Levine ME, Lu AT, Quach A, Chen BH, Assimes TL, Bandinelli S, et al. An epigenetic biomarker of aging for lifespan and healthspan. Aging 2018;10 (4):573–91.
[101] Chen BH, Marioni RE, Colicino E, Peters MJ, Ward-Caviness CK, Tsai PC, et al. DNA methylation-based measures of biological age: meta-analysis predicting time to death. Aging 2016;8(9):1844–65.
[102] Horvath S, Raj K. DNA methylation-based biomarkers and the epigenetic clock theory of ageing. Nat Rev Genet 2018;19(6):371–84.
[103] Westendorp RGJ, Kirkwood TBL. Human longevity at the cost of reproductive success. Nature 1998;396 (6713):743–6.
[104] Seli E. Ovarian aging. Sem Reprod Med 2015;33 (6):375–6.
[105] Grondahl ML, Yding Andersen C, Bogstad J, Nielsen FC, Meinertz H, Borup R. Gene expression profiles of single human mature oocytes in relation to age. Hum Reprod 2010;25(4):957–68.
[106] Hamatani T, Falco G, Carter MG, Akutsu H, Stagg CA, Sharov AA, et al. Age-associated alteration of gene expression patterns in mouse oocytes. Hum Mol Genet 2004;13(19):2263–78.
[107] Manosalva I, Gonzalez A. Aging changes the chromatin configuration and histone methylation of mouse oocytes at germinal vesicle stage. Theriogenology 2010;74(9):1539–47.
[108] van den Berg IM, Eleveld C, van der Hoeven M, Birnie E, Steegers EA, Galjaard RJ, et al. Defective deacetylation of histone 4 K12 in human oocytes is associated with advanced maternal age and chromosome misalignment. Hum Reprod 2011;26 (5):1181–90.
[109] Morin SJ, Tao X, Marin D, Zhan Y, Landis J, Bedard J, et al. DNA methylation-based age prediction and telomere length in white blood cells and cumulus cells of infertile women with normal or poor response to ovarian stimulation. Aging 2018;10 (12):3761–73.
[110] Jenkins TG, Aston KI, Carrell DT. Sperm epigenetics and aging. Transl Androl Urol 2018;7(Suppl. 3): S328–35.
[111] Oakes CC, Smiraglia DJ, Plass C, Trasler JM, Robaire B. Aging results in hypermethylation of ribosomal DNA in sperm and liver of male rats. Proc Natl Acad Sci U S A 2003;100(4):1775–80.
[112] Jenkins TG, Aston KI, Pflueger C, Cairns BR, Carrell DT. Age-associated sperm DNA methylation alterations: possible implications in offspring disease susceptibility. PLoS Genet 2014;10(7):e1004458.
[113] Milekic MH, Xin Y, O'Donnell A, Kumar KK, Bradley-Moore M, Malaspina D, et al. Age-related sperm DNA methylation changes are transmitted to offspring and associated with abnormal behavior and dysregulated gene expression. Mol Psychiatry 2015;20(8):995–1001.
[114] Jenkins TG, Aston KI, Cairns B, Smith A, Carrell DT. Paternal germ line aging: DNA methylation age prediction from human sperm. BMC Genomics 2018;19 (1):763.
[115] Surani MAH, Barton SC, Norris ML. Development of reconstituted mouse eggs suggests imprinting of the genome during gametogenesis. Nature 1984;308 (5959):548–50.
[116] McGrath J, Solter D. Completion of mouse embryogenesis requires both the maternal and paternal genomes. Cell 1984;37(1):179–83.
[117] Devriendt K. Hydatidiform mole and triploidy: the role of genomic imprinting in placental development. Hum Reprod Update 2005;11(2):137–42.
[118] Barlow DP, Bartolomei MS. Genomic imprinting in mammals. Cold Spring Harb Perspect Biol 2014;6(2).
[119] Baran Y, Subramaniam M, Biton A, Tukiainen T, Tsang EK, Rivas MA, et al. The landscape of genomic imprinting across diverse adult human tissues. Genome Res 2015;25(7):927–36.
[120] Court F, Tayama C, Romanelli V, Martin-Trujillo A, Iglesias-Platas I, Okamura K, et al. Genome-wide parent-of-origin DNA methylation analysis reveals the intricacies of human imprinting and suggests a germline methylation-independent mechanism of establishment. Genome Res 2014;24(4):554–69.
[121] Renfree MB, Ager EI, Shaw G, Pask AJ. Genomic imprinting in marsupial placentation. Reproduction 2008;136(5):523–31.
[122] Gkountela S, Zhang KX, Shafiq TA, Liao WW, Hargan-Calvopina J, Chen PY, et al. DNA demethylation dynamics in the human prenatal germline. Cell 2015;161(6):1425–36.
[123] Guo F, Yan L, Guo H, Li L, Hu B, Zhao Y, et al. The transcriptome and DNA methylome landscapes of human primordial germ cells. Cell 2015;161(6):1437–52.
[124] Seisenberger S, Andrews S, Krueger F, Arand J, Walter J, Santos F, et al. The dynamics of genome-wide DNA methylation reprogramming in mouse primordial germ cells. Mol Cell 2012;48(6):849–62.
[125] Yamazaki Y, Mann MR, Lee SS, Marh J, McCarrey JR, Yanagimachi R, et al. Reprogramming of primordial germ cells begins before migration into the genital ridge, making these cells inadequate donors for reproductive cloning. Proc Natl Acad Sci U S A 2003;100(21):12207–12.

[126] Gahurova L, Tomizawa S-I, Smallwood SA, Stewart-Morgan KR, Saadeh H, Kim J, et al. Transcription and chromatin determinants of de novo DNA methylation timing in oocytes. Epigenetics Chromatin 2017;10:25.
[127] Shen L, Inoue A, He J, Liu Y, Lu F, Zhang Y. Tet3 and DNA replication mediate demethylation of both the maternal and paternal genomes in mouse zygotes. Cell Stem Cell 2014;15(4):459–71.
[128] Smith ZD, Chan MM, Mikkelsen TS, Gu H, Gnirke A, Regev A, et al. A unique regulatory phase of DNA methylation in the early mammalian embryo. Nature 2012;484:339.
[129] Smith ZD, Chan MM, Humm KC, Karnik R, Mekhoubad S, Regev A, et al. DNA methylation dynamics of the human preimplantation embryo. Nature 2014;511:611.
[130] Guo H, Zhu P, Yan L, Li R, Hu B, Lian Y, et al. The DNA methylation landscape of human early embryos. Nature 2014;511(7511):606–10.
[131] Monk D, Mackay DJG, Eggermann T, Maher ER, Riccio A. Genomic imprinting disorders: lessons on how genome, epigenome and environment interact. Nat Rev Genet 2019;20(4):235–48.
[132] Holliday R. The inheritance of epigenetic defects. Science 1987;238(4824):163.
[133] Oey H, Whitelaw E. On the meaning of the word 'epimutation'. Trends Genet (TIG) 2014;30(12):519–20.
[134] Buiting K, Gross S, Lich C, Gillessen-Kaesbach G, el-Maarri O, Horsthemke B. Epimutations in Prader-Willi and Angelman syndromes: a molecular study of 136 patients with an imprinting defect. Am J Hum Genet 2003;72(3):571–7.
[135] Court F, Martin-Trujillo A, Romanelli V, Garin I, Iglesias-Platas I, Salafsky I, et al. Genome-wide allelic methylation analysis reveals disease-specific susceptibility to multiple methylation defects in imprinting syndromes. Hum Mutat 2013;34(4):595–602.
[136] Zegers-Hochschild F, Adamson GD, Dyer S, Racowsky C, de Mouzon J, Sokol R, et al. The International Glossary on Infertility and Fertility Care, 2017. Fertil Steril 2017;108(3):393–406.
[137] el Hajj N, Haaf T. Epigenetic disturbances in in vitro cultured gametes and embryos: implications for human assisted reproduction. Fertil Steril 2013;99(3):632–41.
[138] Niemitz EL, Feinberg AP. Epigenetics and assisted reproductive technology: a call for investigation. Am J Hum Genet 2004;74(4):599–609.
[139] Kohda T. Effects of embryonic manipulation and epigenetics. J Hum Genet 2013;58:416.
[140] Santos F, Hyslop L, Stojkovic P, Leary C, Murdoch A, Reik W, et al. Evaluation of epigenetic marks in human embryos derived from IVF and ICSI. Hum Reprod 2010;25(9):2387–95.
[141] Maher ER. Imprinting and assisted reproductive technology. Hum Mol Genet 2005;14(Spec. No. 1):R133–8.
[142] Shufaro Y, Laufer N. Epigenetic concerns in assisted reproduction: update and critical review of the current literature. Fertil Steril 2013;99(3):605–6.
[143] Rinaudo P, Schultz RM. Effects of embryo culture on global pattern of gene expression in preimplantation mouse embryos. Reproduction 2004;128(3):301–11.
[144] Mann MR, Lee SS, Doherty AS, Verona RI, Nolen LD, Schultz RM, et al. Selective loss of imprinting in the placenta following preimplantation development in culture. Development 2004;131(15):3727–35.
[145] Doherty AS, Mann MR, Tremblay KD, Bartolomei MS, Schultz RM. Differential effects of culture on imprinted H19 expression in the preimplantation mouse embryo. Biol Reprod 2000;62(6):1526–35.
[146] Chen SL, Shi XY, Zheng HY, Wu FR, Luo C. Aberrant DNA methylation of imprinted H19 gene in human preimplantation embryos. Fertil Steril 2010;94(6):2356–8 8.e1.
[147] Marin D, Seli E. In vitro fertilization and infertility do not cause a significant alteration in placental gene expression at the end of the first trimester. Fertil Steril 2019;111(3):463–4.
[148] Doornbos ME, Maas SM, McDonnell J, Vermeiden JP, Hennekam RC. Infertility, assisted reproduction technologies and imprinting disturbances: a Dutch study. Hum Reprod 2007;22(9):2476–80.
[149] Marin D, Scott Jr. RT. Extracellular vesicles: a promising tool for assessment of embryonic competence. Curr Opin Obstet Gynecol 2018;30(3):171–8.
[150] Tao X, Zhan Y, Scott KL, Scott R, Seli E. DNA methylation is associated with ploidy status and patient age in human embryos. Fertil Steril 2018;110(4, Suppl.):e80.

Further reading

Capalbo A, Treff N, Cimadomo D, Tao X, Ferrero S, Vaiarelli A, et al. Abnormally fertilized oocytes can result in healthy live births: improved genetic technologies for preimplantation genetic testing can be used to rescue viable embryos in in vitro fertilization cycles. Fertil Steril 2017;108(6):1007–1015.e3.
Grau N, Escrich L, Martin J, Rubio C, Pellicer A, Escriba MJ. Self-correction in tripronucleated human embryos. Fertil Steril 2011;96(4):951–6.

Grau N, Escrich L, Galiana Y, Meseguer M, Garcia-Herrero S, Remohi J, et al. Morphokinetics as a predictor of self-correction to diploidy in tripronucleated intracytoplasmic sperm injection-derived human embryos. Fertil Steril 2015;104(3):728–35.

Marin D, Scott Jr. RT, Treff NR. Preimplantation embryonic mosaicism: origin, consequences and the reliability of comprehensive chromosome screening. Curr Opin Obstet Gynecol 2017;29(3):168–74.

Marin D, Zimmerman R, Tao X, Zhan Y, Scott Jr. RT, Treff NR. Validation of a targeted next generation sequencing-based comprehensive chromosome screening platform for detection of triploidy in human blastocysts. Reprod Biomed Online 2018;36(4):388–95.

PART B

Clinical scenarios

CHAPTER

6

The quest for genetic sequence variants conferring risk of endometriosis

Sun-Wei Guo[1,2]

[1]Shanghai Obstetrics and Gynecology Hospital, Fudan University, Shanghai, P.R. China
[2]Shanghai Key Laboratory of Female Reproductive Endocrine-Related Diseases, Fudan University, Shanghai, P.R. China

Introduction

Endometriosis, characterized by the presence and growth of functional endometrial-like tissues outside the uterine cavity, is an estrogen-dependent disorder affecting 6%–10% of reproductive-age women [1]. As a major contributor to pelvic pain and subfertility, endometriosis impacts negatively on women's quality of life, work productivity, sexual relationships, and self-esteem, mainly because of chronic, debilitating pain and infertility [2–6]. Despite extensive research, its pathogenesis still remains an enigma [7].

Given this state, one simple, brute-force approach, that is, the genetic approach, is very appealing. One does not need to know anything about the molecular genetic mechanisms underlying endometriosis, but through the collection of pedigrees enriched with patients having the disease or large samples of unrelated patients and healthy women, one could use existing genetic signposts [called DNA markers, which are aplenty and scattered throughout the entire human genome with known locations, thanks to the Human Genome Project (HGP)] and localize the responsible gene in a particular chromosomal region(s). Once the gene(s) is(are) identified, one can hope to better understand the pathogenesis of endometriosis, dissect the phenotypic heterogeneity, and make a risk prediction [8]. This is of particular appeal since the entire genome sequence data of a person can be stored on a DVD disc or a flash drive, and, once all susceptibility genes are identified and their risks are quantified, her risk of developing endometriosis could be predicted once she is born.

There were indeed successful stories with the genetic approach. Huntington's disease, for example, was once viewed as a difficult disease with unknown pathogenesis. Using the genetic approach, the gene for Huntington's disease was identified and ultimately cloned [9]. Even for breast cancer, a fairly common cancer, one susceptibility gene was localized on chromosome 17 in 1990 [10] and later cloned [11].

Human Reproductive Genetics
DOI: https://doi.org/10.1016/B978-0-12-816561-4.00006-5

These successes generated enormous enthusiasm in the use of the same genetic approach, with the hope that for many complex diseases such as diabetes, cardiovascular diseases, and endometriosis that invariably have an elusive pathogenesis and collectively contribute to the major health burdens, their pathogenesis could be unveiled by hunting down their susceptibility genes [12]. The simplicity of the study design, called a genetic association study (GAS), is also attractive: simply by comparison of the allelic frequency between women with endometriosis and those without, one can detect genes that confer risk of endometriosis.

This enthusiasm was bolstered even further with the completion of the HGP, which now allows to read the entire DNA sequence of a human genome, touted by many as the "Book of Life." With the advent of high-throughput genotyping technologies, typing of DNA markers, especially the biallelic single-nucleotide polymorphisms (SNPs), has become cheaper and faster, making the scanning of the entire genome more feasible and easier. Such an approach, called a genome-wide GAS or genome-wide association study (GWAS), has gained enormous momentum since the HGP was officially completed in 2003 (Fig. 6.1).

In endometriosis, a deluge of GAS, including GWAS, papers attempting to find DNA variants that might be statistically associated with endometriosis have been published in the last two decades, reflecting the general interest in the use of a GAS/GWAS approach to finding genes for complex diseases (Fig. 6.1). However, despite an impressive list of publications and enormous effort, the quest for genetic variants, either germline mutations or

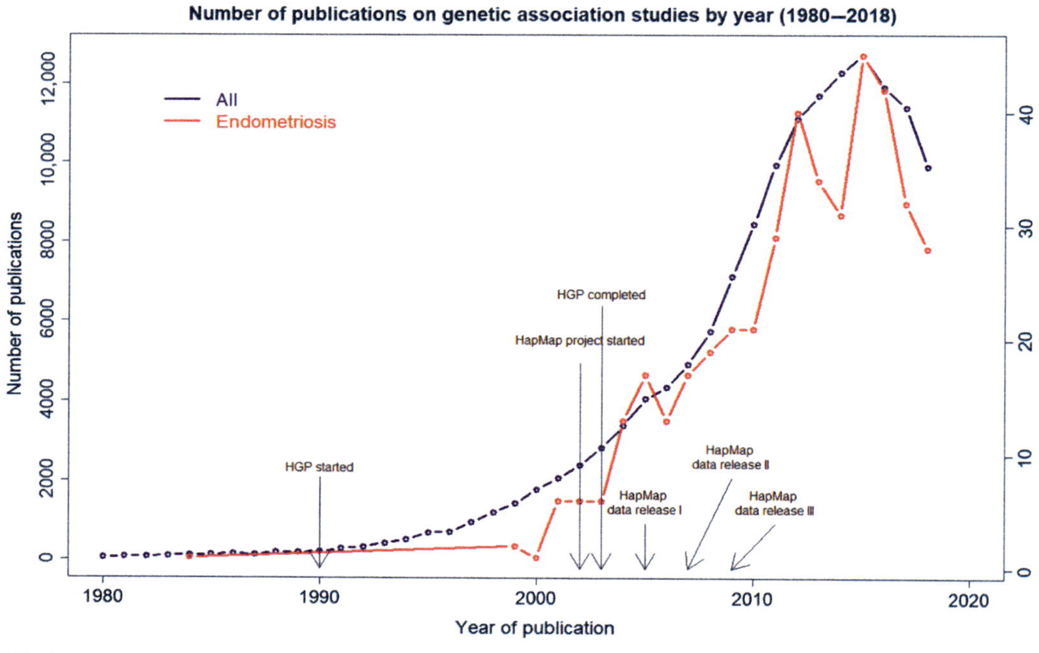

FIGURE 6.1 Number of publications, indexed by PubMed, on genetic association studies (GASs) in general and on endometriosis from 1980 to 2018. The *blue* and *red curves* represent the GASs in general and on endometriosis, respectively. The *y*-axis on the left is for GAS-general, while the *y*-axis on the right is for endometriosis-specific GASs. The occurrences of several important events, such as the start of the Human Genome Project (HGP), are indicated.

polymorphisms, associated with endometriosis has so far borne little, if any, fruit. Frequently, when such associations have been found, the identified polymorphisms appear to be of little predictive value and contribute little to our understanding of the pathogenesis or pathophysiology of the disease. At best, the identified polymorphisms frequently provide tantalizing association with some genes with known functions that may or may not be directly involved in the pathogenesis of endometriosis.

In a recent review on the current status of GWASs on endometriosis, it is reported that the "GWAS SNPs associated with endometriosis to date explain less than 2% of disease risk variability" [8]. The most recent meta-analysis of 15 GWASs and a replication analysis, including 58,115 cases and 733,480 controls, found 27 loci, which collectively explained a paltry 2.2% of the disease risk variability [13]. These findings are in sharp contrast to the estimate that half of the widely quoted estimated 50% heritability (meaning, genetic components contribute to about 50% of endometriosis risk) is due to the common variants that can be captured by GWASs [14]. Some previous meta-analyses on the association of endometriosis and several genetic polymorphisms coding for dioxin detoxification enzymes and for sex steroid biosynthesis and their receptors found no evidence of any association [15–17].

Remarkably, endometriosis is not the only complex disease that has encountered such a problem. A 2012 study, for example, found that incorporating genetic information did not improve clinicians' ability to predict disease risk for many common complex diseases such as breast cancer, type II diabetes, and rheumatoid arthritis [18]. More recently, an analysis of 32 highly relevant traits from five broad disease areas involving 13,436 subjects found that the variance explained by multi-SNP genetic risk scores (GRSs) accounted for a mere 11% of the common-SNP heritability of the 32 traits, indicating that GRSs may not yet be ready for accurate personalized prediction of complex disease traits, and, as such, limiting widespread adoption in clinical practice [19].

As with many other complex diseases or traits, there has been a glaring gap between the estimated heritability of the trait (typically higher than 50%) and the trait (or disease risk) variability that can be explained by the identified SNPs, a phenomenon called "the missing heritability" [20]. Take, for example, height, which is estimated to have a heritability of over 80%, but one GWAS involving 253,288 individuals identified nearly 700 variants that altogether explained merely one-fifth of the heritability for adult height, suggesting that the genetic architecture for human height is characterized by a very large but finite number (thousands) of causal DNA variants [21]. While some investigators claim that the heritability is not missing but "hidden" [22], other researchers find that the resultant heritability estimates are sensitive to the chosen sample and to measurement errors in the phenotype [23].

Advocates of genetic investigations are not deterred by this complexity and think that ever larger sample sizes will solve the problem. With a minimal sample size of 10,000 cases [24], GWASs typically carry a huge price tag. For endometriosis, should we keep on investing in this endeavor? Or should we be more prudent and pause, take stock, reassess what we have, and think hard about what could be done better?

In this chapter, I first provide a primer on genetic studies of complex diseases such as endometriosis, explaining the methods for demonstration of genetic components for a disease, and methods to identify the genes or genetic variants. At the same time, I shall reappraise the evidence for a hereditary component to endometriosis, evaluate the evidence for association of genetic polymorphisms with endometriosis, and discuss the implications of this reappraisal for clinical practice and research. Finally I shall provide explanations as to why the "missing heritability" problem also exists in endometriosis.

A primer on genetic studies of complex diseases and a review of endometriosis genetics

The proof for the existence of a genetic component

In order to identify the genetic variants that predispose people to a disease such as endometriosis, the first step is to demonstrate, with reasonable confidence, that the disease has a genetic component, otherwise any quest for the genetic component is akin to a quixotic endeavor. It is common sense that the first clue that a trait or disease has a genetic component is that it "runs in families." In more technical terms, this is called familial aggregation. However, aside from genes, other, nongenetic factors (beliefs, values, traditions, diet, and lifestyle, etc.) could also be transmitted vertically from parents to offspring just like genetic materials, and many risk factors also "run in families." Remarkably, many diseases are the result of both nature (genes) and nurture (environment and/or meme). Precisely because of this entanglement of nature and nurture, many genetic epidemiological methods, as elaborated below, have been developed to disentangle nature from nurture, but only to a certain extent. In practice, several complementary methods need to be employed collectively in order to show, with certain confidence, that a disease is very likely to have a genetic component.

For many complex traits or complex diseases where no single predisposing gene has ever been unequivocally identified and few risk factors have been consistently reported, we often see studies reporting that for disease X the heritability (meaning, the proportion of the disease risk variability that can attributable to genetic components) is 50% or even 90%. How did they do that?

Well, there is no free lunch. In order to do the calculation, one has to resort, first, to mathematical modeling and make certain assumptions. Quite often, the underlying model for estimating heritability is the so-called "ACE" model, where "A" refers to the *a*dditive genetic contribution to a person's phenotype, "C" is the contribution from environment *c*ommon to or shared by people reared together, and "E" represents *e*nvironmental contributions unique to each person. The phenotype of a person (e.g., the liability to have endometriosis) is $P = A + C + E$, and the data consist of values of P for people either genetically related or otherwise. For example, from parent–offspring and sib–sib correlations (and sometimes correlations between other relatives), the correlation coefficients, representing the "causes" of P, can be estimated under this framework.

In fact, the basis for the entire mathematical set-up was developed in the 1930s, 1940s, and 1950s, framed in the context of Mendelian transmission facilitated by Sir Ronald A. Fisher's view of the way discretely inherited genes [called polygenes, because of their (infinitely) large numbers] determine continuously quantitative phenotypes [25]. The statistical models that are used to estimate and interpret genetic contributions to various phenotypes—including behavioral, cognitive traits—are constructed within this framework. For diseases that are often dichotomous in nature (affected or not), they can be modeled through a quantity called liability that is an unobservable abstract construct/quantity and the probability-based disease risk can be modeled. Variance analysis constitutes the main tool and is used under this framework to characterize genetic inheritance, and hence determination of phenotypes.

Based on the ACE model, the variability of a trait in a population can be calculated by the overall phenotypic variance σ_P^2, which is assumed to be the sum of variability attributable to genetic differences among individuals (additive genetic variance σ_A^2, if no such restriction is imposed, then σ_G^2), the difference in shared environment σ_C^2, and differences in the environment surrounding the individuals (environmental variance σ_E^2), $\sigma_P^2 = \sigma_A^2 + \sigma_C^2 + \sigma_E^2$. Note that this equation entails two very important assumptions, which are (1) there is no epistasis or gene–gene interaction (GXG); and (2) there is no gene–environment interaction (GXE). In controlled experiments, the GXE can be held to be nonexistent, but for human populations this is an assumption that is often difficult to verify at best and frequently violated. In addition, for mathematical convenience the total phenotypic variance is assumed to be the sum of individual variances, even though there is no law that dictates that this should be the case. This is mainly for the purpose of mathematical tractability, otherwise the mathematics would become intractably complex and so preclude any calculation.

It should be noted that there is no reason to believe that the genetic effect has always to be additive and there is no GXG or GXE. Mathematically, the additive form is the most convenient method for mathematical calculation. In reality, genes and environment can interact in a very complex way. Even for simple genetic disorders such as glucose-6-phosphate dehydrogenase deficiency, a diet devoid of fava beans could effectively prevent the disease. Moreover, their actions, individually or interactively, may well be time- or age-dependent. However, once any of these enters into the equation, the mathematics quickly becomes intractable, yielding no theoretical insight at all. The vindication and triumph of Barker's hypothesis, that an adverse environment in the womb and/or during infancy is causally linked to chronic disease risk later in life, is a testimony that the effect of genes and/or environment can be crucially time-dependent.

Given a phenotypic data set comprising individuals with different genetic relatedness [parent–offspring, spousal, siblings, first-cousins, etc., which can be characterized by the probability of gene identity by descent (IBD) [26–28]], and different degrees of shared environment (twins, or nontwins, as long as the amount of shared environment can be specified before calculation), each of the three variance components can be identified and estimated.

The ratio $H^2 = \sigma_G^2/\sigma_P^2$ is called the broad-sense heritability, and shows the proportion of genetic variance in the total phenotypic variance. If the assumption that genes act in an additive manner, that is, no GXG is invoked, then the ratio is called the narrow-sense heritability, and is often denoted by $h^2 = \sigma_A^2/\sigma_P^2$. Almost all estimates of heritability in endometriosis use h^2 based on phenotype correlations among related individuals, in particular, monozygotic (MZ) and dizygotic (DZ) twins. The important assumptions underlying this model are, again, (1) no GXE, (2) no GXG, and (3) all genes act in an additive manner. When GXG exists but is ignored, h^2 often gives inflated heritability [29]. When GXE is present, the overall phenotypic variance becomes $\sigma_P^2 = \sigma_G^2 + \sigma_C^2 + \sigma_{GXC}^2 + \sigma_{GXE}^2 + \sigma_E^2$, and, in this case, neither narrow- nor broad-sense heritability can be clearly defined. In fact, unless *G*, *C*, and *E* can be measured and their interactions can be clearly specified, it is mathematically challenging to even estimate σ_{GXC}^2 or σ_{GXE}^2.

Note that h^2 says nothing about the genes whose sequence variability causes genetic variability of the trait. In addition, heritability has a meaning only in relation to populations, and different populations may have entirely different heritability [30]. For example, the estimated twin-based heritability on cigarette smoking in US adolescents and young adults differs between whites and African-Americans [31]. Moreover, it may change even within the same population at different periods of time. In essence, the heritability concept is built on the mathematical/statistical analytics called variance component analysis and attempts to attribute the genetic contribution to the proportion of variance that can be explained by genetic components in a vastly oversimplified model. As such, it has received much criticism, especially when applied to human population [32]. The most critical argument was that it is impossible to separate hereditary and environmental components in human populations, which are, indeed, intricately entwined and inseparable.

It should be noted that almost all human diseases or disorders have had been shown to have familial aggregation to varying degrees. Scurvy, kuru, and the sudden infant death syndrome (SIDS) were once well-documented to be familially aggregated and were thus suspected to have a genetic component, but were later discredited. Familial aggregation of disease does not necessarily and automatically mean the existence of a hereditary component. Various risk factors for the disease also tend to cluster in families, which can effectively mimic genetic transmission and thus familial aggregation [33]. Indeed, similar to transmission of genes in families, the transmission of memes, which are coded in culture, beliefs, and value systems and manifested in lifestyle and diet, could mimic genetic transmission [34]. In addition, since in many clinical studies it is often difficult to remove reporting and ascertainment biases, these biases often can inflate measures of familial aggregation even in the complete absence of a hereditary and environment/cultural component [35].

Furthermore, there may be traits that are intermediatory to the development of endometriosis. For example, younger age at menarche has been identified as a risk factor for endometriosis [36]. However, ages at menarche in sisters have been shown to be highly correlated [37]. Body mass index (BMI), length of menstrual cycles, and the amount of menses may be risk factors for endometriosis but may also be familially correlated [38]. If there are genetic determinants for some intermediatory factors, such as age at menarche, that are associated with endometriosis, it is possible that endometriosis may also run in families.

Familial aggregation

In genetic epidemiology, the demonstration of familial aggregation for a disease is often taken as the first piece of evidence that the disease has a genetic component. Essentially, by showing an enriched clustering of the disease within a given family, familial aggregation is established.

In practice, the concordance between parent–offspring pairs, sibling pairs, and first-cousin pairs is often estimated to see whether there is familial aggregation. Depending on the genetic relatedness, as determined by probability of gene IBD, the recurrence rate of a relative given that the other relative is affected would increase as the genetic relationship of the pair becomes genetically closer and/or would be much higher than the prevalence of the disease in the general population. For example, the sibling recurrence rate (SRR) is frequently used in genetic epidemiology to demonstrate familial aggregation of a given disease.

Conceptually simple as it may be, however, the actual estimation of SRR in a human population is susceptible to biases of various kinds. For example, a large sibship would be more likely to be ascertained by the investigator and would contain, on average, more affected sibs. It is well documented that SRR is sensitive to ascertainment bias and/or overreporting [35,39]. Inappropriate choice of controls may also result in an inflated SRR estimate [40].

It is common sense that familial aggregation may arise simply because of genetic similarity shared by family members, but also could be attributable to environmental similarities among relatives and to possible transgenerational epigenetic factors [41]. Many risk factors, such as diet and lifestyles, can also run in families. When there are multiple environmental risk factors, each carrying a low disease risk, then the disease can show conspicuous familial aggregation even though it has no genetic component at all [33].

Twin studies

Twin studies are conducted on MZ (identical) and DZ (fraternal) twins. They aim to reveal the importance of environmental and genetic influences for traits, phenotypes, and disorders—if done with care and caution. The major premises of twin studies are: (1) MZ twins share 100% of their genes, while DZ twins share only about 50% (on average) of their genes, and (2) MZ and DZ twins share 100% of their environment. Hence, any difference in disease status between MZ and DZ twins would be likely to be attributable to the difference in shared genes.

While twin studies have been used extensively in human behavioral studies to estimate the contributions of genetic factors to phenotypic variability, the methodology that allows the estimation entails several crucial assumptions. The most critical is that MZ and DZ twins are equally similar environmentally [42,43]. Although MZ twins are genetically more similar than DZ twins, they are often environmentally more similar. It has been shown that, even in the complete absence of any genetic factor and of any biases, the greater environmental similarity alone in MZ twins can result in a higher concordance rate in MZ twins than in DZ twins [44]. This is especially true when there are multiple environmental factors, which may have multiple exposure levels and/or interact strongly, although each of them may be of low risk [44].

In two twin studies that reported the heritability for endometriosis as being in the range of 47%–51% [45,46], which have been widely cited [8,47], both assumed that MZ and DZ twins are equally similar environmentally. In addition, additive genetic action was also assumed [45,46].

This review is not to discredit the published twin studies in endometriosis. Rather, by enumerating explicitly all assumptions and limitations of the statistical methodology, we can better understand what the heritability truly means and what its limitations are. All in all, we cannot rely uncritically on twin studies without checking the validity of the assumptions underlying the methodology.

Adoption studies

Adoption studies are used to estimate the degree to which variation in a trait is due to environmental and genetic influences. The comparison of phenotypic similarity between the adoptees and their biological and adoptive parents, or between the adoptees and their nonbiological siblings, can be a powerful tool to demonstrate how strong the shared genetic or environmental effects are. For example, the comparison between the concordance estimated from data on MZ twins reared apart because of adoption and that from data on MZ twins reared together could help to tease out how much contribution to the phenotypic variability is attributed to the shared environment effect. In endometriosis, unfortunately no adoption study has ever been reported as of the time of writing.

Segregation analysis

Segregation analysis is a statistical technique to determine whether there is evidence that a major gene underlies the distribution of a given trait or disease. In this analysis, only phenotypic information on pedigree members is needed. Given the allelic frequency, the penetrance, or the probability of being affected (or distribution for quantitative traits) given the genotype $P(\mathrm{D} \mid \mathrm{Genotype})$, the analysis—based on the Mendelian law of segregation—provides initial evidence, but not a definitive proof, that a single gene has a major effect on a particular phenotypic trait or disease. In some cases, the penetrance or the mode of inheritance—completely or partially recessive, dominant, or otherwise—can be estimated using the pedigree data. In other cases, segregation analysis can be combined with linkage analysis [48].

In endometriosis, the study that is closest to segregation analysis is that using kinship coefficients and a minimal founder test based on genealogical data [49]. While this study demonstrates familial aggregation of endometriosis, no effort was made to tease out genetic and nongenetic transmission through pedigrees or geneology .

Identification of genes and/or genetic variants: recombination, linkage disequilibrium, and association

The foundation for the identification of genes at chromosomal locations from phenotypic data was laid after the discovery of the phenomenon of genetic linkage in lowly fruit flies in the 1910s by Alfred Sturtevant, then a graduate student of Thomas Morgan, a prominent American geneticist who won the Nobel Prize in Physiology or Medicine in 1933. During meiosis in sexually reproduced organisms (humans included), the genome of each gamete is the result of genetic recombination, a programmed process in which the homologous chromosomes are paired, and DNA strands are cut into segments somewhat randomly and then repaired and rejoined to form new chromosomes. This process allows for the exchange of genetic material (and thus information) from paternal and maternal chromosomes, resulting in a more diverse genetic makeup on the genome.

On average, two genes (called loci) are less likely to break apart if they are physically closer during one round of recombination, hence the haplotype containing a specific combination of alleles at both loci is likely to be transmitted from generation to generation intact if the two loci are in close proximity. However, if the loci are physically distant, they are likely to break apart in just one recombination. If specific haplotypes are persistently present in a population, the two (or more) loci are said to be in linkage disequilibrium when the frequency of association of the different alleles at different loci is higher or lower than would be expected if the loci were independent and associated randomly.

This discovery of genetic linkage was later found to hold universally true in all organisms, including humans, and became a cornerstone and principle in genetics. Basically, if a trait is determined by a gene, then the gene will tend to go hand in hand with its neighboring signposts when transmitted from parents to offspring—thus the term "linkage." In genetics, these signposts are called DNA markers, which are DNA variants with known chromosomal locations, number of alleles, and allele frequencies in a given population. If many relatives in a pedigree having the same trait all carry the same signpost, then there is a good chance that the gene responsible for the trait is near to the signpost. In the human genome, the distance between two loci is measured in centimorgan (cM), and 1 cM means that the alleles on the two loci break apart on average once per 100 meiotic events.

In model organisms such as fruit flies, the identification of genes can be facilitated by various cross-breeding schemes and large samples. In addition, a genetic map, which has a sufficient number of DNA markers, would be needed. In humans, unfortunately, different cross-breedings cannot be made for obvious reasons. Therefore the mapping of disease genes in humans did not take off until the advent and spread of personal computers in the 1980s as many difficulties in calculation of gene segregation and linkage can be offset by statistical computations. In addition, the increased computational power coincided, fortuitously and fortunately, with the discovery of various classes of DNA markers, such as restriction fragment length polymorphisms [50] in the 1980s, variable number of tandem repeats, microsatellites, and short tandem repeats [51] in the 1990s, with increasing heterozygosity and thus informativeness. However, while these markers are very informative, their typing can be labor intensive and, as such, SNPs become more popular due to their abundance and ease of genotyping. The reduced informativeness of a single SNP can be offset by the use of several closely linked SNPs.

Linkage analysis

Linkage analysis is a statistical genetic method that aims to identify chromosomal regions that cosegregate with a disease of interest through pedigrees [52]. In this approach, one does not need to know anything about the molecular genetic mechanisms underlying the disease itself. Through the collection of pedigrees enriched with patients with the disease, one could use an existing genetic map and localize the responsible gene in a particular region. However, while this method is very successful in localizing genes responsible for rare genetic disorders such as cystic fibrosis and Huntington's disease in which (1) there is strong evidence for a major gene (unequivocal Mendelian inheritance), and (2) the mode of inheritance is well-elaborated, it was much less successful for more common diseases such as diabetes and cardiovascular diseases, in which multiple genes are apparently involved and the mode of inheritance is often obscure.

As endometriosis is quite common with no apparent mode of inheritance, the only published linkage analysis of endometriosis attempted to replicate the linkage between endometriosis and galactose-1-phosphate uridyl transferase (GALT) gene and ended with a negative result [53].

Affected sib-pair analysis

Most complex diseases—endometriosis included—have a substantial impact on the public health. Given the failure in linkage analysis of complex diseases, nonparametric methods such as the affected sib-pair method that require no information on the mode of inheritance methods became useful [54]. These methods, computationally simple and easy to apply, use smaller subsets of family members, usually relative pairs, so that sampling family members generally is easier than when extended pedigrees are sought, but often would demand a large number of sib pairs. In endometriosis, however, although the possibility of using the method has been mentioned [55], no such study has ever been published.

Association and genome-wide association studies

Given the failure in mapping complex diseases, scientists found during the mid-1990s that for common diseases, another approach, called "association studies," can be more powerful in gene hunting—at least on paper. Association studies identify disease genes by finding the significant gene frequency differentials between a group of unrelated healthy individuals and another group of unrelated people with the disease of interest. Association studies are thought to be more powerful than affected sib-pair methods for disease gene localization when linkage disequilibrium is present [12,56]—based on the understanding of the genetics of complex diseases at that time.

With the increasing ease of genotyping and the density of the SNP map, and decreasing cost in genotyping SNPs, GWASs become increasingly popular. GWASs essentially perform a genome-wide scanning of numerous SNPs or DNA variants across the entire genome, hoping to find the SNP or variant that is associated with the disease or trait.

However, misclassification of cases and/or controls, insufficient sample size, population stratification, and multiple testing can be problematic for GWASs [57], although some of these factors can be properly controlled if done with care. But GWAS has been plagued with nonreplication, inconsistency [58,59], and inflated initial estimates of the association [60]. And precisely because of its association nature, the identified polymorphism may or may not be the one that is directly responsible for the disease. It is possible that it may be the intermediate factor, such as age at menarche [61], that leads to the increased risk of the disease, a concern initially raised by Di and Guo [62] but later dismissed by Montgomery et al. [63]. Interestingly, however, the most recent GWAS identified SNP rs74485684, which is in close linkage with follicle-stimulating hormone B (FSHB) on chromosome 11 [13]. FSHB has been reported to affect circulating levels of follicle-stimulating hormone and be associated with a shorter menstrual cycle [64,65]. A shorter menstrual cycle has been documented to be a risk factor for endometriosis [66].

Layers of complexity

Multifactorial? Polygenic? Omnigenic?

Endometriosis is widely viewed as a multifactorial disease. It is also viewed frequently as a polygenic disease. From published GWASs, the presence of multiple loci that are associated with endometriosis seems to be certain [13,47,67–70]. In particular, many of the identified polymorphisms are in the intronic, noncoding regions of the genome [13,44], which is in sharp contrast to Mendelian diseases [71], but nonetheless consistent with the notion that complex diseases are driven mainly by noncoding DNA variants that presumably signal the involvement of gene regulation [72–74]. According to the latest study, the 27 identified loci are located on chromosomes 1, 2, 4–12, 14, 15, and 17 [13], spreading across almost the entire genome but not near any genes that are known to be endometriosis-specific, a feature shared by other complex traits [74]. The odds ratio for the identified 27 loci ranged from 1.05 to 1.18 [13], suggesting that each variant contributes a minute portion to the heritability—another conspicious feature of complex traits [74]. Given these features, the "omnigenic model of complex traits" stipulates that the trait/disease can be directly affected by a modest number of genes or gene pathways—called "core genes"—involved in either disease etiology or gene regulation [74]. However, all genes are interconnected, perhaps at different layers, by cell regulatory networks. The core genes may contribute just a small portion to the overall heritability, and most genes expressed in relevant cell types could contribute a small, but nonzero, portion to the heritability [74]. If we accept this model as the likely state for endometriosis, then any gene expressed in any disease-relevant tissues or cells would have a small, but nonzero, effect on regulation of the core genes, contributing, perhaps minutely, to disease risk [74]. In and of itself, the identification of the cell regulatory networks, however, would be a daunting task. If this omnigenic model holds for endometriosis, then making disease predictions would be very challenging.

Genetic architecture

The omnigenic model is just one proposal for complex traits. However, for genetic study of endometriosis, a real question that has been left unaddressed is what the genetic architecture underlying endometriosis is. For one thing, tissue-specific genetic modulation plays a critical role in many complex diseases such as endometriosis. And from our understanding of the pathophysiology of endometriotic lesions, we now know that many cell types, such as platelets [75,76], neutrophils [77], macrophages [78–80], natural killer cells [81,82], other immune cells [83,84], and even sensory nerve fibers [85,86] are involved in the development of endometriosis. It is very likely that the pathogenesis of endometriosis may also involve multiple cell types. So why should a DNA variant in general predispose women to endometriosis?

Remarkably, several groups have demonstrated that disease-associated SNPs are enriched in active chromatin and particularly in chromatin that is active in cell types that are relevant to the disease of interest [87–90], suggesting DNA variants that impact on tissues relevant to the disease are more likely to be the culprit. In addition, signals are clustered around genes that are expressed in relevant cell types [21,91]. All these findings seem to suggest that SNPs in chromatin that is broadly active across most cell types can make substantial contributions to heritability [74].

Compared to these intuitive findings, it is unclear whether the endometriosis-associated SNPs identified so far are in active chromatin or in chromatin that is active in cell types relevant to endometriosis, such as endometrial stromal/epithelial cells and immune cells. Such information may be useful, but unfortunately remains lacking as of now.

Epigenetic transmission

Epigenetics is the meiotically and mitotically heritable potential for gene expression without changes in DNA sequence or content [92]. Epigenetic processes are known to be involved in development, health, disease (including endometriosis), and aging, and are responsible for phenomena such as X-chromosome inactivation and genomic imprinting. The mechanisms involved in epigenetic regulation include DNA methylation, chromatin remodeling, posttranslational histone modification, and RNA-associated gene silencing by noncoding RNAs [41]. In contrast to the life-long stability of genetic sequences (barring acquired mutations and DNA damage), the epigenome is more malleable [93,94]. In particular, it can be modified in response to environmental exposures and lifestyle, such as diet, smoking, and stress [95–97].

Epigenetic changes can lead to subtle alterations in gene expression patterns or to cumulative detrimental effects in a cell, subverting the normal function of a gene and, in turn, increasing the host's susceptibility to a certain disease. While epigenetic plasticity allows for adaptation to environmental and lifestyle conditions, the resultant epigenetic changes or aberrations could also predispose the host to the disease of interest, and possibly transmit the acquired epigenetic codes to her offspring, which could affect the offspring's gene expression patterns and disease susceptibility.

The epigenome appears to be particularly vulnerable to environmental factors during embryogenesis, which becomes evident from numerous studies that have reported serious consequences in later life caused by intrauterine stressors. In animal studies, prenatal stress and prenatal exposure to glucocorticoids (GC) have been shown to have long-term effects on the expression of numerous genes associated with hypothalamus–pituitary axis function and neurologic function [97]. There is growing evidence that the long-term effects of prenatal stress and GC exposure on these genes are mediated through epigenetic mechanisms [98,99].

The first piece of evidence showing postnatal epigenetic programming by postnatal social environments was provided by Weaver et al., who demonstrated that differences in maternal care in rodents after birth determine differences in their offspring behavior in adulthood by epigenetic programming, and, more importantly, programming by maternal care could be reversed in adulthood by cross-fostering as well as epigenetic therapeutics [100]. These studies provide evidence that the epigenome is highly plastic and can be reprogrammed in response to changes in external environment, and can define a consistent phenotype without any changes in the DNA sequence [101]. That is, in addition to the cell type identity, epigenetic processes also provide experiential identity onto the genome [101].

Indeed, in the last two decades, there has been accumulating evidence for nongenetic multigenerational transmission of phenotypic responses to ancestral experiences [102]. A shortage in the food supply during the early life of paternal grandparents has been reported to be associated with high mortality rate (and diabetic deaths) in their grandsons [103,104]. Strikingly, this transmission appears to be sex-specific, such that the food supply of the paternal grandfather was associated with the mortality rate of grandsons only, while the early life food supply of the paternal grandmother was only associated with the mortality rate of granddaughters [103–105].

Children born to mothers who were exposed to the 1944–45 Dutch famine during the last trimester of pregnancy or those who were exposed to the famine in the first few months of life during that time were found to be less obese than controls, whereas exposure in the first half of pregnancy had higher obesity rates than in controls [106]. Further investigation revealed that exposure to famine early in pregnancy is associated with hypermethylation of the imprinted gene insulin-like growth factor 2 receptor 60 years later, suggesting that epigenetic changes might be involved [107]. Examination of the adult offspring (F2 generation) of prenatally exposed F1 fathers, but not mothers, had higher BMI than in offspring of unexposed F1 [108].

The intergenerational transmission also is reported in women prenatally exposed to diethylstilbestrol (DES), a synthetic nonsteroidal estrogen and a known endocrine-disrupting chemical (EDC). Women born to mothers prenatally exposed to DES are found to have increased risk of menstrual aberrations and preterm birth [109]. Incidentally or not, prenatal DES exposure has been reported to increase the risk of endometriosis [110]. Interestingly, exposure to EDCs such as genistein represses enhancer of zeste 2 (EZH2) and reduces levels of the histone 3 lysine 27 trimethylation (H3K27me3) repressive mark through the nongenomic estrogen receptor/phosphatidylinositide 3-kinases/protein kinase B signaling in the developing uterus [111], resulting in increased estrogen signaling [112].

Thus intrauterine exposure to environmental stressors may change the epigenetic patterns after fertilization. However, whether such a change can be transmitted across generations is less clear [41].

However, if endometriosis is caused, in part, by epigenetic aberrations, then conventional DNA sequence-based studies such as GWAS would be difficult, if not impossible, to detect such aberrations. Encouragingly, the epigenome appears to be on the radar screen in endometriosis [113].

Since the first publication reporting that endometriosis is an epigenetic disease in 2005 [114], the number of publications on epigenetics and endometriosis has grown exponentially, similar to the number of papers on epigenetic studies (Fig. 6.2). This seems to be in sharp contrast to genetic association studies, of which the number of publications has tapered off since 2015 (Fig. 6.1).

Heterogeneity and misclassification

Despite a somewhat deceptively simple and straightforward definition, endometriosis is by no means a homogeneous disease. Rather, there are wide variations in location, size, color, depth of invasion, presence or absence of adhesion, the proportion of epithelial/stromal cells, and even the presence or absence of these cell types, as in the well-documented phenomenon of "stromal endometriosis" (i.e., lesions without

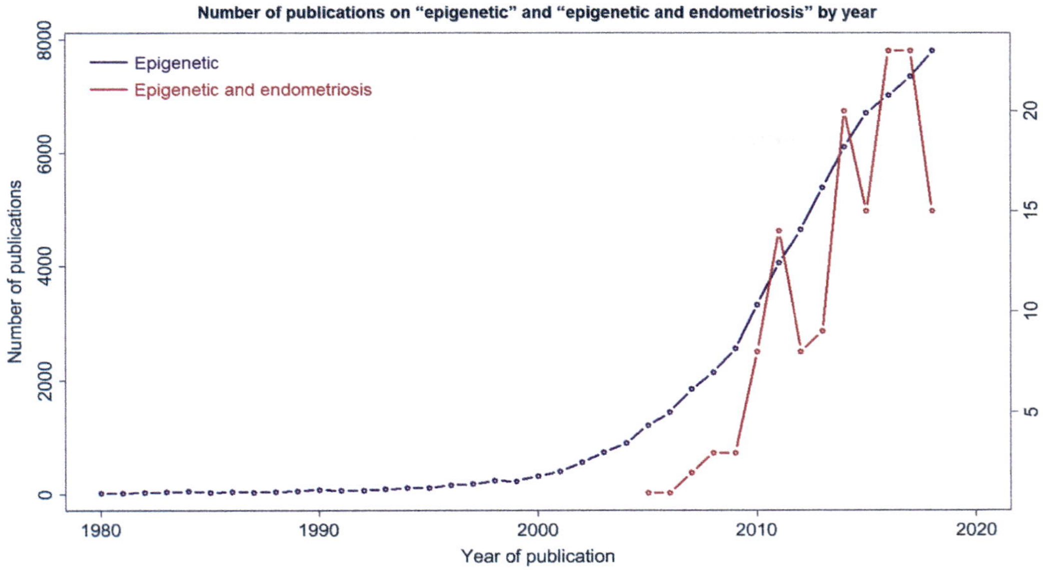

FIGURE 6.2 Number of publications, indexed by PubMed, on "epigenetic" in general and on "epigenetic and endometriosis" from 1980 to 2018. The *dark blue* and *maroon curves* represent "epigenetic" in general and "epigenetic and endometriosis," respectively. The *y*-axis on the left is for "epigenetic," while the *y*-axis on the right is for "epigenetic and endometriosis" papers.

glands) [115,116]. On top of these variations, there is also enormous variation in the symptomatology and severity among patients. Dense fibrotic tissues are often present in and/or surrounding the lesions [115,117–124], especially in deep endometriosis [117,119,121,122]. The fibrosis may result in subsequent adhesion, anatomic distortion, and pelvic pain [119].

There are three major subtypes of endometriosis: ovarian endometriomas, peritoneal endometriosis, and deep endometriosis [119]. These subtypes of endometriosis differ in prevalence, symptomatology, and severity, and have been thought to have different pathogeneses [119]. In GWASs, however, these different subtypes are often undistinguished, and may result in a reduced signal-to-noise ratio if indeed they have different pathogeneses.

In addition, occult or microscopic endometriotic lesions seem to be rather common, although their clinical significance is unclear [125]. Moreover, there is enormous variation in age at onset [126], which can be further complicated by the diagnostic delay [127,128]. Coupled with the lack of a noninvasive diagnostic procedure for endometriosis, these complications increase the possibility of misclassification, labeling women with endometriosis (but undiagnosed yet) as healthy and vice versa. Again, the misclassification would dilute signals while increasing noise, making the identification of DNA variants more difficult.

Conclusion

So far, many GASs and GWASs to identify DNA variants that might be associated with endometriosis have been published and many polymorphisms have been identified. However, each and every one of the identified polymorphisms invariably has a small, even minute, effect, explaining merely a minuscule percentage of the heritability. More disconcertingly, these publications have so far contributed little to our understanding of the pathogenesis or pathophysiology of endometriosis. Granted, the identified polymorphisms are invariably linked with some nearby genes with known functions and much speculation can be made as to what these genes may do to confer the risk of endometriosis. But this can be a fertile ground for "attribution error."

As with other complex traits, this "missing heritability" could be attributable to the inflated heritability estimates in the first place, to various complications specific to endometriosis such as disease heterogeneity, variable age at onset, and misclassification, to the possibility that nongenetic, environmental, and/or epigenetic, factors that may also familially aggregate, and to the possibility that there may be many small-effect genes, each contributing a minuscule but nonzero portion to the heritability. While further increasing the sample sizes may help to identify more DNA variants associated with endometriosis, success is by no means certain or assured.

Fundamentally, no one knows exactly what the genetic underpinning of complex diseases is [20]. At the gene transcriptional level, of course, all diseases are ultimately determined by gene expression patterns and are thus genetic in nature. However, the modulation of gene expression is influenced by genetic variation, environmental exposures, epigenetic regulation, and simply stochastic fluctuations.

Complex diseases such as endometriosis arise over time and are the end result of genetic makeup, lifestyle choices, and a combination of environmental exposures during critical periods of development and epigenetic plasticity. Environmental and lifestyle factors have the potential to change the epigenome, effectively shutting genes down or turning genes on without any alteration in DNA sequence. This could ultimately impact on disease susceptibility. In addition, what we see as familially aggregated is the end result of the totality including DNA variants, environment, lifestyle, and non-DNA machinery (egg cell, and epigenetic factors) [129].

While GWASs could still identify more DNA variants that are associated with endometriosis in the future with increasing sample sizes, there is a real question as to what the potential benefits versus costs would be. Would the identification of, say, 50 DNA variants help to better understand the pathogenesis of endometriosis? Probably not, at least not immediately, since each variant or gene needs to be carefully characterized and its functions delineated, in conjunction with other variants. In addition, the differences in disease risk cannot reveal the totality of functions that a gene may be involved in, since they cannot reveal all the effects that are common to the different alleles [129]. Many believe that all functions and malfunctions of humans at all levels are system properties emerging from the network and interaction of different components [129].

Faced with such complexities and challenges, the GAS/GWAS advocators promise to provide new insights into pathogenesis, classification, and comorbidity, if with ever increasing larger sample sizes with detailed phenotypic and clinical information [130]. Will they ever deliver?

Acknowledgment

This research was supported in part by grants 81530040 and 81771553 from the National Science Foundation of China, and a grant for Shanghai Medical Center for Female Reproductive Disease (2017ZZ01016) from the Science and Technology Commission of Shanghai Municipality.

References

[1] Giudice LC, Kao LC. Endometriosis. Lancet 2004;364:1789–99.

[2] Denny E, Mann CH. Endometriosis-associated dyspareunia: the impact on women's lives. J Fam Plann Reprod Health Care 2007;33:189–93.

[3] Fourquet J, Baez L, Figueroa M, Iriarte RI, Flores I. Quantification of the impact of endometriosis symptoms on health-related quality of life and work productivity. Fertil Steril 2011;96:107–12.
[4] Nnoaham KE, Hummelshoj L, Webster P, d'Hooghe T, de Cicco Nardone F, de Cicco Nardone C, et al. Impact of endometriosis on quality of life and work productivity: a multicenter study across ten countries. Fertil Steril 2011;96:366–373.e8.
[5] Culley L, Law C, Hudson N, Denny E, Mitchell H, Baumgarten M, et al. The social and psychological impact of endometriosis on women's lives: a critical narrative review. Hum Reprod Update 2013;19:625–39.
[6] Lovkvist L, Bostrom P, Edlund M, Olovsson M. Age-related differences in quality of life in Swedish women with endometriosis. J Womens Health (Larchmt) 2016.
[7] Garry R. Is insulin resistance an essential component of PCOS?: the endometriosis syndromes: a clinical classification in the presence of aetiological confusion and therapeutic anarchy. Hum Reprod 2004;19:760–8.
[8] Zondervan KT, Rahmioglu N, Morris AP, Nyholt DR, Montgomery GW, Becker CM, et al. Beyond endometriosis genome-wide association study: from genomics to phenomics to the patient. Semin Reprod Med 2016;34:242–54.
[9] Snell RG, MacMillan JC, Cheadle JP, Fenton I, Lazarou LP, Davies P, et al. Relationship between trinucleotide repeat expansion and phenotypic variation in Huntington's disease. Nat Genet 1993;4:393–7.
[10] Hall JM, Lee MK, Newman B, Morrow JE, Anderson LA, Huey B, et al. Linkage of early-onset familial breast cancer to chromosome 17q21. Science 1990;250:1684–9.
[11] Miki Y, Swensen J, Shattuck-Eidens D, Futreal PA, Harshman K, Tavtigian S, et al. A strong candidate for the breast and ovarian cancer susceptibility gene BRCA1. Science 1994;266:66–71.
[12] Risch N, Merikangas K. The future of genetic studies of complex human diseases. Science 1996;273:1516–17.
[13] Rahmioglu N, Banasik K, Christofidou P, Danning R, Galarneau G, Giri A, et al. Large-scale genome-wide association meta-analysis of endometriosis reveals 13 novel loci and genetically-associated comorbidity with other pain conditions. In, 2018. BioRxiv: Avaliable from: https://doi.org/10.1101/406967.
[14] Lee SH, Harold D, Nyholt DR, Goddard ME, Zondervan KT, Williams J, et al. Estimation and partitioning of polygenic variation captured by common SNPs for Alzheimer's disease, multiple sclerosis and endometriosis. Hum Mol Genet 2013;22:832–41.
[15] Guo SW. Glutathione S-transferases M1 (GSTM1)/T1 (GSTT1) gene polymorphisms and endometriosis: a meta-analysis of genetic association studies. Mol Hum Reprod 2005;11:729–43.
[16] Guo SW. Association of endometriosis risk and genetic polymorphisms involving sex steroid biosynthesis and their receptors: a meta-analysis. Gynecol Obstet Invest 2005;61:90–105.
[17] Wu Y, Strawn E, Basir Z, Wang YD, Halverson G, Jailwala P, et al. Genomic alterations in the ectopic and eutopic endometrium of women with endometriosis. Gynecol Obstet Invest 2006;62:148–59.
[18] Aschard H, Chen J, Cornelis MC, Chibnik LB, Karlson EW, Kraft P. Inclusion of gene-gene and gene-environment interactions unlikely to dramatically improve risk prediction for complex diseases. Am J Hum Genet 2012;90:962–72.
[19] Nolte IM, van der Most PJ, Alizadeh BZ, de Bakker PI, Boezen HM, Bruinenberg M, et al. Missing heritability: is the gap closing? An analysis of 32 complex traits in the Lifelines Cohort Study. Eur J Hum Genet (EJHG) 2017;25:877–85.
[20] Maher B. Personal genomes: the case of the missing heritability. Nature 2008;456:18–21.
[21] Wood AR, Esko T, Yang J, Vedantam S, Pers TH, Gustafsson S, et al. Defining the role of common variation in the genomic and biological architecture of adult human height. Nat Genet 2014;46:1173–86.
[22] Yang J, Benyamin B, McEvoy BP, Gordon S, Henders AK, Nyholt DR, et al. Common SNPs explain a large proportion of the heritability for human height. Nat Genet 2010;42:565–9.
[23] Krishna Kumar S, Feldman MW, Rehkopf DH, Tuljapurkar S. Limitations of GCTA as a solution to the missing heritability problem. Proc Natl Acad Sci USA 2016;113:E61–70.
[24] Visscher PM, Wray NR, Zhang Q, Sklar P, McCarthy MI, Brown MA, et al. 10 Years of GWAS discovery: biology, function, and translation. Am J Hum Genet 2017;101:5–22.
[25] Feldman MW, Ramachandran S. Missing compared to what? Revisiting heritability, genes and culture. Philos Trans R Soc Lond Ser B Biol Sci 2018;373:20170064.
[26] Guo SW. Gametogenesis processes and multilocus gene identity by descent. Am J Hum Genet 1996;58:408–19.
[27] Guo SW. Computation of identity-by-descent proportions shared by two siblings. Am J Hum Genet 1994;54:1104–9.
[28] Guo SW. Proportion of genome shared identical by descent by relatives: concept, computation, and applications. Am J Hum Genet 1995;56:1468–76.
[29] Zuk O, Hechter E, Sunyaev SR, Lander ES. The mystery of missing heritability: genetic interactions create phantom heritability. Proc Natl Acad Sci USA 2012;109:1193–8.
[30] Feldman MW, Lewontin RC. The heritability hang-up. Science 1975;190:1163–8.

[31] Bares CB, Kendler KS, Maes HH. Racial differences in heritability of cigarette smoking in adolescents and young adults. Drug Alcohol Depend 2016;166:75–84.
[32] Lewontin RC. Annotation: the analysis of variance and the analysis of causes. Am J Hum Genet 1974;26:400–11.
[33] Guo SW. Familial aggregation of environmental risk factors and familial aggregation of disease. Am J Epidemiol 2000;151:1121–31.
[34] Cavalli-Sforza LL, Feldman MW. Cultural transmission and evolution. Princeton, NJ: Princeton University Press; 1981.
[35] Guo SW. Inflation of sibling recurrence-risk ratio, due to ascertainment bias and/or overreporting. Am J Hum Genet 1998;63:252–8.
[36] Moen MH, Schei B. Epidemiology of endometriosis in a Norwegian county. Acta Obstet Gynecol Scand 1997;76:559–62.
[37] Salces I, Rebato EM, Susanne C, San Martin L, Rosique J. Familial resemblance for the age at menarche in Basque population. Ann Hum Biol 2001;28:143–56.
[38] Salces I, Rebato E, Slachmuylder JL, Vercauteren M, Rosique J, Susanne C. Genetic and environmental sources on familial transmission in Basque families. II. Stature, weight and body mass index. Ann Hum Biol 2003;30:176–90.
[39] Guo SW. Sibling recurrence risk ratio as a measure of genetic effect: caveat emptor!. Am J Hum Genet 2002;70:818–19.
[40] Guo SW. Chapter 6. The relevance of genetics in endometriosis research. In: Garcia-Velasco JA, Rizk B, editors. Endometriosis: current management and future trends. New York: Jaypee Brothers Medical Publishers; 2009. p. 40–9.
[41] van Otterdijk SD, Michels KB. Transgenerational epigenetic inheritance in mammals: how good is the evidence? FASEB J 2016;30:2457–65.
[42] Phillips DI. Twin studies in medical research: can they tell us whether diseases are genetically determined? Lancet 1993;341:1008–9.
[43] Pam A, Kemker SS, Ross CA, Golden R. The "equal environments assumption" in MZ-DZ twin comparisons: an untenable premise of psychiatric genetics? Acta Genet Med Gemellol 1996;45:349–60.
[44] Guo SW. Does higher concordance in monozygotic twins than in dizygotic twins suggest a genetic component? Hum Hered 2001;51:121–32.
[45] Saha R, Pettersson HJ, Svedberg P, Olovsson M, Bergqvist A, Marions L, et al. Heritability of endometriosis. Fertil Steril 2015;104:947–52.
[46] Treloar SA, O'Connor DT, O'Connor VM, Martin NG. Genetic influences on endometriosis in an Australian twin sample. Fertil Steril 1999;71:701–10.
[47] Fung JN, Montgomery GW. Genetics of endometriosis: state of the art on genetic risk factors for endometriosis. Best Pract Res Clin Obstet Gynaecol 2018;50:61–71.
[48] Guo SW, Jenisch S, Stuart P, Lange EM, Kukuruga D, Nair R, et al. Combined segregation and linkage analysis of HLA markers in familial psoriasis. Eur J Hum Genet (EJHG) 2002;10:327–33.
[49] Stefansson H, Geirsson RT, Steinthorsdottir V, Jonsson H, Manolescu A, Kong A, et al. Genetic factors contribute to the risk of developing endometriosis. Hum Reprod 2002;17:555–9.
[50] Botstein D, White RL, Skolnick M, Davis RW. Construction of a genetic linkage map in man using restriction fragment length polymorphisms. Am J Hum Genet 1980;32:314–31.
[51] Weber JL, Polymeropoulos MH, May PE, Kwitek AE, Xiao H, McPherson JD, et al. Mapping of human chromosome 5 microsatellite DNA polymorphisms. Genomics 1991;11:695–700.
[52] Morton NE. Sequential tests for the detection of linkage. Am J Hum Genet 1955;7:277–318.
[53] Stefansson H, Einarsdottir A, Geirsson RT, Jonsdottir K, Sverrisdottir G, Gudnadottir VG, et al. Endometriosis is not associated with or linked to the GALT gene. Fertil Steril 2001;76:1019–22.
[54] Penrose LS. The detection of autosomal linkage in a data which consist of pairs of brothers and sisters of unspecified parentage. Ann Eugene 1935;6:133–8.
[55] Kennedy S, Bennett S, Weeks DE. Affected sib-pair analysis in endometriosis. Hum Reprod Update 2001;7:411–18.
[56] Xiong M, Guo SW. The power of linkage detection by the transmission/disequilibrium tests. Hum Hered 1998;48:295–312.
[57] Pearson TA, Manolio TA. How to interpret a genome-wide association study. JAMA 2008;299:1335–44.
[58] Ioannidis JP. Non-replication and inconsistency in the genome-wide association setting. Hum Hered 2007;64:203–13.
[59] Ioannidis JP, Ntzani EE, Trikalinos TA, Contopoulos-Ioannidis DG. Replication validity of genetic association studies. Nat Genet 2001;29:306–9.
[60] Kraft P. Curses—winner's and otherwise—in genetic epidemiology. Epidemiology 2008;19:649–51 discussion 57–8.
[61] Nnoaham KE, Webster P, Kumbang J, Kennedy SH, Zondervan KT. Is early age at menarche a risk factor for endometriosis? A systematic review and meta-analysis of case-control studies. Fertil Steril 2012;98:702–712.e6.
[62] Di W, Guo SW. The search for genetic variants predisposing women to endometriosis. Curr Opin Obstet Gynecol 2007;19:395–401.
[63] Montgomery GW, Nyholt DR, Zhao ZZ, Treloar SA, Painter JN, Missmer SA, et al. The search for genes contributing to endometriosis risk. Hum Reprod Update 2008;14:447–57.

[64] Ruth KS, Beaumont RN, Tyrrell J, Jones SE, Tuke MA, Yaghootkar H, et al. Genetic evidence that lower circulating FSH levels lengthen menstrual cycle, increase age at menopause and impact female reproductive health. Hum Reprod 2016;31:473–81.

[65] Rull K, Grigorova M, Ehrenberg A, Vaas P, Sekavin A, Nommemees D, et al. FSHB -211 G>T is a major genetic modulator of reproductive physiology and health in childbearing age women. Hum Reprod 2018;33:954–66.

[66] Wei M, Cheng Y, Bu H, Zhao Y, Zhao W. Length of menstrual cycle and risk of endometriosis: a meta-analysis of 11 case-control studies. Medicine (Baltimore) 2016;95:e2922.

[67] Uno S, Zembutsu H, Hirasawa A, Takahashi A, Kubo M, Akahane T, et al. A genome-wide association study identifies genetic variants in the CDKN2BAS locus associated with endometriosis in Japanese. Nat Genet 2010;42:707–10.

[68] Nyholt DR, Low SK, Anderson CA, Painter JN, Uno S, Morris AP, et al. Genome-wide association meta-analysis identifies new endometriosis risk loci. Nat Genet 2012;44:1355–9.

[69] Painter JN, Anderson CA, Nyholt DR, Macgregor S, Lin J, Lee SH, et al. Genome-wide association study identifies a locus at 7p15.2 associated with endometriosis. Nat Genet 2011;43:51–4.

[70] Albertsen HM, Chettier R, Farrington P, Ward K. Genome-wide association study link novel loci to endometriosis. PLoS One 2013;8:e58257.

[71] Botstein D, Risch N. Discovering genotypes underlying human phenotypes: past successes for mendelian disease, future approaches for complex disease. Nat Genet 2003;33(Suppl.:):228–37.

[72] Welter D, MacArthur J, Morales J, Burdett T, Hall P, Junkins H, et al. The NHGRI GWAS catalog, a curated resource of SNP-trait associations. Nucleic Acids Res 2014;42:D1001–6.

[73] Li YI, van de Geijn B, Raj A, Knowles DA, Petti AA, Golan D, et al. RNA splicing is a primary link between genetic variation and disease. Science 2016;352:600–4.

[74] Boyle EA, Li YI, Pritchard JK. An expanded view of complex traits: from polygenic to omnigenic. Cell 2017;169:1177–86.

[75] Ding D, Liu X, Duan J, Guo SW. Platelets are an unindicted culprit in the development of endometriosis: clinical and experimental evidence. Hum Reprod 2015;30:812–32.

[76] Zhang Q, Duan J, Liu X, Guo SW. Platelets drive smooth muscle metaplasia and fibrogenesis in endometriosis through epithelial-mesenchymal transition and fibroblast-to-myofibroblast transdifferentiation. Mol Cell Endocrinol 2016;428:1–16.

[77] Takamura M, Koga K, Izumi G, Urata Y, Nagai M, Hasegawa A, et al. Neutrophil depletion reduces endometriotic lesion formation in mice. Am J Reprod Immunol 2016;76:193–8.

[78] Haber E, Danenberg HD, Koroukhov N, Ron-El R, Golomb G, Schachter M. Peritoneal macrophage depletion by liposomal bisphosphonate attenuates endometriosis in the rat model. Hum Reprod 2009;24:398–407.

[79] Bacci M, Capobianco A, Monno A, Cottone L, Di Puppo F, Camisa B, et al. Macrophages are alternatively activated in patients with endometriosis and required for growth and vascularization of lesions in a mouse model of disease. Am J Pathol 2009;175:547–56.

[80] Duan J, Liu X, Guo S-W. The M2a macrophage subset may be critically involved in fibrogenesis of endometriosis in mouse. Reprod Biomed Online 2018;37:254–68.

[81] Du Y, Liu X, Guo SW. Platelets impair natural killer cell reactivity and function in endometriosis through multiple mechanisms. Hum Reprod 2017;32:794–810.

[82] Guo SW, Du Y, Liu X. Platelet-derived TGF-beta1 mediates the down-modulation of NKG2D expression and may be responsible for impaired natural killer (NK) cytotoxicity in women with endometriosis. Hum Reprod 2016;31:1462–74.

[83] Binda MM, Donnez J, Dolmans MM. Targeting mast cells: a new way to treat endometriosis. Expert Opin Ther Targets 2017;21:67–75.

[84] Osuga Y, Koga K, Hirota Y, Hirata T, Yoshino O, Taketani Y. Lymphocytes in endometriosis. Am J Reprod Immunol 2011;65:1–10.

[85] Liu X, Yan D, Guo SW. Sensory nerve-derived neuropeptides accelerate the development and fibrogenesis of endometriosis. Hum Reprod 2019;34:452–68.

[86] Yan D, Liu X, Guo S-W. Neuropeptides substance P and calcitonin gene related peptide accelerate the development and fibrogenesis of endometriosis. Sci Rep 2019;9:2698.

[87] Finucane HK, Bulik-Sullivan B, Gusev A, Trynka G, Reshef Y, Loh PR, et al. Partitioning heritability by functional annotation using genome-wide association summary statistics. Nat Genet 2015;47:1228–35.

[88] Trynka G, Sandor C, Han B, Xu H, Stranger BE, Liu XS, et al. Chromatin marks identify critical cell types for fine mapping complex trait variants. Nat Genet 2013;45:124–30.

[89] Farh KK, Marson A, Zhu J, Kleinewietfeld M, Housley WJ, Beik S, et al. Genetic and epigenetic fine mapping of causal autoimmune disease variants. Nature 2015;518:337–43.

[90] Roadmap Epigenomics C, Kundaje A, Meuleman W, Ernst J, Bilenky M, Yen A, et al. Integrative analysis of 111 reference human epigenomes. Nature 2015;518:317–30.

[91] Hu X, Kim H, Stahl E, Plenge R, Daly M, Raychaudhuri S. Integrating autoimmune risk loci with gene-expression data identifies specific pathogenic immune cell subsets. Am J Hum Genet 2011;89:496–506.
[92] Waterland RA, Michels KB. Epigenetic epidemiology of the developmental origins hypothesis. Annu Rev Nutr 2007;27:363–88.
[93] Thompson RF, Atzmon G, Gheorghe C, Liang HQ, Lowes C, Greally JM, et al. Tissue-specific dysregulation of DNA methylation in aging. Aging Cell 2010;9:506–18.
[94] Gautrey HE, van Otterdijk SD, Cordell HJ, Newcastle 85+ Study Core Team, Mathers JC, Strathdee G. DNA methylation abnormalities at gene promoters are extensive and variable in the elderly and phenocopy cancer cells. FASEB J 2014;28:3261–72.
[95] Mathers JC, Strathdee G, Relton CL. Induction of epigenetic alterations by dietary and other environmental factors. Adv Genet 2010;71:3–39.
[96] Talikka M, Sierro N, Ivanov NV, Chaudhary N, Peck MJ, Hoeng J, et al. Genomic impact of cigarette smoke, with application to three smoking-related diseases. Crit Rev Toxicol 2012;42:877–89.
[97] Cao-Lei L, de Rooij SR, King S, Matthews SG, Metz GAS, Roseboom TJ, et al. Prenatal stress and epigenetics. Neurosci Biobehav Rev 2017; May 18 [Online ahead of print].
[98] Mueller BR, Bale TL. Sex-specific programming of offspring emotionality after stress early in pregnancy. J Neurosci Off J Soc Neurosci 2008;28:9055–65.
[99] Mulligan CJ, D'Errico NC, Stees J, Hughes DA. Methylation changes at NR3C1 in newborns associate with maternal prenatal stress exposure and newborn birth weight. Epigenetics 2012;7:853–7.
[100] Weaver IC, Cervoni N, Champagne FA, D'Alessio AC, Sharma S, Seckl JR, et al. Epigenetic programming by maternal behavior. Nat Neurosci 2004;7:847–54.
[101] Szyf M, Tang YY, Hill KG, Musci R. The dynamic epigenome and its implications for behavioral interventions: a role for epigenetics to inform disorder prevention and health promotion. Transl Behav Med 2016;6:55–62.
[102] Szyf M. Nongenetic inheritance and transgenerational epigenetics. Trends Mol Med 2015;21:134–44.
[103] Pembrey ME. Male-line transgenerational responses in humans. Hum Fertil (Camb) 2010;13:268–71.
[104] Pembrey ME, Bygren LO, Kaati G, Edvinsson S, Northstone K, Sjostrom M, et al. Sex-specific, male-line transgenerational responses in humans. Eur J Hum Genet (EJHG) 2006;14:159–66.
[105] Grossniklaus U, Kelly WG, Kelly B, Ferguson-Smith AC, Pembrey M, Lindquist S. Transgenerational epigenetic inheritance: how important is it? Nat Rev Genet 2013;14:228–35.
[106] Ravelli GP, Stein ZA, Susser MW. Obesity in young men after famine exposure in utero and early infancy. N Engl J Med 1976;295:349–53.
[107] Heijmans BT, Tobi EW, Stein AD, Putter H, Blauw GJ, Susser ES, et al. Persistent epigenetic differences associated with prenatal exposure to famine in humans. Proc Natl Acad Sci USA 2008;105:17046–9.
[108] Seisenberger S, Andrews S, Krueger F, Arand J, Walter J, Santos F, et al. The dynamics of genome-wide DNA methylation reprogramming in mouse primordial germ cells. Mol Cell 2012;48:849–62.
[109] Titus L, Hatch EE, Drake KM, Parker SE, Hyer M, Palmer JR, et al. Reproductive and hormone-related outcomes in women whose mothers were exposed in utero to diethylstilbestrol (DES): a report from the US National Cancer Institute DES Third Generation Study. Reprod Toxicol 2019;84:32–8.
[110] Upson K, Sathyanarayana S, Scholes D, Holt VL. Early-life factors and endometriosis risk. Fertil Steril 2015;104:964–971.e5.
[111] Sandovici I, Hammerle CM, Ozanne SE, Constancia M. Developmental and environmental epigenetic programming of the endocrine pancreas: consequences for type 2 diabetes. Cell Mol Life Sci 2013;70:1575–95.
[112] Prusinski L, Al-Hendy A, Yang Q. Developmental exposure to endocrine disrupting chemicals alters the epigenome: identification of reprogrammed targets. Gynecol Obstet Res Open J 2016;3:1–6.
[113] Rahmioglu N, Drong AW, Lockstone H, Tapmeier T, Hellner K, Saare M, et al. Variability of genome-wide DNA methylation and mRNA expression profiles in reproductive and endocrine disease related tissues. Epigenetics 2017;12:897–908.
[114] Wu Y, Halverson G, Basir Z, Strawn E, Yan P, Guo SW. Aberrant methylation at HOXA10 may be responsible for its aberrant expression in the endometrium of patients with endometriosis. Am J Obstet Gynecol 2005;193:371–80.
[115] Clement PB. The pathology of endometriosis: a survey of the many faces of a common disease emphasizing diagnostic pitfalls and unusual and newly appreciated aspects. Adv Anat Pathol 2007;14:241–60.
[116] Mai KT, Yazdi HM, Perkins DG, Parks W. Pathogenetic role of the stromal cells in endometriosis and adenomyosis. Histopathology 1997;30:430–42.
[117] Cornillie FJ, Oosterlynck D, Lauweryns JM, Koninckx PR. Deeply infiltrating pelvic endometriosis: histology and clinical significance. Fertil Steril 1990;53:978–83.

[118] Stovall DW, Anners JA, Halme J. Immunohistochemical detection of type I, III, and IV collagen in endometriosis implants. Fertil Steril 1992;57:984–9.

[119] Nisolle M, Donnez J. Peritoneal endometriosis, ovarian endometriosis, and adenomyotic nodules of the rectovaginal septum are three different entities. Fertil Steril 1997;68:585–96.

[120] Matsuzaki S, Canis M, Darcha C, Dechelotte P, Pouly JL, Bruhat MA. Fibrogenesis in peritoneal endometriosis. A semi-quantitative analysis of type-I collagen. Gynecol Obstet Invest 1999;47:197–9.

[121] Bonte H, Chapron C, Vieira M, Fauconnier A, Barakat H, Fritel X, et al. Histologic appearance of endometriosis infiltrating uterosacral ligaments in women with painful symptoms. J Am Assoc Gynecol Laparosc 2002;9:519–24.

[122] Khare VK, Martin DC, Eltorky M. A comparative study of ovarian and pelvic wall-infiltrating endometriosis. J Am Assoc Gynecol Laparosc 1996;3:235–9.

[123] Itoga T, Matsumoto T, Takeuchi H, Yamasaki S, Sasahara N, Hoshi T, et al. Fibrosis and smooth muscle metaplasia in rectovaginal endometriosis. Pathol Int 2003;53:371–5.

[124] Guo SW, Ding D, Shen M, Liu X. Dating endometriotic ovarian cysts based on the content of cyst fluid and its potential clinical implications. Reprod Sci 2015;22:873–83.

[125] Khan KN, Fujishita A, Kitajima M, Hiraki K, Nakashima M, Masuzaki H. Occult microscopic endometriosis: undetectable by laparoscopy in normal peritoneum. Hum Reprod 2014;29:462–72.

[126] Liu X, Yuan L, Shen F, Guo SW. Patterns of and factors potentially influencing the age at first surgery for women with ovarian endometriomas. Gynecol Obstet Invest 2008;66:76–83.

[127] Arruda MS, Petta CA, Abrao MS, Benetti-Pinto CL. Time elapsed from onset of symptoms to diagnosis of endometriosis in a cohort study of Brazilian women. Hum Reprod 2003;18:756–9.

[128] Hudelist G, Fritzer N, Thomas A, Niehues C, Oppelt P, Haas D, et al. Diagnostic delay for endometriosis in Austria and Germany: causes and possible consequences. Hum Reprod 2012;27:3412–16.

[129] Noble D. Genes and causation. Philos Trans Ser A Math Phys Eng Sci 2008;366:3001–15.

[130] Montgomery GW, Zondervan KT, Nyholt DR. The future for genetic studies in reproduction. Mol Hum Reprod 2014;20:1–14.

CHAPTER

7

Genetics of polycystic ovarian syndrome

Yvonne V. Louwers and Joop S.E. Laven

Division of Reproductive Endocrinology and Infertility, Erasmus University Medical Center, Rotterdam, The Netherlands

Introduction

Polycystic ovarian syndrome (PCOS) is the most common endocrine disorder in women, and is characterized by ovulatory dysfunction, hyperandrogenism, and polycystic ovarian morphology (PCOM) [1]. The diagnosis is made according to the so-called 2003 Rotterdam consensus criteria. Oligomenorrhea is defined as a menstrual cycle interval being less than 21 days or more than 35 days. Amenorrhea is defined as absent menstrual cycles or a cycle interval exceeding 199 days. Biochemical hyperandrogenism is defined as either free testosterone, free androgen index [FAI: total testosterone × 100/ serum sex hormone binding globulin (SHBG) levels] or calculated bioavailable testosterone. Laboratory reference ranges should be used to interpreter the androgen levels. Clinical hyperandrogenism is defined as modified a Ferriman–Gallwey score of seven or higher. PCOM is defined as having more than 12 follicles per ovary, or an ovarian volume exceeding 10 mL [2–5]. Due to the fact that only two out of three criteria are needed to be diagnosed as having PCOS there are basically four different phenotypes. The recently published international PCOS guidelines endorse the 2003 Rotterdam criteria in adults. The first phenotype is the full-blown clinical picture suffering from ovulatory dysfunction, hyperandrogenism, either clinical, biochemical, or both, and having PCOM. The second phenotype is the one with ovulatory dysfunction and either clinical or biochemical hyperandrogenism. Hyperandrogenism can also be accompanied by PCOM, constituting the third possible phenotype, whereas ovulatory dysfunction together with PCOM constitutes the fourth subphenotype of PCOS. Hence PCOS is a very heterogeneous syndrome made up of four different phenotypes [2–5].

The prevalence varies between 5% and 20%, depending on which population is assessed. The incidence is generally lower in unselected population-based samples compared to hospital-referred patients [6]. The PCOS phenotype might change with increasing age or changes in body mass. In general, menstrual cycle length decreases with increasing age in women with PCOS. Similarly, androgen levels decrease with increasing age. Although PCOM seems to be a relatively constant phenomenon over the years, women might experience an amelioration of the symptoms and ovarian

Human Reproductive Genetics
DOI: https://doi.org/10.1016/B978-0-12-816561-4.00007-7

dysfunction as indicated by an increase in the number of regular menstrual cycles, and a decrease in serum androgen levels may occur [7].

The syndrome is also associated with other distressing phenomena such as depression, negative self-esteem, and metabolic dysfunction characterized by insulin resistance and compensatory hyperinsulinemia. PCOS increases the risk for type II diabetes mellitus, gestational diabetes, and other pregnancy-related complications. Women with PCOS also more often have hypertension, hence they are at risk for cerebrovascular and cardiovascular events although data on the latter are scarce. Finally, if left untreated, due to unopposed estrogen exposure, women with PCOS are at increased risk of developing endometrial cancer [1].

Heritability

PCOS appears to run in families. The first papers describing this familial aggregation of hyperandrogenism in PCOS kindreds was from the group of Legro and coworkers. They found that although 50% of all sisters were affected, only 25% had a similar phenotype compared to the proband, whereas the remaining 25% suffered from hyperandrogenemia per se [8]. In subsequent studies it was shown that brothers of women with PCOS have dyslipidemia as well as evidence of insulin resistance, similar to that of their proband sisters with PCOS. These findings are consistent with the hypothesis that some metabolic abnormalities in PCOS are heritable and not sex specific [9]. More recently evidence has emerged indicating clustering of metabolic syndrome, hypertension, and dyslipidemia in mothers, fathers, sisters, and brothers of women with PCOS [10].

Twin studies revealed similar results, indicating a familial component in PCOS due to genetic factors. Data from a large Dutch cohort of monozygotic (MZ) twins were compared with a similarly large cohort of dizygotic (DZ) twins. PCOS was defined as less than nine menstrual cycles and acne or hirsutism, in agreement with the 2003 Rotterdam consensus. The results point to a strong contribution of familial factors to PCOS. The resemblance in MZ twin sisters for PCOS was about twice as large as in DZ twin pairs, indicating a high degree of heritability. Univariate analyses indicated a strong contribution of genetic factors to the variance in PCOS. Moreover, a subsequent trivariate genetic analysis of oligomenorrhea, acne, and hirsutism confirmed that the familial component in PCOS is due to genetic factors [11]. In a more recent study this Dutch group showed that the prevalence of PCOS was not different in women from opposite-sex and same-sex twin pairs, singleton sisters, or spouses. This indicates that possible androgen exposure of the female fetus, caused by a shared intrauterine environment with a male fetus, does not result in PCOS-like traits [12].

Candidate gene studies

Candidate gene association studies are the most commonly used approach among current genetic studies for human diseases. Candidate gene studies rely on the hypothesis that the gene of interest is involved in the pathogenesis of the disease or trait under study. In PCOS, candidate genes have been studies that were involved in the biosynthesis and trafficking of androgens, genes related to metabolic aspects of PCOS, and genes correlated with inflammatory cytokines. Currently more than 200 studies have been reported on single-nucleotide polymorphisms (SNPs) in genes involved in these pathways. Numerous studies have reported on other SNPs in genes that are associated with either the risk of having PCOS or one of its characteristic features. However, the majority of these studies are small and lack proper replication studies and should therefore be interpreted with caution [1].

One of the first identified risk factors for PCOS was a so-called dinucleotide marker of the fibrillin gene, that is, D19S884. A recent association analysis in Chinese women showed that PCOS women were significantly different from controls in the distribution of D19S884 allele frequencies. Moreover, instead of the well-known allele 8, the most common allele in the Chinese population was proved to be allele 7, whose allele frequencies were statistically different between cases and controls. A subsequent metaanalysis of both alleles 7 and 8 only identified the latter as a significant allelic association at the D19S884 marker in all combined samples. Hence a potential association of the D19S884 marker in the fibrillin gene with PCOS in Chinese Han women was found. This metaanalysis identified that allele 8 may increase a woman's susceptibility to PCOS [13].

Genes involved in androgen metabolism have been studied extensively. For instance, *CYP17A1* encodes the enzyme P450c17a (17-α-hydroxylase and 17-lyase), which is a rate-limiting enzyme that transforms progesterone into testosterone, has been studied in detail. Two SNPs in the promotor region of the genes encoding for *CYP17A1* and *CYP11A1* were associated with serum androgen levels in a subset of Indian women [14]. However, a recent metaanalysis failed to verify this relationship [15].

The androgen receptor (AR) has also been studied in relation to PCOS susceptibility and the associated hyperandrogenism. Again several studies revealed discordant findings and hence the role of the trinucleotide CAG repeats and their role in PCOS remains controversial. However, a recent metaanalysis including 1536 PCOS patients and 1807 controls revealed that the lengths of CAG repeats contributed to hyperandrogenism in PCOS [16].

Another candidate gene that has been repeatedly studied is the fat mass and obesity associated (FTO) gene. In a recent metaanalysis including 12 studies only a single-nucleotide polymorphism (rs9939609) in the FTO gene significantly increased the risk of PCOS in women. However, two other SNPs (rs8050136 and rs1421085) were associated with PCOS only in a recessive model [17].

Taking the increased risk for type II diabetes and the insulin resistance frequently encountered in women with PCOS into account the insulin receptor (*INSR*) gene also has been studied frequently. In a recent metaanalysis a total of 20 case–control studies, including 23,845 controls and 17,460 PCOS cases, were analyzed. Ninety-eight SNPs distributed in 23 exons and the flanking regions of INSR were investigated, among which 17 SNPs were found to be associated with PCOS. Only three SNPs detected in more than three studies were selected for further analyses. Twelve studies, including 1158 controls and 1264 PCOS cases, entered the analysis of rs1799817, but no significant association was found for every genotype ($P>.05$). Further subgroup stratification by ethnicity and weight did not lead to the discovery of a significant correlation. For another SNP, rs2059806, four studies including 442 controls and 524 PCOS cases qualified for metaanalysis, and no significant association with PCOS was found for any genotype. Four studies including 12,830 controls and 11,683 PCOS cases investigated the correlation between rs2059807 and PCOS, and five of the six cohorts indicated a significant impact. The current metaanalysis suggests no significant correlation between both SNPs rs1799817/rs2059806 and the susceptibility for PCOS. In contrast, the rs2059807 SNP could be a promising candidate SNP that might be involved in susceptibility to PCOS [18].

Insulin receptor substrates (IRSs) are functionally plausible candidates for PCOS susceptibility. A number of studies on polymorphisms of IRSs have been conducted, but the results are controversial. Among those studies *IRS1* is the most commonly studied IRS. Although significantly associated with PCOS in Japanese and Greek populations, a recent metaanalysis of 11 studies did not reveal a significant association between IRS 1 SNPs and the risk of developing PCOS [19].

The minisatellite variable number of tandem repeats (VNTR) locus on chromosome 11p15.5 in the promoter of the *INS* gene is nearly 600 base pairs (bp) upstream of the translation initiation site. The polymorphism arises from a tandem repetition of 14–15 bp. The variation in VNTR was shown to influence the transcriptional activity of the gene in vitro and regulates *INS* transcription levels. A recent metaanalysis revealed no significant association between *INS VNTR* polymorphisms and the risk of PCOS in the overall population. However, variance in the *INS VNTR* was shown to be associated with susceptibility to the anovulatory PCOS subphenotype [20].

There are several follicle-stimulating hormone (FSH) receptor polymorphisms located in the follicle-stimulating hormone receptor (FSHR) gene. The two most common are the Thr307Ala and Asn680Ser polymorphisms. A total of 11 studies were included in a recent metaanalysis. The random-effect analysis showed Asn680Ser to be significantly associated with the reduced susceptibility to PCOS in a dominant model (Asn/Asn + Asn/Ser vs Ser/Ser, OR = 0.83, 95% CI: 0.69–1.00) as well as in a recessive model (Asn/Asn vs Asn/Ser + Ser/Ser, OR = 0.84, 95% CI: 0.72–0.98). Moreover, the homozygote comparison (Asn/Asn vs Ser/Ser, OR = 0.79, 95% CI: 0.63–0.98) and the allele contrast comparison (Asn vs Ser, OR = 0.87, 95% CI: 0.79–0.97) both showed that these FSHR SNPs were protective factors for PCOS. Finally, no significant associations were found between Thr307Ala and PCOS [21].

More recently, based on the fact that anti-Müllerian hormone (AMH) serum levels are increased in women with PCOS SNPs in the *AMH* gene as well as in the AMH Type II Receptor (*AMHR2*) gene, these genes have been studied. Five studies, involving a total of 2042 PCOS cases and 1071 controls, were included in a recent metaanalysis. This study concluded that neither SNPs in the *AMH* gene nor those in the *AMHR2* conferred a heightened risk for PCOS [22].

The results of a metaanalysis, including 13 studies, assessing the role of different tumor necrosis factor-alpha (TNF-α) SNPs and PCOS susceptibility suggests a positive association between one TNF-α SNP (1031T > C and IL-6-174G > C) and the risk of PCOS. However, no associations were detected between another nine SNPs in the TNF-α gene and the risk for PCOS. However, due to the heterogeneity and low quality of the studies related to PCOS polymorphisms in the metaanalysis, the results should be interpreted with caution according to these authors [23].

Another metaanalysis, including a total of 14 studies, investigated the association of SNPs in the interleukins IL-6 and IL-1β and did not find a significant relationship between these SNPs and the susceptibility for PCOS [24]. In the same year a second metaanalysis confirmed these results for the IL-6 SNP [25].

Genome-wide association studies

The transition to genome-wide association studies (GWAS) has provided a new conceptual framework in the search for variants underlying common disorders. Rather than focusing on biological candidate genes as described in the previous section, in GWAS the whole genome is screened without any prior predilection for specific regions, genes, or variants of interest. Therefore GWAS is generally characterized as a "hypothesis-free" or an "agnostic" approach. This "hypothesis-free" basis of GWAS offered the opportunity to overcome difficulties and obstacles imposed by the incomplete understanding of the pathophysiology of the disease or trait under study.

The first GWAS in PCOS was performed by a group based at Shandong University in China. The discovery set included 744 PCOS cases and 895 controls and subsequent replications involved two independent large cohorts of Han Chinese women with PCOS and controls. Three genome-wide significant loci were identified showing strong associations with PCOS located at chromosome 2 (2p16.3 and 2p21) and chromosome 9 (9q33.3) [26]. In a second GWAS published a year later they identified nine new loci that were significantly associated with PCOS. The PCOS-associated signals showed evidence of enrichment for candidate genes related to insulin signaling, gonadotropic hormone function, and type II diabetes. Other candidate genes were related to calcium signaling and endocytosis [27].

A few years later a study in American women of European descent was published identifying two new loci mapping to chromosome 8 (8p23.1) and chromosome 11 (11p14.1), and a known locus on chromosome 9 (9q22.32) previously found in Chinese GWAS. The SNP on chromosome 11 in the region of the follicle-stimulating hormone B polypeptide (*FSHB*) gene was strongly associated with the former PCOS NIH diagnosis as well as with luteinizing hormone (LH) levels [28]. In the same year a large European collaboration produced another GWAS on PCOS. That study was performed in up to 5184 self-reported cases of white European ancestry and 82,759 controls, with follow-up in a further approximately 2000 clinically validated cases and approximately 100,000 controls. Six signals for PCOS in or near known genes (*ERBB4/HER4*, *YAP1*, *THADA*, *FSHB*, *RAD50*, and *KRR1*) were identified. Variants in/near three of the four epidermal growth factor receptor genes were associated with PCOS at or near genome-wide significance. Mendelian randomization analyses indicate causal roles in PCOS etiology for higher body mass index, higher insulin resistance, and lower serum SHBG concentrations. Furthermore, genetic susceptibility to later menopause is significantly associated with higher PCOS risk and PCOS-susceptibility alleles are significantly associated with higher serum anti-Mullerian hormone concentrations in girls. This large-scale study implicates an etiological role of the epidermal growth factor receptors, infers causal mechanisms relevant to clinical management and prevention, and suggests balancing selection mechanisms involved in PCOS risk [29].

Another GWAS in Korean women consisted of 976 PCOS cases and 946 controls, with a replication cohort including 249 PCOS cases and 778 controls. One novel locus with genome-wide significance and seven moderately associated loci for PCOS were identified. The strongest association was on chromosome 8 (8q24.2). The latter signal was located upstream of the *KHDRBS3* gene, which is associated with telomerase activity, and could drive PCOS and related phenotypes [30].

Another GWAS compared patients with PCOS with women from infertile couples due to tubal occlusion or male factor infertility who were used as controls. By primary selection and secondary verification at two stages in the experiment, three SNPs were found to contain significantly different allele frequencies between the patient and control groups. Genes involved were the known *THADA*, *DENND1A*, and a new locus in the *TOX3* gene. The average expression levels at the three discovered SNP sites were significantly different between the patient and control groups, indicating their possible functional role in the pathogenesis of PCOS [31].

A recent metaanalysis of the cross-ethnic effects through GWAS identified genetic variants for 12 of 17 genetic variants mapping to the Chinese PCOS loci that had similar effect sizes and identical directions with PCOS patients from northern European ancestry, indicating a common genetic risk profile for PCOS across populations. Therefore it is expected that a large GWAS in PCOS patients with northern European ancestry will partly identify similar loci as the GWAS in Chinese PCOS patients [32].

Indeed, the most recent study of over 10,000 cases of PCOS and over 100,000 controls of European ancestry identified only three novel loci (near the *PLGRKT*, *ZBTB16*, and *MAPRE1* genes) and replicated 11 previously reported loci (see Fig. 7.1). Only one locus differed significantly in its association by diagnostic criteria; otherwise the genetic architecture was similar between PCOS diagnosed by self-report and PCOS diagnosed by NIH or non-NIH Rotterdam criteria across common variants at 13 loci. Identified variants were associated with hyperandrogenism, gonadotropin regulation, and testosterone levels in affected women. Moreover, linkage disequilibrium score regression analysis revealed genetic correlations with obesity, fasting insulin, type II diabetes, lipid levels, and coronary artery disease, indicating a shared genetic architecture between metabolic traits and PCOS. Finally, Mendelian randomization analyses suggested that all loci associated with body mass index, fasting insulin, menopause timing, depression, and male-pattern balding play a causal role in PCOS. These data clearly demonstrate three novel loci associated with PCOS and similar genetic architecture for all diagnostic criteria. The data also provide the first genetic evidence for a male phenotype for PCOS and a causal link to depression, a previously hypothesized comorbid disease. Thus genetics provide a comprehensive view of PCOS that encompasses multiple diagnostic criteria, gender, reproductive potential, and mental health [33].

Functional studies

The ultimate proof that SNPs in or near genes are involved in the pathogenesis of PCOS is finally derived from functional studies showing that gene products really influence phenotypical features, response to treatment, and long-term health. Several studies have been performed to address whether identified SNPs really play such a role in PCOS.

The first two studies looked at RNA expression profiles in ovarian tissue and theca cells. The microarray analysis of PCOS and normal ovaries identifies dysregulated expression of

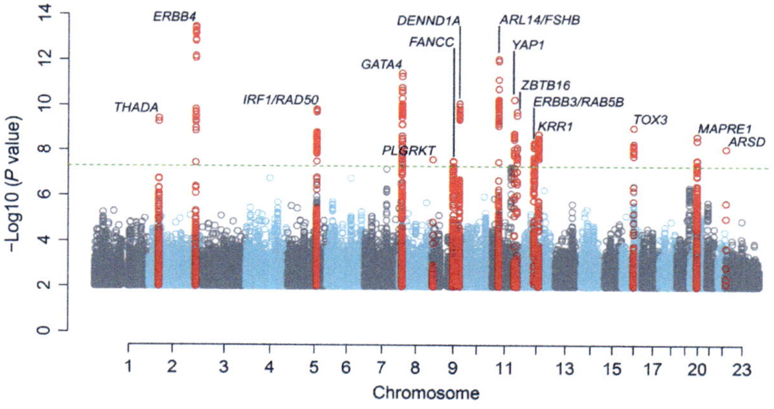

FIGURE 7.1 Manhattan plot showing the results of a metaanalysis for polycystic ovarian syndrome (PCOS) status, adjusting for age. On the *Y* axis the inverse log10 of the *P* value [−log10 (*P*)] is plotted. The *green dashed line* designates the minimum *P* value for genome-wide significance ($<5.0 \times 10^{-8}$). Genome-wide significant loci are denoted with a label showing the nearest gene to the index single-nucleotide polymorphism (SNP) at each locus. SNPs with *P* values $\leq 1.0 \times 10^{-2}$ are not depicted. Source: *Day F, Karaderi T, Jones MR, Meun C, He C, Drong A, et al. Large-scale genome-wide meta-analysis of polycystic ovary syndrome suggests shared genetic architecture for different diagnosis criteria, PLoS Genet 2018;14. Used with permission of the authors.*

genes encoding components of several biological pathways or systems such as Wnt signaling, extracellular matrix components, and immunological factors. Analyses of whole ovarian tissue mounts and those only harboring theca cells were surprisingly similar [34,35]. Surprisingly there is not much of an overlap between the expression array findings and the risk loci discovered through GWAS. Focusing on granulosa cells, another study demonstrated that genes linked to diabetes mellitus, inflammation, cardiovascular diseases, and infertility are of importance in women suffering from PCOS. It is of interest that most of the identified dysregulated genes were also involved in oxidative stress, lipid metabolism, and insulin signaling. This might indicate that these genes may be involved in follicular growth arrest as well as in the metabolic disorders associated with PCOS [36].

A more recent study demonstrated that a splice variant (DENND1A.V2) derived from the *DENND1A* gene identified in all GWAS up till now plays a functional role in controlling theca cell steroidogenesis. This particular study showed that overexpression of DENND1A.V2 is sufficient to convert normal theca cells into a PCOS biochemical phenotype characterized by increased *CYP17A1* and *CYP11A1* gene expression and augmented androgen and progestin production. Moreover, suppression of DENND1A.V2 function pushes PCOS theca cells toward a normal phenotype, non-PCOS phenotype in terms of steroidogenic enzyme gene expression, and steroid production [37].

In a more recent study from the same group the functional roles of strong PCOS candidate loci focusing on FSHR, *LHCGR*, *INSR*, and *DENND1A* were reviewed. They proposed that these candidate genes comprise a hierarchical signaling network by which *DENND1A*, *LHCGR*, *INSR*, *RAB5B*, adapter proteins, and associated downstream signaling cascades converge to regulate theca cell androgen biosynthesis. Moreover, other genetic variants identified in earlier GWAS including *YAP1*, *RAB5B*, *C9orf3*, *TOX3*, and *HMGA2* genes also fit into this model [38].

In one Chinese study it was shown that by applying a recessive model certain *THADA* variants were associated with increased serum LH as well as increased testosterone levels in subjects with PCOS. The LH/FSH ratio was also significantly higher in those women homozygous for the A allele. In case they used a recessive model the homozygous C allele genotype was significantly associated with increased levels of low-density lipoprotein. Similarly, in a dominant model variants in *DENND1A* were significantly associated with elevated serum insulin levels in patients with PCOS [39].

A very recent study looking at the expression levels of several of GWASs identified genetic variants in adipose tissue biopsies. Subsequently these women were treated with metformin for some time. A variant in the *THADA* locus was associated with a response to metformin and metformin was a predicted upstream regulator at the same locus. Moreover, the *FSHB* locus was associated with serum LH levels. Genes near the PCOS risk loci demonstrated differences in expression as a function of genotype in adipose women, including *BLK* and *NEIL2* (*GATA4* locus), and *GLIPR1* and *PHLDA1* (*KRR1* locus). By combining data on the phenotype, expression quantitative trait loci and upstream regulatory and pathway analyses these authors hypothesized that there are several genetically determined PCOS subphenotypes. Hence, *FSHB*, *FHSR*, and *LHR* loci may influence PCOS risk based on their relationship to gonadotropin levels. In contrast *THADA*, *GATA4*, *ERBB4*, *SUMO1P1*, *KRR1*, and *RAB5B* loci appear to confer risk through metabolic mechanisms whilst the*IRF1*, *SUMO1P1*, and *KRR1* loci may confer PCOS risk in development. Finally, the *TOX3* and *GATA4* loci appear to be involved in inflammation and its consequences. These data suggest the potential that, based on the genetic findings in women with PCOS, certain subphenotypes can be distinguished, offering opportunities for personalized treatment [40].

Several other PCOS risk loci have promising functional candidate genes mapped to signals at 2p16.3 (*LHCGR, FSHR*) and 11p14.1 (*FSHB*). These genes play important roles in ovarian follicle development and ovulation, making them clear candidate susceptibility genes for PCOS. Data on the role of *FSHR* polymorphisms in PCOS are conflicting. It seems that in large Chinese studies *FSHR* polymorphisms are not associated with either PCOS risk or with PCOS treatment outcome. However, in large-scale studies in Caucasians these polymorphisms seem to influence the risk of having PCOS. Moreover, these studies also showed that some polymorphisms might affect some clinical features of PCOS as well as treatment outcome. Although most research has focused on the role of *FSHR* polymorphisms there seems to be also some evidence showing that SNPs in the *LHCGR* as well as those in the *FSHB* gene might also alter the phenotype of PCOS [41].

AMH serum levels are increased in most women with PCOS [1]. Moreover, there seems to be a genetic predisposition for this phenomenon because fathers as well as brothers of women with PCOS also have higher levels of AMH [42]. Earlier studies were not able to show that genetic variants in the AMH and AMH type II receptor gene were associated with PCOS susceptibility, however, a later study did reveal that the AMH Ile(49)Ser polymorphism contributes to the severity of the PCOS phenotype [43]. Interestingly, a recent report identified 24 rare genetic variants in a case–control study. Eighteen of these variants were specific for PCOS patients and nearly all were associated with decreased AMH signaling. This might increase androgen biosynthesis due to decreased AMH-mediated inhibition of CYP17 activity [44]. Of note in this context is the fact that recent studies identified that gonadotropin-releasing hormone neurons (GnRH) also harbor AMHR2 and the same GnRH neurons respond to AMH administration by increasing LH secretion with a concomitant decrease in FSH secretion [45]. Furthermore, genetic susceptibility to later menopause is associated with higher PCOS risk and PCOS-susceptibility alleles are associated with higher serum anti-Mullerian hormone concentrations in girls [29]. These findings were recently validated in another study demonstrating some genetic variants determining age at menopause that are also associated with the risk for developing PCOS. These data also suggest opposing influences of the genetic variants on both menopausal age and PCOS [46]. Indeed women with PCOS do enter menopause at a later age compared to healthy controls [47].

Similarly, reduced methylation in the LHCGR locus and increased methylation in the INSR locus have been described in detail, suggesting that local genetic variation plays an important role in gene regulation. For instance nonobese PCOS women possess significant alterations in LH receptor expression, resulting in increased androgen secretion from the ovaries [48,49]. Moreover, in obese women with PCOS the insulin receptor is underexpressed in metabolic tissues and overexpressed in the ovaries, resulting in peripheral insulin resistance and excess ovarian androgen production. These studies provide a genetic and molecular basis for the reported clinical heterogeneity of PCOS [49].

Recently, epigenetic mechanisms have been involved in the pathogenesis of PCOS. Several studies have shown that methylation in DNA and miRNAs is altered in women with PCOS in blood, serum, adipose tissue, granulosa cells, and theca. This evidence indicates that women with PCOS have a different epigenetic regulation, which might be triggered by an adverse intrauterine environment or by postnatal environmental elements such as diet and/or obesity [50].

Conclusion

PCOS is a complex genetic disorder which runs within families of affected women and has a high degree of heritability. Several hundreds of candidate genes have been studied, however, the majority of these genetic variants have not been replicated in sufficiently large case–control studies. Genetic variants in the *Fibrillin* gene, the AR, FTO gene, the insulin receptor, the *FSHR* gene, the *TNF alpha* gene, and some variants in the *IL-6* gene confer a certain risk for PCOS and have been replicated in sufficiently large studies or metaanalyses. More recently, GWASs have identified up to 20 genetic variant genes involved in neuroendocrine, metabolic, and reproductive pathways. Cross-ethnic analyses indicate a common genetic risk profile for PCOS across populations. These studies also provided evidence for shared biologic pathways between PCOS and a number of metabolic disorders, menopause, depression, and male-pattern balding, a putative male phenotype. There is not much overlap between GWAS findings and most functional molecular studies. However, most of the identified SNPs seem to play a role in a pathway responsible for trafficking and recycling of large protein transmembrane receptors. Moreover, some promising SNPs involved in gonadotropin action have been identified which not only constitute risk factors for PCOS but also seem to influence the response to ovulation induction treatment. Last but not least, evidence is accumulating that epigenetic mechanisms might also play a role in the pathogenesis of PCOS, either during fetal programming or in later life through factors as obesity and diet composition.

References

[1] Azziz R, Carmina E, Chen Z, Dunaif A, Laven JS, Legro RS, et al. Polycystic ovary syndrome. Nat Rev Dis Prim 2016;2:16057.

[2] Rotterdam ESHRE/ASRM-Sponsored PCOS Consensus Workshop Group. Revised 2003 Consensus on diagnostic criteria and long-term health risks related to polycystic ovary syndrome (PCOS). Hum Reprod (Oxford, Engl) 2004;19:41–7.

[3] Teede HJ, Misso ML, Costello MF, Dokras A, Laven J, Moran L, et al. Recommendations from the international evidence-based guideline for the assessment and management of polycystic ovary syndrome. Clin Endocrinol 2018;89:251–68.

[4] Teede HJ, Misso ML, Costello MF, Dokras A, Laven J, Moran L, et al. Recommendations from the international evidence-based guideline for the assessment and management of polycystic ovary syndrome. Fertil Steril 2018;110:364–79.

[5] Teede HJ, Misso ML, Costello MF, Dokras A, Laven J, Moran L, et al. Recommendations from the international evidence-based guideline for the assessment and management of polycystic ovary syndrome. Hum Reprod (Oxford, Engl) 2018;33:1602–18.

[6] Lizneva D, Kirubakaran R, Mykhalchenko K, Suturina L, Chernukha G, Diamond MP, et al. Phenotypes and body mass in women with polycystic ovary syndrome identified in referral versus unselected populations: systematic review and meta-analysis. Fertil Steril 2016;106:1510–1520.e2.

[7] Brown ZA, Louwers YV, Fong SL, Valkenburg O, Birnie E, de Jong FH, et al. The phenotype of polycystic ovary syndrome ameliorates with aging. Fertil Steril 2011;96:1259–65.

[8] Legro RS, Driscoll D, Strauss III JF, Fox J, Dunaif A. Evidence for a genetic basis for hyperandrogenemia in polycystic ovary syndrome. Proc Natl Acad Sci USA 1998;95:14956–60.

[9] Sam S, Coviello AD, Sung YA, Legro RS, Dunaif A. Metabolic phenotype in the brothers of women with polycystic ovary syndrome. Diabetes Care 2008;31:1237–41.

[10] Yilmaz B, Vellanki P, Ata B, Yildiz BO. Metabolic syndrome, hypertension, and hyperlipidemia in mothers, fathers, sisters, and brothers of women with polycystic ovary syndrome: a systematic review and meta-analysis. Fertil Steril 2018;109:356–364.e32.

[11] Vink JM, Sadrzadeh S, Lambalk CB, Boomsma DI. Heritability of polycystic ovary syndrome in a Dutch twin-family study. J Clin Endocrinol Metab 2006;91:2100–4.

[12] Kuijper EA, Vink JM, Lambalk CB, Boomsma DI. Prevalence of polycystic ovary syndrome in women from opposite-sex twin pairs. J Clin Endocrinol Metab 2009;94:1987–90.

[13] Xie GB, Xu P, Che YN, Xia YJ, Cao YX, Wang WJ, et al. Microsatellite polymorphism in the fibrillin 3

gene and susceptibility to PCOS: a case-control study and meta-analysis. Reprod Biomed Online 2013;26:168–74.

[14] Pusalkar M, Meherji P, Gokral J, Chinnaraj S, Maitra A. CYP11A1 and CYP17 promoter polymorphisms associate with hyperandrogenemia in polycystic ovary syndrome. Fertil Steril 2009;92:653–9.

[15] Zhao H, Lv Y, Li L, Chen ZJ. Genetic studies on polycystic ovary syndrome. Best Pract Res Clin Obstet Gynaecol 2016;37:56–65.

[16] Peng CY, Xie HJ, Guo ZF, Nie YL, Chen J, Zhou JM, et al. The association between androgen receptor gene CAG polymorphism and polycystic ovary syndrome: a case-control study and meta-analysis. J Assist Reprod Genet 2014;31:1211–19.

[17] Liu Y, Chen Y. Fat mass and obesity associated gene polymorphism and the risk of polycystic ovary syndrome: a meta-analysis. Iran J Public Health 2017;46:4–11.

[18] Feng C, Lv PP, Yu TT, Jin M, Shen JM, Wang X, et al. The association between polymorphism of INSR and polycystic ovary syndrome: a meta-analysis. Int J Mol Sci 2015;16:2403–25.

[19] Ioannidis A, Ikonomi E, Dimou NL, Douma L, Bagos PG. Polymorphisms of the insulin receptor and the insulin receptor substrates genes in polycystic ovary syndrome: a Mendelian randomization meta-analysis. Mol Genet Metab 2010;99:174–83.

[20] Song LY, Luo JR, Peng QL, Wang J, Xie L, He Y, et al. Lack of association of INS VNTR polymorphism with polycystic ovary syndrome: a meta-analysis. J Assist Reprod Genet 2014;31:675–81.

[21] Qiu L, Liu J, Hei QM. Association between two polymorphisms of follicle stimulating hormone receptor gene and susceptibility to polycystic ovary syndrome: a meta-analysis. Chin Med Sci J (Chung-kuo i hsueh k'o hsueh tsa chih) 2015;30:44–50.

[22] Wang F, Niu WB, Kong HJ, Guo YH, Sun YP. The role of AMH and its receptor SNP in the pathogenesis of PCOS. Mol Cell Endocrinol 2017;439:363–8.

[23] Wu H, Yu K, Yang Z. Associations between TNF-alpha and interleukin gene polymorphisms with polycystic ovary syndrome risk: a systematic review and meta-analysis. J Assist Reprod Genet 2015;32:625–34.

[24] Guo R, Zheng Y, Yang J, Zheng N. Association of TNF-alpha, IL-6 and IL-1beta gene polymorphisms with polycystic ovary syndrome: a meta-analysis. BMC Genet 2015;16:5.

[25] Wang Q, Tong X, Ji Y, Li H, Lu W, Song Z. Meta-analysis of the correlation between IL-6 -174 G/C polymorphism and polycystic ovarian syndrome. J Obstet Gynaecol Res 2015;41:1087–92.

[26] Chen ZJ, Zhao H, He L, Shi Y, Qin Y, Shi Y, et al. Genome-wide association study identifies susceptibility loci for polycystic ovary syndrome on chromosome 2p16.3, 2p21 and 9q33.3. Nat Genet 2011;43:55–9.

[27] Shi Y, Zhao H, Shi Y, Cao Y, Yang D, Li Z, et al. Genome-wide association study identifies eight new risk loci for polycystic ovary syndrome. Nat Genet 2012;44:1020–5.

[28] Hayes MG, Urbanek M, Ehrmann DA, Armstrong LL, Lee JY, Sisk R, et al. Genome-wide association of polycystic ovary syndrome implicates alterations in gonadotropin secretion in European ancestry populations. Nat Commun 2015;6:7502.

[29] Day FR, Hinds DA, Tung JY, Stolk L, Styrkarsdottir U, Saxena R, et al. Causal mechanisms and balancing selection inferred from genetic associations with polycystic ovary syndrome. Nat Commun 2015;6:8464.

[30] Lee H, Oh JY, Sung YA, Chung H, Kim HL, Kim GS, et al. Genome-wide association study identified new susceptibility loci for polycystic ovary syndrome. Hum Reprod (Oxford, Engl) 2015;30:723–31.

[31] Chen L, Hu LM, Wang YF, Yang HY, Huang XY, Zhou W, et al. Genome-wide association study for SNPs associated with PCOS in human patients. Exp Ther Med 2017;14:4896–900.

[32] Louwers YV, Stolk L, Uitterlinden AG, Laven JS. Cross-ethnic meta-analysis of genetic variants for polycystic ovary syndrome. J Clin Endocrinol Metab 2013;98:E2006–12.

[33] Day F, Karaderi T, Jones MR, Meun C, He C, Drong A, et al. Large-scale genome-wide meta-analysis of polycystic ovary syndrome suggests shared genetic architecture for different diagnosis criteria. PLoS Genet 2018;14:e1007813.

[34] Jansen E, Laven JS, Dommerholt HB, Polman J, van Rijt C, van den Hurk C, et al. Abnormal gene expression profiles in human ovaries from polycystic ovary syndrome patients. Mol Endocrinol (Baltimore, Md) 2004;18:3050–63.

[35] Wood JR, Nelson-Degrave VL, Jansen E, McAllister JM, Mosselman S, Strauss III JF. Valproate-induced alterations in human theca cell gene expression: clues to the association between valproate use and metabolic side effects. Physiol Genomics 2005;20:233–43.

[36] Kaur S, Archer KJ, Devi MG, Kriplani A, Strauss III JF, Singh R. Differential gene expression in granulosa cells from polycystic ovary syndrome patients with and without insulin resistance: identification of susceptibility gene sets through network analysis. J Clin Endocrinol Metab 2012;97:E2016–21.

[37] McAllister JM, Modi B, Miller BA, Biegler J, Bruggeman R, Legro RS, et al. Overexpression of a DENND1A isoform produces a polycystic ovary

syndrome theca phenotype. Proc Natl Acad Sci USA 2014;111:E1519–27.
[38] McAllister JM, Legro RS, Modi BP, Strauss III JF. Functional genomics of PCOS: from GWAS to molecular mechanisms. Trends Endocrinol Metab (TEM) 2015;26:118–24.
[39] Cui L, Zhao H, Zhang B, Qu Z, Liu J, Liang X, et al. Genotype-phenotype correlations of PCOS susceptibility SNPs identified by GWAS in a large cohort of Han Chinese women. Hum Reprod (Oxford, Engl) 2013;28:538–44.
[40] Pau CT, Mosbruger T, Saxena R, Welt CK. Phenotype and tissue expression as a function of genetic risk in polycystic ovary syndrome. PLoS One 2017;12:e0168870.
[41] Laven JSE. Follicle stimulating hormone receptor (FSHR) polymorphisms and polycystic ovary syndrome (PCOS). Front Endocrinol (Lausanne). 2019;10:23.
[42] Torchen LC, Kumar A, Kalra B, Savjani G, Sisk R, Legro RS, et al. Increased antimullerian hormone levels and other reproductive endocrine changes in adult male relatives of women with polycystic ovary syndrome. Fertil Steril 2016;106:50–5.
[43] Kevenaar ME, Laven JS, Fong SL, Uitterlinden AG, de Jong FH, Themmen AP, et al. A functional antimullerian hormone gene polymorphism is associated with follicle number and androgen levels in polycystic ovary syndrome patients. J Clin Endocrinol Metab 2008;93:1310–16.
[44] Gorsic LK, Kosova G, Werstein B, Sisk R, Legro RS, Hayes MG, et al. Pathogenic anti-Mullerian hormone variants in polycystic ovary syndrome. J Clin Endocrinol Metab 2017;102:2862–72.
[45] Cimino I, Casoni F, Liu X, Messina A, Parkash J, Jamin SP, et al. Novel role for anti-Mullerian hormone in the regulation of GnRH neuron excitability and hormone secretion. Nat Commun 2016;7:10055.
[46] Saxena R, Bjonnes AC, Georgopoulos NA, Koika V, Panidis D, Welt CK. Gene variants associated with age at menopause are also associated with polycystic ovary syndrome, gonadotrophins and ovarian volume. Hum Reprod (Oxford, Engl) 2015;30:1697–703.
[47] Mulders AG, Laven JS, Eijkemans MJ, de Jong FH, Themmen AP, Fauser BC. Changes in anti-Mullerian hormone serum concentrations over time suggest delayed ovarian ageing in normogonadotrophic anovulatory infertility. Hum Reprod (Oxford, Engl) 2004;19:2036–42.
[48] Wang P, Zhao H, Li T, Zhang W, Wu K, Li M, et al. Hypomethylation of the LH/choriogonadotropin receptor promoter region is a potential mechanism underlying susceptibility to polycystic ovary syndrome. Endocrinology 2014;155:1445–52.
[49] Jones MR, Brower MA, Xu N, Cui J, Mengesha E, Chen YD, et al. Systems genetics reveals the functional context of PCOS loci and identifies genetic and molecular mechanisms of disease heterogeneity. PLoS Genet 2015;11:e1005455.
[50] Concha CF, Sir PT, Recabarren SE, Perez BF. [Epigenetics of polycystic ovary syndrome]. Rev Med Chil 2017;145:907–15.

CHAPTER

8

Male factor infertility: genetic and epigenetic aspects

Brent M. Hanson[1] *and James M. Hotaling*[2]

[1]RMA New Jersey, Sidney Kimmel Medical College at Thomas Jefferson University, Basking Ridge, NJ, United States [2]Department of Surgery – Urology, University of Utah Center for Reconstructive Urology and Men's Health, Salt Lake City, UT, United States

Introduction

Male factor infertility affects approximately 7% of the male population and impacts 15% of couples worldwide [1,2]. It has long been recognized that a complex relationship exists between male infertility, biologic factors, and environmental factors [3]. More recently, publications have focused specifically on the intrinsic link between infertility and genetic or epigenetic aspects. Despite significant efforts, an identifiable pathophysiologic cause for male factor infertility is lacking in nearly half of cases [4]. Dysregulation of either genetic or epigenetic factors has emerged as a potential etiology for previously unexplained cases of infertility. Genetic anomalies or epigenetic changes, which include alterations in DNA methylation and histone modifications, can have sweeping detrimental effects on fertility. This chapter discusses the commonly identified genetic anomalies associated with male factor infertility and provides a background for recent discoveries which relate to genetics and infertility. The following pages also provide a summary of the current understanding of the role of epigenetics in male fertility.

Gene mutations and alterations in chromosomes can result in abnormal spermatogenesis (Table 8.1). Nearly 15% of the male genome is involved in male reproduction, but only a handful of genes have been identified as clinically useful in the evaluation of male infertility [5]. Genetic abnormalities such as Klinefelter syndrome, Y chromosome microdeletions, and single gene mutations are known to impact a man's ability to reproduce [6]. The frequency of chromosomal anomalies and microdeletions of the azoospermia factor (AZF) region of the Y chromosome is directly correlated with the severity of spermatogenic defects and approaches 30% in men with azoospermia (15% karyotype abnormalities, 15% AZF microdeletions) [7]. It is also believed that a significant proportion of idiopathic male infertility cases can be attributed to underlying genetic

Human Reproductive Genetics
DOI: https://doi.org/10.1016/B978-0-12-816561-4.00008-9

TABLE 8.1 Genetic causes of male infertility.

Condition	Category	Frequency	Diagnosis	Clinical presentation and comments
Klinefelter syndrome	Sex chromosome (X)	• 0.1%–0.2% of males in the general population • 3%–4% of male infertility cases • 11% of nonobstructive azoospermia cases	Karyotype 47,XXY (90%) 46,XY/47,XXY 48,XXXY 49,XXXXY	• Hypergonadotropic hypogonadism • Impaired spermatogenesis • Progressive destruction of seminiferous tubules • High degree of phenotypic variation • Tall stature, small testes, gynecomastia, broad hips, sparse body hair, and signs of androgen deficiency • Linked to diabetes, dyslipidemia, and cardiovascular disease • Frequently underdiagnosed
Y chromosome microdeletion of the azoospermia factor (AZF) region	Sex chromosome (Y)	• 4% of male infertility cases • 10%–15% of idiopathic azoospermia and severe oligozoospermia cases	Polymerase chain reaction (PCR) AZFc deletion: 75% AZFb + c deletion: 14% AZFb deletion: 7% AZFa deletion: 2% Partial deletions: 2%	• Severe spermatogenic defects • Hypergonadotropic hypogonadism • Extremely poor prognosis with AZFa and AZFb deletions. Prognosis improved for AZFc deletions • Sperm retrieval success rates via microTESE 30%–50% with AZFc deletions • Vertical transmission of microdeletion to male offspring
Polymorphisms in various autosomal genes (*LOC203413*, *BRDT*, *OR2W3*, *GRTH*, *FKBP6*, *MSY2*, *TSSK2*, and *SOD2*)	Autosomal	• Each polymorphism unlikely to contribute to a significant proportion of the infertile male population	Whole-genome testing (genome-wide association studies, GWAS) Next-generation sequencing (NGS) Single-nucleotide polymorphism (SNP) array and copy number variant (CNV) studies	• Discordant data within the literature (controversial) • Low degree of clinical applicability • Low frequency of specific mutations • Wide range of clinical phenotypes

XX male DSDs	Sex chromosome (X)	• 1 in 20,000 newborn males	Karyotype 90% possess SRY region on X chromosome	• Hypergonadotropic hypogonadism • Degeneration of seminiferous tubules, testicular failure • Arise from translocations of segment of the Y chromosome to the X chromosome during paternal meiosis • Often with normal male external genitalia and small testes • Increased prevalence of hypospadias and micropenis
X-linked androgen receptor (AR) defects	Sex chromosome (X)	• 1.7% of infertile male patients • Very rare in general population	PCR amplification of coding region of AR gene (longer CAG repeats in exon 1 associated with infertility)	• Located at Xq11-12 • Presence of longer CAG trinucleotide repeats on AR can cause infertility and neuromuscular disease • Contradictory results (higher association with infertility in Asian populations and less in European) • Phenotype ranges from mild defect of virilization to complete female phenotype
TEX11 gene defect	Sex chromosome (X)	• 1% of azoospermic men	PCR amplification and Sanger sequencing	• Encodes a vital protein for male germ cell meiotic DNA recombination • TEX11 protein normally expressed in sperm and testes • Higher rates of absence of TEX11 activity in azoospermic men
Kallmann syndrome	Sex chromosome (X)	• 1 in 30,000 males	Next-generation sequencing *ANOS1* gene mutation (X-linked recessive) Autosomal dominant forms (*FGFR1*, *PROKR2*, *PROK2*, *CHD7*, and *FGF8*)	• Delayed or absent puberty and anosmia • Failure of GnRH neurons to migrate via olfactory placode • Hypogonadotropic hypogonadism • Micropenis, cryptorchidism, and lack of sexual development • Associated with unilateral renal agenesis, cleft lip/palate, and hearing loss

anomalies. The analysis of polymorphisms in genes involved in spermatogenesis is an area of tremendous research potential, and polymorphisms in several genes such as the androgen receptor (*AR*), DNA polymerase gamma (*POLG*), 5-methylenetetrahydrofolate reductase, deleted-in-azoospermia-like, follicle-stimulating hormone receptor, estrogen receptor alpha, and protamine 1 and 2 genes have been investigated for potential roles in male infertility [7,8]. While publications have yielded conflicting results regarding the impact of each polymorphism on overall male fertility, developing a better understanding of underlying genetic abnormalities associated with male infertility is crucial. The use of genetically compromised spermatozoa in assisted reproductive technology (ART) may be associated with adverse outcomes such as abnormal embryo development, implantation failure, or increased risk of miscarriage and birth defects [9]. Identifying genetic abnormalities which result in infertility could serve as a key to avoiding adverse reproductive outcomes going forward.

Epigenetic modifications are responsible for controlling a number of processes within the human body, and they serve a regulatory role within the male reproductive system [10]. Epigenetic modifications involve changes to the phenotype of an individual which arise separately and distinctly from the DNA sequence itself. The two major molecular modifications which fall under the classification of epigenetics are DNA methylation and post-translational histone modification [11,12]. Altered epigenetic profiles in sperm have been identified in men with oligozoospermia and oligoasthenoteratozoospermia. The extensive epigenetic reprogramming pathways which establish the functional qualities of spermatozoa can be altered by numerous environmental or lifestyle factors. Abnormalities in epigenetics may have detrimental effects on semen analysis parameters, fertilization, implantation, placentation, and fetal growth [10,13]. Due to the fact that epigenetic modifications do not induce changes in the gene sequence or copy number, epigenetics could provide a plausible explanation for at least a portion of cases of male infertility in which no genetic anomalies are detected using conventional techniques of genetic analysis [14]. In addition to changes within the spermatozoa, epigenetic changes which affect the seminal fluid may impact postejaculatory sperm survival and competence, and may result in disruptions to normal cytokine regulation involved with early embryogenesis [15]. It has also been shown that epigenetic alterations in men may have downstream effects on metabolic and reproductive function in offspring [16,17]. The male epigenome represents an area which could serve as a potential diagnostic or prognostic tool in the context of male infertility, and a significant number of previously unidentified causes of male infertility may, in fact, relate to epigenetic abnormalities.

Genetic aspects of male infertility

Underlying genetic abnormalities are common in infertile men. In a study published in 2017, it was found that 27.3% of men with nonobstructive azoospermia and 15.9% of men with severe oligospermia had underlying genetic abnormalities. As a comparison, only 1.3% of normozoospermic controls possessed an underlying genetic abnormality [18]. Among men with nonobstructive azoospermia, the most frequently observed genetic conditions include sex chromosome disorders such as Klinefelter syndrome and Y chromosome microdeletions. Together, Y chromosome microdeletions and Klinefelter syndrome account for 10%–20% of severe spermatogenic failure cases [19]. Autosomal translocations and inversions can also be seen, but these genetic mutations are present in a relatively small proportion of cases. A Chinese study published in 2012, which evaluated 1056 infertile men, demonstrated that male factor infertility was attributed to chromosomal translocations in only 2.1% of patients (0.7% of patients possessed Robertsonian translocations, 1.0% had autosome–autosome reciprocal translocations, and 0.4% demonstrated gonosome–autosome reciprocal translocations) [20].

Men with known genetic syndromes may also face issues related to fertility. While Klinefelter syndrome may be the most well-known genetic syndrome associated with infertility, patients with Kallman syndrome, sickle cell anemia, cystic fibrosis (*CFTR* gene mutations), Kartagener syndrome, myotonic dystrophy, Fanconi anemia, and beta thalassemia exhibit diminished fertility potential as well as elevated somatic health risks related to their specific disease processes [21]. Prior to the advent of ART, infertility associated with genetic syndromes likely limited the natural transmission of genetic abnormalities to future generations. The use of techniques such as microdissection testicular sperm extraction (microTESE) and intracytoplasmic sperm injection (ICSI) in modern fertility practice has now made it possible for many infertile men with genetic abnormalities to ultimately father children. However, this situation increases the risk of passing genetic aberrations to future generations and necessitates the implementation of genetic screening protocols for partners as well as embryos [18,22].

In recent years, the use of genomic microarray testing has been applied to the entire male genome in genome-wide association studies to assist in identifying previously unrecognized genetic causes of infertility [19]. Initial studies have targeted the most severe phenotypes of male infertility, including nonobstructive azoospermia and complete globozoospermia. In the future, variations in multiple genes and regulatory regions may be identified which could characterize less severe forms of abnormal spermatogenesis on the spectrum of male infertility and subfertility [19]. Much work remains to be done in this area, and studies are ongoing which utilize next-generation sequencing and copy number variant techniques to explore the link between genetics and male infertility [23,24].

Klinefelter syndrome

Klinefelter syndrome is identified as the underlying etiology of infertility in an estimated 3%–4% of infertile men [25]. Among men with nonobstructive azoospermia, reported prevalence is much higher, approaching 11% [26]. Klinefelter syndrome results in primary testicular failure early in the reproductive years and affects somewhere between 0.1% and 0.2% of males in the general population [26]. This disease process results from an additional X chromosome in men, most commonly presenting as a 47,XXY karyotype. Men with this condition generally have severely reduced sperm counts and underdeveloped testes. This abnormality is associated with significant health comorbidities and a life expectancy which is shortened by somewhere between 2 and 5 years [27]. Klinefelter syndrome has been well characterized since its initial description in 1942 and phenotypically presents with a constellation of findings that includes tall stature, small testes, gynecomastia in late puberty, gynoid aspect of the hips (broad hips), sparse body hair, signs of androgen deficiency, findings consistent with low serum testosterone, and elevated gonadotropins. Azoospermia, oligospermia, and hyalinization or fibrosis of the seminiferous tubules are also commonly observed [28,29].

Despite its common nature, Klinefelter syndrome remains underdiagnosed. Only 25% of men with Klinefelter syndrome are diagnosed during their lifetimes, and fewer than 10% of patients are diagnosed before puberty [30].

Variations exist in the clinical phenotype of Klinefelter syndrome, but men with this disorder nearly universally suffer from absolute or relative hypergonadotropic hypogonadism and impaired spermatogenesis. Testicular function is negatively impacted in childhood, and young boys with Klinefelter syndrome display low testicular volumes when compared to age-matched controls [31]. From a fertility standpoint, men with infertility related to Klinefelter syndrome often require surgical sperm extraction to obtain spermatozoa to be used for fertilization. In a 2012 publication evaluating 16 studies which looked at sperm retrieval rates among men with Klinefelter syndrome, the average overall sperm retrieval rate was 51%, with a range of 28%–69% at various centers using different surgical techniques. When microTESE was used, higher retrieval rates were noted when compared to nonmicrodissection TESE (61% vs 47%) [26]. Younger age at the time of sperm retrieval has been correlated with higher success rates for surgical sperm extraction procedures, highlighting the progressive destruction which occurs as a result of this disease process [32]. While only 8% of adults with Klinefelter syndrome have sperm in the ejaculate, approximately 70% of males 12–20 years of age had sperm present in ejaculated semen samples [26].

From a genetic standpoint, Klinefelter syndrome has been successfully identified for decades. Initially, diagnosis for both Klinefelter syndrome and Y chromosome deletions was achieved through cytogenetic techniques [19]. The specific chromosomal abnormality which is present in Klinefelter syndrome is due to either meiotic or mitotic nondisjunction, which results in the observed sex chromosomal aneuploidy. Approximately 90% of cases present with the pure form of the disease, a 47,XXY karyotype. The remaining 10% of cases are the result of mosaicism (46,XY/47,XXY), higher grade aneuploidy (48,XXXY; 49,XXXXY), and structurally abnormal X chromosomes [33,34]. In men with Klinefelter syndrome, the extra X chromosome typically undergoes inactivation, but studies have shown that certain genes escape the inactivation process. The genes which remain active are thought to be either directly or indirectly responsible for the clinical manifestations of Klinefelter syndrome [33].

The high degree of phenotypic variation seen in patients with Klinefelter syndrome directly relates to the underlying genetics. For instance, not all patients display the classic finding of tall stature associated with Klinefelter syndrome. The presence or absence of tall stature is believed to relate to the short stature homeobox-containing gene, which resides in the pseudoautosomal region of the X chromosome. This gene is not subject to X chromosomal inactivation [35]. Variations in the presence or absence of mature spermatozoa in the testes of men with Klinefelter syndrome are likely related to the associated degree of gonosomal mosaicism. In patients with mosaicism, 46,XY spermatogonia which have lost the additional X chromosome and have returned to the normal diploid state are able to avoid cellular destruction and can proceed through meiosis I and meiosis II as well as spermatogenesis. It is theorized that these healthy spermatogonia come to reside in a scattered fashion within the seminiferous tubules. The distribution of normal and abnormal cells is thought to be random, which explains the often haphazard nature of healthy seminiferous tubules within the testes [26]. The process by which a 47,XXY spermatogonial stem cell loses its supernumerary X chromosome is likely related to anaphase lag during mitotic renewal or differentiation [36]. Regardless of the underlying mechanism, a man's ability to produce adequate spermatozoa is directly influenced by the number of normal 46,XY germ cells present.

Abnormalities in sperm production may begin in utero for patients with Klinefelter syndrome. Two studies published by Winge et al.

which utilized RNA sequencing technology demonstrated that the testes of male fetuses with Klinefelter syndrome express alterations in transcription profiles even prior to birth. Specifically, these fetal testes had a significant enrichment of X chromosomal transcripts and long noncoding RNAs, which suggested that the failure of gonocyte differentiation into pre-spermatogonia in the fetal testes was a direct precursor to abnormal spermatogenesis and abnormal maturation of Sertoli and Leydig cells in the adult testes of men with Klinefelter syndrome [37,38]. Klinefelter syndrome is one of the most heavily studied areas of male infertility. However, despite its history, researchers continue to make new discoveries related to the genetic aspects of Klinefelter syndrome.

Y chromosome microdeletions

Approximately 10%–15% of idiopathic azoospermia and severe oligozoospermia cases can be attributed to Y chromosome microdeletions [39]. The AZFa, b, and c regions on the long arm of the Y chromosome are the specific areas which have been found to play a role in spermatogenesis [40]. Y chromosome microdeletions are preferentially associated with severe defects in spermatogenesis, so testing for Y chromosome microdeletions is a standard component in the evaluation of azoospermic men [41]. A 2019 study from the United Kingdom evaluated 1473 men with infertility and sought to describe the prevalence of Y chromosome microdeletions among men with varying degrees of semen analysis abnormalities. In this study, the overall incidence of microdeletions was 4%. Microdeletions were most commonly observed on the c region of the long arm of the Y chromosome. Frequency by region of deletion was as follows: AZFc microdeletion (75%), AZFb + c (13.8%), AZFb (6.9%), AZFa (1.7%), and partial AZFa (1.7%). A high follicle-stimulating hormone (FSH) level ($P < .001$) and a low sperm concentration ($P < .05$) were both found to be significantly predictive of the presence of a microdeletion [42]. The AZFc subregion is located at the distal end of AZF and appears to be one of the primary drivers for genetic variation in the Y chromosome [43].

While Klinefelter syndrome can easily be detected on karyotype, the Y chromosome microdeletions which result in infertility are frequently too small for detection by this method. Advanced molecular techniques such as polymerase chain reaction (PCR) are required to confirm the diagnosis of a Y chromosome microdeletion [44]. The specific region which possesses the microdeletion often dictates the prognosis for men with Y chromosome microdeletions. Deletions of the AZFa or AZFb regions predict poor clinical outcomes, and even with the use of surgical sperm extraction, it is extremely unlikely for mature spermatozoa to be isolated [45]. Therefore surgical sperm extraction is not recommended for men who carry microdeletions of the AZFa or AZFb regions. Men with AZFc microdeletions have comparatively better outcomes, and successful surgical sperm extraction procedures are often able to be performed. It is of note that, if a man with an AZFc microdeletion has mature spermatozoa isolated, outcomes with ICSI appear to be unaffected [46]. A 2018 study evaluating sperm retrieval rates via microTESE in men with AZFc microdeletions reported successful sperm retrievals in 36.3% of the azoospermic patients [47].

The AZFc subregion has been the subject of extensive research during recent years. The AZFc subregion is an area on the long arm of the Y chromosome which is 3.5 Mb in size. This subregion consists of repeated DNA amplicons and is prone to structural variation in men. While some variation is clinically insignificant, certain disruptions in this portion of the chromosome result in infertility [48]. Partial deletions have recently gained scientific attention, and four partial deletions which adversely impact spermatogenesis have been identified (b2/b4, gr/gr, b2/b3, and b1/b3) [43,49–51]. The gr/gr deletion is the most common deletion of these and occurs as a result of recombination [52].

One of the most important clinical implications of Y chromosome microdeletions within the AZFc subregion is the fact that male offspring of men with AZFc deletions will inherit the same deletion and will likely be severely oligospermic or azoospermic [53]. The detection of Y chromosome microdeletions of individual subregions prior to assisted reproductive interventions allows for clinical risk stratification and can potentially prevent the transmission of an AZFc microdeletion to future generations. Methods by which AZFc partial deletions are identified include two sequence-tagged sites (STSs) for the AZFc subregion (sY254 and sY255) which is specific to the *DAZ* gene in the P2 and P1 palindromes, an sY160 STS marker, and STS-PCR [54,55]. Several commercial kits are available to test for Y chromosome microdeletions. As a result, screening for AZF subregion microdeletions has become a more mainstream component of the male fertility evaluation. In the years to come, increased identification of Y chromosome microdeletions, specifically AZFc deletions, will likely assume a more prominent role in the screening process of infertile men and in research related to overall population genetics.

Gene polymorphisms as a cause of male infertility

As previously stated, Klinefelter syndrome and Y chromosome microdeletions constitute a significant proportion of the genetic causes of male infertility. Investigations into alternative genetic etiologies of male factor infertility are much less clear and have produced conflicting results. Several studies have explored the possible relationship between autosomally located genes and their potential impact on spermatogenesis. For example, a 2009 Dutch study evaluated five autosomal genes (*SYCP3*, *MSH4*, *DNMT3L*, *STRA8*, and *ETV5*) and found that changes in *STRA8* and *ETV5* were detected in a population of infertile men but not in a control group of men with normozoospermia. While this finding was initially promising, a functional analysis subsequently revealed that alterations in these genes were unlikely to be the cause of fertility issues in this population of men [56].

Similarly, a 2007 publication evaluated the relationship between the catalytic subunit of human mitochondrial DNA POLG which is encoded by a gene located on chromosome 15q24. This gene contains a polymorphic CAG repeat and was suggested to be a contributing factor in cases of idiopathic male subfertility [57,58]. In a comparison of 225 infertile or subfertile men and 123 men with proven paternity, homozygous mutations of *POLG* were found in both groups (1.8% of controls and 1.6% of infertile or subfertile men). This study concluded that polymorphisms of the *POLG* gene were unlikely to be associated with male infertility [58]. A 2012 publication investigated the possible association of nine single-nucleotide polymorphisms (SNPs) located on eight different genes (*FASLG*, *JMJDIA*, *LOC203413*, *TEX15*, *BRDT*, *OR2W3*, *INSR*, and *TAS2R38*) with male infertility [59]. This study included a population of 136 men with idiopathic infertility (60 men with azoospermia and 76 men with oligozoospermia) and 161 fertile controls. Using multiplex PCR /SNaPshot analyses followed by capillary electrophoresis, the study authors found that three of the nine SNPs were significantly associated ($P < .05$) with male infertility (rs5911500 in LOC203413, rs3088232 in *BRDT*, and rs11204546 in *OR2W3*) [59].

Further studies evaluating SNPs of the gonadotropin-regulated testicular helicase gene, the *FKBP6* gene, the *MSY2* gene, the *TSSK2* gene, and several other genes have suggested that these polymorphisms may be associated with human spermatogenesis impairment and male factor infertility [60–63]. SNP studies have predominantly evaluated populations of men with previously unexplained infertility in an attempt to uncover subtle genetic defects which may result in diminished fertility outcomes. While several polymorphisms have shown promising associations with infertility, others have not. For example, a 2017 case–control study of 380 male patients with idiopathic infertility and 398 normal fertile controls failed to demonstrate an association between the *TP53* gene and male infertility [64]. Similarly, a SNP of rs4880 of the *SOD2* gene was found to have no association with male infertility in a study of 519 men with idiopathic infertility and 338 fertile controls [65].

Polymorphisms in antioxidant genes are believed to be more susceptible to sperm DNA damage and male infertility, therefore these genes have been an area of ongoing research. A 2012 Chinese publication examined 11 SNPs from six antioxidant genes (*GPX1, CAT, PON1, NQO1, SOD2/MnSOD*, and *SOD3*) in 580 men with infertility and 580 controls. This study reported that individuals with abnormalities in the *PON1* and *SOD2* genes had significantly higher levels of sperm DNA fragmentation and an increased risk of male infertility [66]. Overall, studies involving the role of SNPs in male infertility are highly contradictory. While many of these genetic mutations may play a role in male fertility, each individual polymorphism likely contributes to a very small percentage of cases within the infertile male population. To date, testing for SNPs in the general infertile population has not gained clinical applicability although it remains an exciting area of future research.

The X chromosome and male infertility

Despite being one of the most genetically stable human chromosomes from an evolutionary standpoint, the X chromosome has numerous areas of rapidly evolving genes which are expressed in the testes [67]. There is a growing body of evidence that X-linked genes may play an important role in male infertility and spermatogenesis [68]. Genes within pseudoautosomal regions (PAR1 and PAR2) located at the distal ends of the X and Y chromosomes behave in an autosomal fashion and are capable of recombination during meiosis. This allows for genes associated with the X chromosome to carry out important functions related to male reproduction [69,70]. A supernumerary X chromosome resulting in a 47,XXY karyotype (Klinefelter syndrome) has clear reproductive consequences in men. Klinefelter syndrome has been discussed in detail previously in this chapter. However, other abnormalities involving the X chromosome can also result in male factor infertility.

Nonsyndromic 46,XX testicular disorders of sex development (XX male DSDs) are rare, with a reported incidence of 1 in 20,000 newborn males [71]. Most cases of 46,XX testicular DSD males arise from translocations of portions of the short arm of the Y chromosome to one of the X chromosomes, resulting in male external genitalia and testicular differentiation, despite the lack of a Y chromosome [72]. Males with this condition are infertile and exhibit azoospermia as a result of degeneration of the seminiferous tubules and testicular failure. Hormonally, 46,XX testicular DSD males have decreased serum testosterone levels and elevations in luteinizing hormone andFSH, consistent with hypergonadotropic hypogonadism [67,73]. Approximately 90% of males with this disorder possess the sex-determining region of the Y chromosome, and translocation of this segment of the Y chromosome generally takes place during paternal meiosis [74]. This specific disorder of sex development does not represent a significant proportion of male factor infertility cases, but it does serve as an interesting example of the genetic mechanisms which determine the roles of the X and Y chromosomes as they relate to fertility.

The relationship between the X-linked *AR* gene, located at Xq11-12, and male infertility is somewhat controversial [75]. Certain studies have demonstrated that the presence of longer AR-CAG trinucleotide repeats is associated with an increased risk of male infertility. It has also been reported that AR-CAG sequences of greater than 40 repeats give rise to Kennedy disease, a fatal neuromuscular disease which is accompanied by abnormal semen parameters [76]. A 2016 metaanalysis which evaluated 44 publications determined that increased AR-CAG length can result in an increased susceptibility to male infertility [75]. While increased rates of male factor infertility related to CAG repeats were statistically significant, the clinical significance of these relatively small absolute increases in male infertility remains uncertain [67,77]. Defects in the AR are also involved in androgen insensitivity syndrome, which can manifest as a female phenotype in karyotypic males. These individuals are also infertile [78].

X-linked genes such as the testis-expressed 11 (*TEX11*) gene, human reproductive homeobox (*RHOX*) genes, the *ANOS1/KAL1* gene, the *USP26* gene, and the *TAF7L* gene have also been explored as possible causes of male factor infertility [67]. The *TEX11* gene encodes a protein which is vital for male germ cell meiotic DNA recombination [79]. *TEX11* deficiency has been shown to result in meiotic arrest and male infertility and has the potential to serve as a genetic marker for men with idiopathic infertility [80,81]. Several mutations in the *RHOX* gene cluster, specifically *RHOXF1* and *RHOXF2/2B* aberrations, impair transcription factors and result in severe oligozoospermia [82]. *ANOS1/KAL1*, located on Xp22.31, is involved with the neuronal migration of gonadotropin-releasing hormone-producing cells within the hypothalamus and is associated with Kallmann syndrome, a well-documented cause of hypogonadotropic hypogonadism [67,83]. The *USP26* gene on Xp26 assembles the AR and is involved in this receptor's ubiquitination. Defects in this gene result in infertility related to AR dysfunction, described above [84]. Finally, the *TAF7L* gene has been extensively studied in knockout mice and results in reduced sperm count and motility, and diminished fertility potential in mouse models [85]. Currently, the role of *TAF7L* in humans and its relationship to male infertility are a matter of speculation, and further studies are needed [67].

Epigenetic aspects of male infertility

The phenotypic characteristics of individuals are derived from both genetic composition and epigenetic modifications. The term epigenetics was originally developed by Conrad Waddington in the 1940s to describe interactions between genes and the environment that could not be explained through classic genetics [86]. Since that time, the definition of epigenetics has evolved as scientific understanding of the concept has developed. Today, the study of epigenetics focuses primarily on the two major epigenetic modifications that occur in chromatin: DNA methylation and posttranslational histone modifications [10]. DNA methylation involves the addition of a methyl group ($-CH_3$) to the 5′ position of the cytosine pyrimidine ring typically located in a CpG dinucleotide. Methylation occurs due to activity of the enzyme DNA methyltransferase [12,87]. Histones are proteins that package the DNA into nucleosomes. Posttranslational histone modifications include acetylation, methylation, ubiquitination, and phosphorylation. Acetylation of histones typically correlates with transcriptionally active regions, whereas hypoacetylation patterns are commonly associated with inactivated regions [88]. Patterns of epigenetic modification regulate the specific genes that are active at various stages of life. During development, the epigenetic profile of germ cells is dynamic, undergoing an orchestrated sequence of changes as gametogenesis progresses (Table 8.2) [89]. The finely tuned epigenetic environment has been found to regulate chromatin modifications that are required for proper meiosis and appropriate maturation of gametes [90].

The relationship between epigenetics and male infertility is a rapidly growing area of study. It is believed that aberrant epigenetic modifications may underlie certain cases of male factor infertility [91]. In oligozoospermic men, there appears to be an increased incidence of hypermethylation in several maternally imprinted gametic differentially methylated regions (DMRs) as well as elevated rates of hypomethylation of paternally imprinted DMRs [92]. Abnormal methylation profiles of the insulin-like growth factor 2 gene and the H19 DMR have been shown to cause abnormalities during the mitosis phase of spermatogenesis

TABLE 8.2 Epigenetic changes during spermatogenesis.

Stage of cellular division	Stage of spermatogenesis	Epigenetic modifications	Epigenetic abnormalities
Mitosis	• Primordial germ cells	• DNA and histone demethylation (specific histones involved: H3K4 and H3K9) • Imprint erasure • Histone deacetylation • Expression of DNA methyltransferases	• Abnormal DNA methylation • Altered expression of mRNAs and other noncoding RNAs
	• Spermatogonia (A and B)	• Progressive methylation of DNA • Establishment of paternal methylation	
Meiosis	• Primary spermatocyte (meiosis I) • Secondary spermatocyte (meiosis II)	• Histone methylation (via H3K9 and H3K4)	• Double strand breaks • Chromosome nondisjunction • Abnormal histone modification
Postmeiotic differentiation	• Round spermatid	• Hyperacetylation of histones and global remodeling • Some histone markers (such as H3K9me2) on the inactive X chromosome are retained • Testis-specific linker histone variant HIT2 is crucial to chromatin condensation • Histones replaced by heterogeneous group of nuclear proteins known as transition proteins • Expression of DNA methyltransferase	• Abnormal histone modification
	• Elongated spermatid	• Maintenance of DNA methylation • Demethylation of H3K9 • Replacement of transition proteins to protamine (mostly P2) • Expression of histone-I-like protein	• Abnormal protamine replacement and centrosome formation
	• Mature spermatozoa	• Maintenance of genomic imprinting	• DNA fragmentation problems

and can result in oligoasthenoteratozoospermia or oligozoospermia [93]. These findings are in concordance with the results of additional publications which demonstrate abnormal methylation of the paternal DNA at H19 and GTL2 in infertile men. Epigenetic abnormalities of the DMRs LIT1, PEG1/MEST, PEG3, SNRPN, and ZAC, responsible for encoding a zinc finger protein which regulates apoptosis and cell cycle arrest, have also been reported in oligozoospermic patients [4]. Taken as a whole, a wide array of disordered epigenetic methylation patterns appears to result in diminished sperm quality. Consistently, studies evaluating epigenetic patterns among men with infertility have demonstrated dysfunctional acetylation and alterations in methylation when compared to normozoospermic controls [94,95]. A comprehensive meta-regression analysis published in 2017 demonstrated a dramatic 50%–60% decline in sperm counts in men in North America, Europe, Australia, and New Zealand between 1973 and 2011. While this downward trend in sperm counts has not been fully explained, lifestyle factors and epigenetic changes may play a large role in the overall reduction in male fertility in recent decades [96].

In order to accurately determine the impact of epigenetics on male factor infertility, precise technologies are essential to test for epigenetic mutations. High-resolution technologies are beginning to emerge, such as the RNA sequencing technique Drop-Seq [17,97]. This method allows for single-cell resolution of complete transcriptomes through the use of a novel microfluidics approach which isolates and develops library preparations for individual cells at low cost. This kind of technology lends itself to countless opportunities from both a research and a diagnostic perspective. Current scientific research is limited by the fact that many modern technologies cannot fully test the clinical impact of each epigenetic alteration. However, the identification of specific epigenetic signatures which are highly associated with spermatogenic abnormalities has broadened the present understanding of epigenetics as a whole and has provided a strong foundation for future research [17,98].

The roles of environment and lifestyle and transgenerational inheritance of epigenetic mutations

The fact that many epigenetic causes of infertility are induced by lifestyle factors differentiates epigenetic abnormalities from genetic etiologies of infertility. Studies have demonstrated that exposure to environmental toxins, stress, and dietary substances early in development may have a significant impact on human somatic and reproductive health [99,100]. Ongoing exposure to certain aggravating factors throughout adulthood is also likely to contribute to the epigenetic changes which impact male fertility. Smoking, stress, level of physical activity, diet, alcohol intake, and sleep disturbances such as shift work have been associated with male factor infertility and have been implicated in epigenetic changes [101,102]. Substances with recognized antiandrogenic effects such as air pollutants, soil pollutants, and plasticizers have been shown to have a negative impact on steroidogenesis and testosterone levels, resulting in male factor infertility [103]. Phthalates and other endocrine disruptors are commonly used for industrial purposes and are virtually unavoidable in consumer products. These compounds interfere with the normal cell cycle, may affect apoptosis signaling, and alter the epigenetic regulation of target cells. All of these mechanisms may serve as explanations for how specific substances can ultimately diminish a man's fertility potential [104].

It has been demonstrated that epigenetic factors may not only result in undesirable consequences for male fertility and paternal health, but may also negatively impact the health of future generations [105]. Exposures that provoke altered epigenetic programming within the paternal germ line have been shown to transmit epigenetically altered patterns and phenotypes to subsequent generations. These alterations can be found in offspring even in the absence of ongoing environmental exposures [105,106]. During germ cell development, there are several time periods where high degrees of epigenetic programming naturally occurs. These time frames represent critical windows of sensitivity to environmental factors. Exposure to toxins or endocrine disruptors during these periods can result in lasting epigenetic effects for offspring [107,108]. The period of gonadal sex determination during early testicular development and the time of fertilization appear to be two crucial points at which epigenetic factors are highly influenced by environmental insults [109].

There are several examples of environmental exposures which may result in epigenetic changes that ultimately lead to health ramifications in offspring. Paternal exposure to pesticides may result in nervous system tumors in children, cigarette smoking may result in increased rates of childhood leukemia, and chemicals related to woodwork and wood processing may increase rates of leukemia in children [110–112]. Exposure to ionizing radiation may result in increased DNA methylation and impaired DNA repair processes, which can lead to persistent instability of the male germ line and a predisposition to various cancers in offspring [113]. There is also some evidence that cardiovascular mortality in offspring may be related to epigenetic changes in the spermatozoa, although this effect may take multiple generations to manifest itself [114].

Paternal diet is another area which has been studied as a potential source of epigenetic changes. In developed nations, access to high-fat diets is frequently associated with obesity. In the United States, obesity currently affects 33.9% of the population greater than 20 years of age and is increasing at an alarming rate [16,115]. Aside from the known association between obesity and infertility in adult men, studies evaluating the impact of paternal obesity on epigenetics have demonstrated altered methylation patterns in offspring. These findings support the notion that developing sperm are susceptible to environmental insults related to diet and that obesity-related epigenetic abnormalities can be passed on to children [16]. Nonhuman animal model studies have discovered altered metabolic processing in the offspring of obese fathers [116]. In women, children born to mothers who underwent gastric bypass surgery and experienced weight reduction prior to pregnancy had markedly improved epigenetic profiles of receptor signaling in insulin, leptin, and glucoregulatory pathways compared to their siblings born prior to the bariatric surgery and weight loss [117]. This suggests that weight loss and dietary modification can reverse some of the abnormal epigenetic patterns seen in obese patients and potentially prevent vertical transmission of epigenetic aberrations.

Epigenetics and outcomes of assisted reproductive technology

Specific epigenetic aberrations can affect early embryonic development and success rates with ART [118]. It has been previously discussed in this chapter that epigenetic changes may lead to diminished fertility. However, it has been suggested that the use of ART can also induce epigenetic changes which may impact pregnancy outcomes and the health of offspring (Fig. 8.1). Studies analyzing the methylation status of CpG sites within gene promoters of the placenta and umbilical cord blood have been compared between children conceived spontaneously and those conceived through in vitro fertilization (IVF). The group of children conceived via IVF appeared

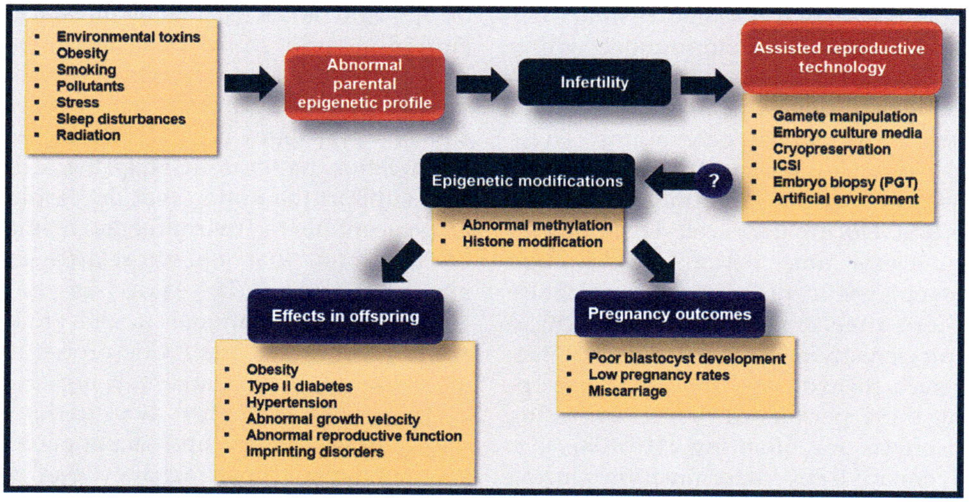

FIGURE 8.1 The relationship between epigenetics and assisted reproductive technology (ART).

to possess epigenetic alterations in genes involved in chronic metabolic disorders such as obesity, type II diabetes, and high blood pressure [119]. These findings are consistent with other studies which have reported an increased risk of obesity, changes in blood pressure, and increased late infancy growth velocity in children conceived via ART [120]. A higher prevalence of imprinting disorders such as Beckwith–Wiedemann syndrome and Angelman syndrome has also been reported in children born after ART when compared to children born following spontaneous conception [14,121–123].

Reported mechanisms by which ART results in epigenetic disturbances include gamete handling, embryonic exposure to culture media, cryopreservation, and procedures such as ICSI and embryo biopsy for purposes of preimplantation genetic testing [124,125]. Studies which proport ART as a cause of epigenetic remodeling claim that the nonphysiologic processes involved in the majority of infertility treatments lead to changes within the embryo which have downstream effects on health. Given the extensive gamete manipulation that occurs under artificial conditions, it is reasonable to hypothesize that ART creates alterations in the epigenetic profiles of embryos. However, it remains unclear whether observed epigenetic differences in embryos and offspring are entirely due to the ART procedures or to the underlying parental subfertility, which may itself be caused by epigenetic modifications [126].

From a paternal perspective, reports have suggested that the epigenetic defects that arise in embryos achieved via ART protocols are a consequence of the use of epigenetically abnormal sperm. Several authors have suggested that DNA methylation changes at imprinted loci are inherited from the sperm of men with oligozoospermia and do not arise from ART interventions [93,127]. Additionally, in a population of men with unexplained infertility, epigenetic alterations (decreased methylation) in histone-retained CpG sites impacted numerous genes involved in embryonic development. These epigenetic differences which originated from the sperm were associated with poor blastocyst development during IVF cycles [128]. Further supporting this idea, a 2017 study found that blastocysts derived from couples with a diagnosis of male factor infertility displayed transcription alterations with enrichment for genes involved in cancer processes. The transcription alterations which were observed were believed to be the result of epigenetic dysfunction of paternal origin [129].

A cross-sectional study evaluating the issue of paternal epigenetic modifications and IVF outcomes analyzed urinary phthalate concentrations in men prior to IVF cycles. As mentioned previously, phthalates are endocrine-disrupting compounds which are pervasive in the environment due to widespread industrial and commercial use [130]. A higher degree of phthalate exposure was associated with epigenetic change, demonstrated by abnormalities in sperm DMRs related to genes involved in growth and development, cell movement, and cytoskeleton structure. Epigenetic changes related to phthalate exposures were associated with lower quality blastocyst-stage embryos following IVF [131]. Importantly, not all studies support a direct relationship between male epigenetic dysfunction and poorer ART outcomes. A 2013 analysis of 119 normospermic men and 175 oligozoospermic men evaluated the methylation profiles of study participants and found that epimutations in the H19 DMR and PEG1/MEST DMR were more common in oligozoospermic men, but these epimethylations did not negatively impact ART outcome [132]. Despite conflicting evidence within the medical literature, the relationship between epigenetics and ART outcomes is an area which has a high level of clinical impact, and further studies will hopefully shed clarity on this topic.

Implications

The relationship between male infertility, genetics, and epigenetics is a subject of ongoing research. Numerous genetic and epigenetic factors are known to be involved in proper functioning of the male reproductive system, and in recent years, there has been a dramatic surge in scientific focus related to this area. To date, the most common identifiable genetic causes of male factor infertility remain Klinefelter syndrome and Y chromosome microdeletions of the AZF subregions. Unfortunately, a significant percentage of cases of male factor infertility remain unexplained. Efforts to identify genetic polymorphisms and defects related to the X chromosome which potentially underlie idiopathic cases of male infertility are under way. Men with severe spermatogenic defects have been the primary population of interest for current research. Going forward, studies may uncover more subtle genetic abnormalities which contribute to less severe forms of male factor infertility.

Investigations related to epigenetics have demonstrated that DNA methylation patterns and histone modifications play an important role in semen analysis parameters and the functional capacity of sperm. Environmental exposures and lifestyle appear to have a profound impact on the epigenetic landscape that is closely linked to male fertility. Through transgenerational inheritance, alterations in epigenetic programming appear to have consequences for both male fertility and the health of offspring. The effect of epigenetics on ART, early embryo development, and pregnancy outcomes is a controversial topic. As utilization of ART increases, it will be important to have a clear understanding of how underlying parental subfertility or ART interventions relate to observed epigenetic changes.

As technology advances, researchers and clinicians will likely have the ability to more precisely test for novel genetic and epigenetic disturbances which may negatively influence fertility. As etiologies that result in male infertility become clearer, researchers and physicians will hopefully be able to tailor fertility interventions and provide improved reproductive outcomes for men with a variety of genetic or epigenetic abnormalities. Overall, it is clear that the role of both genetics and epigenetics is a complex yet vital aspect of male reproductive health.

References

[1] Krausz C, Riera-Escamilla A. Genetics of male infertility. Nat Rev Urol 2018;15::369–84.
[2] Rives N. Y chromosome microdeletions and alterations of spermatogenesis, patient approach and genetic counseling. Ann Endocrinol 2014;75(2):112–14.
[3] Bendayan M, Alter L, Swierkowski-Blanchard N, Caceres-Sanchez L, Selva J, Robin G, et al. Environment and lifestyle: impacts on male fertility? Gynecol Obstet Fertil Senol 2018;46(1):47–56.
[4] Gunes S, Arslan MA, Hekim GNT, Asci R. The role of epigenetics in idiopathic male infertility. J Assist Reprod Genet 2016;33(5):553–69.
[5] Eisenberg M. Relationship between semen production and medical comorbidity. Fertil Steril 2015;103 (1):66–71.
[6] McLachlan R. Genetic causes of male infertility, <https://andrologyaustralia.org> [Accessed 20.02.19].
[7] Plaseska-Karanfilska D, Noveski P, Plaseski T, Maleva I, Madjunkova S, Moneva Z. Genetic causes of male infertility. BJMG 2012;Suppl. 15::31–4.
[8] Krausz C, Giachini C. Genetic risk factors in male infertility. Arch Androl 2007;53(3):125–33.
[9] Aitken RJ, Koopman P, Lewis SE. Seeds of concern. Nature., 432:. 2004. p. 48–52.
[10] Dada R, Kumar M, Jesudasan R, Fernandez JL, Gosalvez J, Agarwal A. Epigenetics and its role in male infertility. J Assist Reprod Genet 2012;29 (3):213–23.
[11] Li E. Chromatin modification and epigenetic reprogramming in mammalian development. Nat Rev Genet 2002;3(9):662–73.
[12] Talbert PB, Henikoff S. Spreading of silent chromatin: inaction at a distance. Nat Rev Genet 2006;7 (10):793–803.
[13] Emery BR, Carrell D. The effect of epigenetic sperm abnormalities on early embryogenesis. Asian J Androl 2006;8(2):131–42.
[14] Stuppia L, Franzago M, Ballerini P, Gatta V, Antonucci I. Epigenetics and male reproduction: the consequences of paternal lifestyle on fertility, embryo development, and children lifetime health. Clin Epigenetics 2015;7::120.
[15] Robertson S. Seminal plasma and male factor signalling in the female reproductive tract. Cell Tissue 2005;322:43–52.
[16] Craig J. Obesity, male infertility, and the sperm epigenome. Fertil Steril 2017;107(4):848–59.
[17] Jenkins TG, Aston K, James ER, Carrell DT. Sperm epigenetics in the study of male fertility, offspring health, and potential clinical applications. Syst Biol Reprod Med 2017;63(2):69–76.
[18] Xie C. Multicenter study of genetic abnormalities associated with severe oligospermia and non-obstructive azoospermia. J Int Med Res 2017;46(1):107–14 epub ahead of print.
[19] Aston K. Genetic susceptibility to male infertility: news from genome-wide association studies. Andrology 2014;2(3):1–7.
[20] Dong Y, Du RC, Jiang YT, Wu J, Li LL, Liu RZ. Impact of chromosomal translocations on male infertility, semen quality, testicular volume, and reproductive hormone levels. J Int Med Res 2012;40(6):2274–83.
[21] Zorrilla M. The genetics of infertility: current status of the field. Curr Genet Med Rep 2013;1(4):247–60.
[22] Balkan M. Cytogenetic and Y chromosome microdeletion screening studies in infertile males with oligozoospermia and azoospermia in southeast Turkey. J Assist Reprod Genet 2008;25(11–12):559–65.
[23] Lopes AM, Aston K, Thompson E, Carvalho F, Goncalves J, Huang N. Human spermatogenic failure purges deleterious mutation load from the autosomes and both sex chromosomes, including the gene DMRT1. PLoS Genet, 9. 2013. p. e1003349.
[24] Stouffs K, Vandermaelen D, Massart A, Menten B, Vergult S, Tournaye H. Array comparative genomic hybridization in male infertility. Hum Reprod 2012;27:921–9.
[25] Paduch DA, Bolyakov A, Cohen P, Travis A. Reproduction in men with Klinefelter syndrome: the past, the present, and the future. Semin Reprod Med 2009;27::137–48.
[26] Mehta A. Klinefelter syndrome: an argument for early aggressive hormonal and fertility management. Fertil Steril 2012;98(2):274–83.
[27] Calogero A. Klinefelter syndrome: cardiovascular abnormalities and metabolic disorders. J Endocrinol Invest 2017;40(7):705–12.
[28] Lanfranco F, Kamischke A, Zitzmann M, Nieschlag E. Klinefelter's syndrome. Lancet 2004;364(9430):273–83.
[29] Groth KA, Skakkebaek A, Host C, Gravholt CH, Bojesen A. Clinical review: Klinefelter syndrome—a clinical update. J Clin Endocrinol Metab 2013;98(1):20–30.
[30] Bojesen A, Juul S, Gravholt CH. Prenatal and postnatal prevalence of Klinefelter syndrome: a national registry study. J Clin Endocrinol Metab 2003;88::622–6.

[31] Aksglaede L, Skakkebaek NE, Almstrup K, Juul A. Clinical and biological parameters in 166 boys, adolescents and adults with nonmosaic Klinefelter syndrome: a Copenhagen experience. Acta Paediatr 2011;100:793–806.
[32] Ramasamy R, Ricci J, Palermo GD, Gosden LV, Rosenwaks Z, Schlegel PN. Successful fertility treatment for Klinefelter's syndrome. J Urol 2009;182::1108–13.
[33] Bearelly P, Oates R. Recent advances in managing and understanding Klinefelter syndrome. F1000Res. 2019;8:112.
[34] Rajender A, Oates R. Evaluation and management of Klinefelter syndrome. Update Series (Lesson 24). Linthicum: American Urological Association; 2018.
[35] Ottesen AM, Aksglaede L, Garn I. Increased number of sex chromosomes affects height in a nonlinear fashion: a study of 305 patients with sex chromosome aneuploidy. Am J Med Genet 2017;55(33):9557–61.
[36] Bonomi M, Rochira V, Pasquali D. Klinefelter syndrome (KS): genetics, clinical phenotype and hypogonadism. J Endocrinol Invest 2017;40(2):123–34.
[37] Winge SB, Dalgaard MD, Jensen JM. Transcriptome profiling of fetal Klinefelter testis tissue reveals a possible involvement of long non-coding RNAs in gonocyte maturation. Hum Mol Genet 2018;27(3):430–9.
[38] Winge SB, Dalgaard MD, Belling KG. Transcriptome analysis of the adult human Klinefelter testis and cellularity-matched controls reveals disturbed differentiation of Sertoli- and Leydig cells. Cell Death Dis 2018;9(6):586.
[39] Foresta C, Ferlin A, Moro E, Scandellari C. Y Chromosome. Lancet. 2000;355(9199):234–5.
[40] Zaimy MA, Kalantar SM, Sheikhha MH. The frequency of Yq microdeletion in azoospermic and oligospermic Iranian infertile men. Iran J Reprod Med 2013;11::453–8.
[41] ASRM. Management of nonobstructive azoospermia: a committee opinion. Fertil Steril 2018;110(7):1239–45.
[42] Johnson M, Raheem A, DeLuca F, Hallerstrom M, Zainal Y, Poselay S, et al. An analysis of the frequency of Y-chromosome microdeletions and the determination of a threshold sperm concentration for genetic testing in infertile men. BJU Int 2019;123(2):367–72.
[43] Nailwal M, Chauhan JB. Azoospermia factor C subregion of the Y chromosome. J Hum Reprod Sci 2017;10 (4):256–60.
[44] ASRM. Evaluation of the azoospermic male: a committee opinion. Fertil Steril 2018;109::777–82.
[45] Hopps CV, Mielnik A, Goldstein M, Palermo GD, Rosenwaks Z, Schlegel PN. Detection of sperm in men with Y chromosome microdeletions of the AZFa, AZFb and AZFc regions. Hum Reprod 2003;18 (8):1660–5.
[46] Oates RD, Silber S, Brown LG, Page DC. Clinical characterization of 42 oligospermic or azoospermic men with microdeletion of the AZFc region of the Y chromosome, and of 18 children conceived via ICSI. Hum Reprod 2002;17(11):2813–24.
[47] Sabbaghian M, Mohseni Meybodi A, Rafaee A, Saba S, Zamanian M, Sadighi-Gilani MA. Sperm retrieval rate and reproductive outcome of infertile men with azoospermia factor c deletion. Andrologia 2018;50(7):e13052.
[48] Navarro-Costa P, Gonçalves J, Plancha CE. The AZFc region of the Y chromosome: at the crossroads between genetic diversity and male infertility. Hum Reprod Update 2010;16::525–42.
[49] Fernandes S, Paracchini S, Meyer LH, Floridia G, Tyler-Smith C, Vogt PH. A large AZFc deletion removes DAZ3/DAZ4 and nearby genes from men in Y haplogroup. N Am J Hum Genet 2004;74::180–7.
[50] Kuroda-Kawaguchi T, Skaletsky H, Brown LG, Minx PJ, Cordum HS, Waterston RH. The AZFc region of the Y chromosome features massive palindromes and uniform recurrent deletions in infertile men. Nat Genet 2001;29::279–86.
[51] Visser L, Westerveld GH, Korver CM, Van Daalen SK, Hoving SE, Rozen S. Y chromosome gr/gr deletions are a risk factor for low semen quality. Hum Reprod 2009;24::2667–73.
[52] Bansal SK, Jaiswal D, Gupta N, Singh K, Dada R, Sankhwar SN. Gr/gr deletions on Y-chromosome correlate with male infertility: an original study, meta-analyses, and trial sequential analyses. Sci Rep 2016;6::19798.
[53] Lee SH, Ahn SY, Lee KW, Kwack K, Jun HS, Cha KY. Intracytoplasmic sperm injection may lead to vertical transmission, expansion, and de novo occurrence of Y-chromosome microdeletions in male fetuses. Fertil Steril 2006;85::1512–15.
[54] Nailwal JC. Screening of Y-chromosome microdeletion in the AFZc sub-region of infertile men, Gujarat, India. IJBPAS 2016;5:2828–39.
[55] Sathyanarayana SH, Malini SSN. Impact of Y chromosome AZFc subdeletion shows lower risk of fertility impairment in Siddi tribal men, Western Ghats, India. Basic Clin Androl 2015;25::1.
[56] Stouffs K, Vandermaelen D, Tournaye H, Liebaers I, VanSteirteghem A, Lissens W. Genetics and male infertility. Verh K Acad Geneeskd Belg 2009;71 (3):115–39.
[57] Jensen M, Leffers H, Petersen JH, Nyboe-Andersen A, Jorgensen N, Carlsen E, et al. Frequent polymorphism of the mitochondrial DNA polymerase gamma gene (POLG) in patients with normal spermiograms and unexplained subfertility. Hum Reprod 2004;19 (1):65–70.

[58] Plaseski T, Noveski P, Dimitrovski C, Efremov GD, Plaseska-Karanfilska D. CAG repeat polymorphism of the mitochondrial DNA polymerase gamma gene in Macedonian infertile and fertile men. BJMG 2007;10 (2):37–42.
[59] Plaseski T, Noveski P, Popeska Z, Emremov GD, Plseska-Karanfilska D. Association study of single-nucleotide polymorphisms in FASLG, JMJDIA, LOC203413, TEX15, BRDT, OR2W3, INSR, and TAS2R38 genes with male infertility. J Androl 2012;33 (4):675–83.
[60] Z A, Zhang S, Yang Y, Ma Y, Lin L, Zhang W. Single nucleotide polymorphisms of the gonadotrophin-regulated testicular helicase (GRTH) gene may be associated with human spermatogenesis impairment. Hum Reprod 2006;21(3):755–9.
[61] Zhang W, Zhang S, Xiao C, Yang Y, Zhoucun A. Mutation screening of the FKBP6 gene and its association study with spermatogenic impairment in idiopathic infertile men. Reproduction. 2007;133(2):511–16.
[62] Deng Y, Zhang W, Su D, Yang Y, Ma Y, Zhang H, et al. Some single nucleotide polymorphisms of MSY2 gene might contribute to susceptibility to spermatogenic impairment in idiopathic infertile men. Urology 2008;71(5):878–82.
[63] Zhang H, Su D, Yang Y, Zhang W, Liu Y, Bai G, et al. Some single-nucleotide polymorphisms of the TSSK2 gene may be associated with human spermatogenesis impairment. J Androl 2010;31(4):388–92.
[64] Ni MX, Zhi H, Liu SM, Zhu PR, Zhang J, Wu QY, et al. Single nucleotide polymorphism of the TP53 gene is not correlated with male infertility. Zhonghua Nan Ke Xue 2017;23(2):142–6.
[65] Zhu PR, Wu Q, Yu MM, Zhang MC, Ni MX, Liu SM, et al. Nucleotide polymorphism rs4880 of the SOD2 gene and the risk of male infertility. Zhonghua Nan Ke Xue 2017;23(2):137–41.
[66] Ji G, Gu A, Wang Y, Huang C, Hu F, Zhou Y, et al. Genetic variants in antioxidant genes are associated with sperm DNA damage and risk of male infertility in a Chinese population. Free Radic Biol Med 2012;52 (4):775–80.
[67] Ropke A, Tüttelmann F. Mechanisms in endocrinology: aberrations of the X chromosome as cause of male infertility. Eur J Endocrinol 2017;177(5):R250–9.
[68] Mueller JL, Skaletsky H, Brown LG, Zaghlul S, Rock S, Graves T, et al. Independent specialization of the human and mouse X chromosomes for the male germ line. Nat Genet 2013;45::1083–7.
[69] Burgoyne P. Genetic homology and crossing over in the X and Y chromosomes of mammals. Hum Genet 1982;61::85–90.
[70] Helena-Mangs A, Morris Brian J. The human pseudoatosomal region (PAR): origin, function and future. Curr Genomics 2007;8::129–36.
[71] Anik A, Çatl G, Abaci A, Bober E. 46,XX male disorder of sexual development: a case report. J Clin Res Pediatr Endocrinol 2013;5(4):258–60.
[72] Ma Rigola MC, Ribas I, Egozcue J, Miro R, Fuster C. A comparative genomic hybridization study in a 46,XX male. Fertil Steril 2002;78::186–8.
[73] Verona E, Zitzmann M, Gromoll J, Churing AN, Nieschlag E. Clinical, endocrinological, and epigenetic features of the 46,XX male syndrome, compared with 47,XXY Klinefelter patients. J Clin Endocrinol Metab 2007;92::3458–65.
[74] Weil D, Wang I, Dietrich A, Poustka A, Weissenbach J, Petit C. Highly homologous loci on the X and Y chromosomes are hotspots for ectopic recombinations leading to XX maleness. Nat Genet 1994;7::414–19.
[75] Pan B, Li R, Chen Y, Tang Q, Wu W, Chen L, et al. Genetic association between androgen receptor gene CAG repeat length polymorphism and male infertility: a meta-analysis. Medicine (Baltimore) 2016;95(10): e2878.
[76] Brooks BP, Fischbeck KH. Spinal and bulbar muscular atrophy: a trinucleotide-repeat expansion neurodegenerative disease. Trends Neurosci 1995;18::459–61.
[77] Tut TG, Ghadessy F, Trifiro MA, Pinsky L, Young EL. Long polyglutamine tracts in the androgen receptor are associated with reduced trans-activation, impaired sperm production, and male infertility. J Clin Endocrinol Metab 1997;82::3777–82.
[78] Hughes IA, Davies JD, Bunch TI, Pasterski V, Mastroyannopoulou K, MacDougall J. Androgen insensitivity syndrome. Lancet. 2012;380 (9851):1419–28.
[79] Adelman CA, Petrini J. ZIP4H (TEX11) deficiency in the mouse impairs meiotic double strand break repair and the regulation of crossing over. PLoS Genet 2008;4::e1000042.
[80] Yatsenko AN, Georgiadis AP, Ropke A, Berman AJ, Jaffe T, Olszewska M, et al. X-linked TEX11 mutations, meiotic arrest, and azoospermia in infertile men. NEJM 2015;372:2097–107.
[81] Sha Y, Zheng Liangkai, Ji Z, Mei L, Ding L, Lin S, et al. A novel TEX11 mutation induces azoospermia: a case report of infertile brothers and literature review. BMC Med Genet 2018;19(1):63.
[82] Borgmann J, Tüttelmann F, Dworniczak B, Ropke A, Song HW, Kliesch S, et al. The human RHOX gene cluster: target genes and functional analysis of gene variants in infertile men. Hum Mol Genet 2016;25::4898–910.

[83] Young J, Xu C, Papadakis GE, Acierno JS, Maione L, Hietamaki J, et al. Clinical management of congenital hypogonadotropic hypogonadism. Endocr Rev 2019;40(2):669–710 epub ahead of print.

[84] Dirac AMG, Bernards R. The deubiquitinating enzyme USP26 is a regulator of androgen receptor signaling. Mol Cancer Res 2010;8::844–54.

[85] Zhou H, Grubisic I, Zheng K, He Y, Wang PJ, Kaplan T, et al. Taf7l cooperates with Trf2 to regulate spermiogenesis. Proc Natl Acad Sci USA 2013;110::16886–91.

[86] Waddington C. The epigenotype. Endeavour 1942;1::18–20.

[87] Bestor T, Laudano A, Mattaliano R, Ingram V. Cloning and sequencing of a cDNA encoding DNA methyltransferase of mouse cells. The carboxyl-terminal domain of the mammalian enzymes is related to bacterial restriction methyltransferases. J Mol Biol 1988;203(4):971–83.

[88] Lachner M, O'Sullivan RJ, Junewein T. An epigenetic road map for histone lysine methylation. J Cell Sci 2003;116(Pt11):2117–24.

[89] Allegrucci C, Thurston A, Lucas E, Young L. Epigenetics and the germline. Reproduction. 2005;129 (2):137–49.

[90] Kimmins S, Sassone-Corsi P. Chromatin remodelling and epigenetic features of germ cells. Nature 2005;434(7033):583–9.

[91] Kitamura A, Miyauchi N, Hamada H, Hiura H, Chiba H, Okae H, et al. Epigenetic alterations in sperm associated with male infertility. Congenit Anom 2015;55::133–44.

[92] Sato A, Hiura H, Okae H. Assessing loss of imprint methylation in sperm from subfertile men using novel methylation polymerase chain reaction Luminex analysis. Fertil Steril 2011;95::129–34.

[93] Kobayashi H. DNA methylation errors at imprinted loci after assisted conception originate in the parental sperm. Eur J Hum Genet 2009;17(12):1582–91.

[94] Schon SB, Luense L, Wang X, Bartolomei MS, Coutifaris C, Garcia BA, et al. Histone modification signatures in human sperm distinguish clinical abnormalities. J Assist Reprod Genet 2018;36 (2):267–75 Epub ahead of print.

[95] Tang Q, Pen F, Yang J, Fu Z, Lu Y, Wu X, et al. Idiopathic male infertility is strongly associated with aberrant DNA methylation of imprinted loci in sperm: a case-control study. Clin Epigenetics 2018;10::134.

[96] Levine H, Jørgensen N, Martino-Andrade A, Mendiola J, Weksler-Derri D, Mindlis I, et al. Temporal trends in sperm count: a systematic review and meta-regression analysis. Hum Reprod Update 2017;23(6):646–59.

[97] Macosko EZ, Basu A, Satija R, Nemesh J, Shekhar K, Goldman M. Highly parallel genome-wide expression profiling of individual cells using nanoliter droplets. Cell Biochem Biophys 2015;161:1202–14.

[98] Aoki VW, Emery BR, Liu L, Carrell DT. Protamine levels vary between individual sperm cells of infertile human males and correlate with viability and DNA integrity. J Androl 2006;27::890–8.

[99] Guillette LJ, Iguchi T. Life in a contaminated world. Science 2012;337:1614–15.

[100] Guerrero-Bosagna C, Skinner MK. Environmentally induced epigenetic transgenerational inheritance of phenotype and disease. Mol Cell Endocrinol 2012;354::3–8.

[101] Alegria-Torres J. Epigenetics and lifestyle. Epigenomics. 2011;3::267–77.

[102] Sharma R. Lifestyle factors and reproductive health: taking control of your fertility. Reprod Biol Endocrinol 2013;11:66.

[103] DiNisio A, Foresta C. Water and soil pollution determinant of water and food quality/contamination and its impact on male fertility. Reprod Biol Endocrinol 2019;17(4):1–13.

[104] Sifakis S, Androutsopoulos VP, Tsatsakis AM, Spandidos DA. Human exposure to endocrine disrupting chemicals: effects on the male and female reproductive systems. Environ Toxicol Pharmacol 2017;40::241–58.

[105] Schagdarsurengin U, Steger K. Epigenetics in male reproduction: effect of paternal diet on sperm quality and offspring health. Nat Rev Urol 2016;13 (10):584–95.

[106] Skinner M. Environmental epigenetic transgenerational inheritance and somatic epigenetic mitotic stability. Epigenetics 2011;6::838–42.

[107] Jirtle RL, Skinner M. Environmental epigenomics and disease susceptibility. Nat Rev Genet 2007;8::253–62.

[108] Nilsson EE, Skinner MK. Environmentally induced epigenetic transgenerational inheritance of reproductive disease. Biol Reprod 2015;93(6):145–52.

[109] Messerschmidt DM, Knowles BB, Solter D. DNA methylation dynamics during epigenetic reprogramming in the germline and preimplantation embryos. Genes Dev 2014;28::812–28.

[110] Feychting M. Paternal occupational exposures and childhood cancer. Environ Health Perspect 2001;109::193–6.

[111] Reid A. Parental occupational exposure to exhausts, solvents, glues and paints, and risk of childhood leukemia. Cancer Causes Control 2011;22::1575–85.

[112] Liu R. Paternal smoking and risk of childhood acute lymphoblastic leukemia: systematic review and meta-analysis. J Oncol 2011;2011:1–16.
[113] Dubrova Y. Transgenerational mutation by radiation. Nature 2000;405:37.
[114] Bygren L. Change in paternal grandmothers early food supply influenced cardiovascular mortality of the female grandchildren. BMC Genet 2014;15:12.
[115] NCHS. National Center for Health Statistics: Health, United States, 2008, with chartbook. National Center for Health Statistics; 2009.
[116] DeCastro-Barbosa T, Ingerslev LR, Alm PS, Versteyhe S, Massart J, Rasmussen M. High-fat diet reprograms the epigenome of rat spermatozoa and transgenerationally affects metabolism of the offspring. Mol Metab 2016;5:184–97.
[117] Berglind D, Müller P, Willmer M, Sinha I, Tynelius P, Naslund E. Differential methylation in inflammation and type 2 diabetes genes in siblings born before and after maternal bariatric surgery. Obesity. 2016;24::250–61.
[118] Giacone F, Cannarella R, Mongioi LM, Alamo A, Condorelli RA, Calogero AE, et al. Epigenetics of male fertility: effects on assisted reproductive techniques. World J Mens Health 2018;37(2):148–56.
[119] Katari S, Turan N, Bibikova M, Erinle O, Chalian R, Foster M. DNA methylation and gene expression differences in children conceived in vitro or in vivo. Hum Mol Genet 2009;18::3769–78.
[120] Ceelen M, van Weissenbruch MM, Vermeiden JP, Van Leeuwen FE, Delemarre-Vande Waal HA. Cardiometabolic differences in children born after in vitro fertilization. J Clin Endocrinol Metab 2008;93:1682–8.
[121] Gosden R, Trasler J, Lucifero D, Faddy M. Rare congenital disorders, imprinted genes, and assisted reproductive technology. Lancet. 2003;361:1975–7.
[122] DeBaun MR, Niemitz EL, Feinberg AP. Association of in vitro fertilization with Beckwith-Wiedemann syndrome and epigenetic alterations of LIT1 and H19. Am J Hum Genet 2003;73::156–60.
[123] Gicquel C, Gaston V, Mandelbaum J, Siffroi JP, Flahault A, LeBouc Y. In vitro fertilization may increase the risk of Beckwith-Wiedemann syndrome related to the abnormal imprinting of the KCN1OT gene. Am J Hum Genet 2003;72::1338–41.
[124] Jiang Z, Wang Y, Lin J, Xu J, Ding G, Huang H. Genetic and epigenetic risks of assisted reproduction. Best Pract Res Clin Obstet Gynaecol 2017;44::90–104.
[125] Niemitz EL, Feinberg AP. Epigenetics and assisted reproductive technology: a call for investigation. Am J Hum Genet 2004;74:599–609.
[126] Litzky JF, Deyssenroth MA, Everson TM, Armstrong DA, Lambertini L, Chen J, et al. Placental imprinting variation associated with assisted reproductive technologies and subfertility. Epigenetics 2017;12 (8):653–61.
[127] Marques CJ, Costa P, Vaz B, Carvalho F, Fernandes S, Barros A. Abnormal methylation of imprinted genes in human sperm is associated with oligozoospermia. Mol Hum Reprod 2008;14::67–74.
[128] Denomme MM, McCallie BR, Parks JC, Schoolcraft WB, Katz-Jaffe MG. Alterations in the sperm histone-retained epigenome are associated with unexplained male factor infertility and poor blastocyst development in donor oocyte IVF cycles. Hum Reprod 2017;32(12):2443–55.
[129] McCallie BR, Parks JC, Griffin DK, Schoolcraft WB, Katz-Jaffe MG. Infertility diagnosis has a significant impact on the transcriptoms of developing blastocysts. Mol Hum Reprod 2017;23(8):549–56.
[130] Sedha S, Kumar S, Shukla S. Role of oxidative stress in male reproductive dysfunctions with reference to phthalate compounds. Urol J 2015;12(5):2304–16.
[131] Wu H, Estill MS, Shershebnev A, Suvorov A, Krawetz SA, Whitcomb BW, et al. Preconception urinary phthalate concentrations and sperm DNA methylation profiles among men undergoing IVF treatment: a cross-sectional study. Hum Reprod 2017;32(11):2159–69.
[132] Montjean D, Ravel C, Benkhalifa M, Cohen-Bacrie P, Berthaut I, Bashamboo A. Methylation changes in mature sperm deoxyribonucleic acid from oligozoospermic men: assessment of genetic variants and assisted reproductive technology outcome. Fertil Steril 2013;100::1241–7.

CHAPTER

9

Mitochondrial genetics

Elpida Fragouli[1,2]

[1]IVI RMA Global, Magdalen Centre, Oxford Science Park, Oxford, United Kingdom

[2]Nuffield Department of Obstetrics and Gynaecology, University of Oxford, John Radcliffe Hospital, Oxford, United Kingdom

Introduction

Mitochondria are among the more interesting cellular organelles. They are key regulators of several critical cellular processes, such as the buffering of cytosolic calcium, apoptosis via the mitochondrial permeability transition pore, and other signaling pathways [1]. Their main role, however, is the generation of energy in the form of adenosine triphosphate (ATP) via the biochemical reaction of oxidative phosphorylation (OXPHOS) [2,3]. OXPHOS takes place in the electron transport chain (ETC), which is located in the inner mitochondrial membrane [4]. Mitochondria originated from bacteria which were endosymbionts in the eukaryotic cell [5]. They are unique, compared to other cellular organelles, because they contain one or more copies of their own genome, the mitochondrial DNA (mtDNA).

The human mitochondrial genome is a circular double-stranded molecule of 16.6 kb in size, encoding for 37 genes [6]. Of these, 13 are responsible for the ETC complexes I, III, IV, and V subunit construction, and the remaining encode for 22 tRNAs and two rRNAs [7]. The genes involved in the construction of the subunits of all other ETC complexes, and those responsible for the rest of the mitochondrial transcriptional and translational machinery are encoded by the nuclear genome [6,7]. Similar to the ETC, the mtDNA is located in the inner mitochondrial membrane. The mtDNA's location, as well as its lack if histones, leave it vulnerable to the deleterious effects of reactive oxygen species (ROS), generated during OXPHOS, and make it particularly prone to mutations [8].

The mitochondrial genome consists of different polymorphic variant combinations, which are associated with populations from specific regions or continents. The polymorphic variants determine an individual's mitochondrial haplotype [9]. Human mtDNA haplogroups are classified into several categories, each of which has been given a letter of the alphabet (A–Z). The origin of the mtDNA haplogroups traces back to the most recent common maternal ancestor for all living humans, known as Mitochondrial Eve (reviewed in Ref. [10]). It is thought that mitochondrial haplogroups may be capable of influencing

DOI: https://doi.org/10.1016/B978-0-12-816561-4.00009-0

processes such as spermatogenesis [11], the incidence of meiotic chromosome errors during oogenesis [12], and predisposition to age-associated disorders [1].

As mitochondria are the main providers of energy in the form of ATP, they can be considered to be the powerhouses of the cell. The generation of mitochondrial energy is necessary to support a multitude of cellular processes, including several associated with reproduction and embryogenesis. This chapter covers different aspects related to mitochondrial genetics during gametogenesis and preimplantation embryo development.

Mitochondrial inheritance and replication

Mitochondria and their genome have a non-Mendelian pattern of inheritance, and they are passed from a mother to her children [13]. The inherited mtDNA molecules are genetically homogeneous, or homoplasmic. Cases in which a subpopulation of the mtDNA molecules within a cell carry a sequence variation that may end up affecting mitochondrial function are generally infrequent. The subpopulation of the variant mtDNA molecules is characterized as heteroplasmic. The likelihood of clinically significant heteroplasmy being present through generations is reduced by a mechanism known as the genetic bottleneck [14]. The genetic bottleneck regulates mitochondrial segregation during oogenesis, through the elimination of most of the egg's mtDNA molecules, with only a small population ultimately being passed to the next generation [15]. The result of this regulatory mechanism is either the removal of mutated mtDNA molecules, or their increase above a critical level of heteroplasmy, potentially leading to mitochondrial disease. It is thought that the genetic bottleneck takes place toward the end of oogenesis, and can be influenced by different mutations [15].

Sperm mitochondria enter the oocyte after fertilization, but are lost during early embryogenesis through a ubiquitination and autophagy process ([16,17]). Elimination of sperm mitochondria is thought to take place for two different reasons: to avoid transmission of mtDNA mutations acquired due to ROS exposure during spermatogenesis, and to protect the embryo from potentially pathogenic levels of heteroplasmy [17–19]. There have been some recent reports of paternally derived mitochondria persisting in individuals of some families [20], however, such cases are rare.

Mitochondrial organelle replication starts after implantation [21]. Hence, the early embryo is supported energetically by the oocyte's mitochondria. It should be noted that the timing of the mitochondrial genome replication differs from that of the actual organelle. Specifically, during the initial embryonic cleavage divisions, the oocyte provides the newly formed blastomeres with its own mitochondria and mtDNA [22–24], and this means that the amounts of mtDNA remain stable. mtDNA replication begins after the embryo has differentiated into a blastocyst, and it is first observed in the trophectoderm (TE) part [2,3,25–27], due to the advanced differentiation state of this tissue, which is destined to give rise to the fetal placenta (i.e., pluripotency loss). Conversely, the inner cell mass (ICM) part needs to maintain pluripotency until later in fetal development. Therefore ICM mtDNA replication is initiated once cellular tissues of different fetal parts are formed [3].

mtDNA replication is under strict regulatory control by several nuclear-encoded genes, such as the transcription factor TFAM which stabilizes mtDNA, and Peo1/SSbp1 which unwinds it. Moreover, the role of the polymerase POLGA/B is critical for the maintenance of the efficiency and fidelity of mtDNA replication [28], while the mitochondrial helicase Twinkle and the mitochondrial single-stranded binding protein are also very important [29,30]. These proteins along with the transcription factors TFB1M, TFB2M, the mtRNA polymerase, and mTERF1 constitute the core mtDNA nucleoid and ensure the correct transcription, replication, and packaging of the mitochondrial genome [31]. Mitochondrial biogenesis is regulated by the nuclear genome also, via the AMP-activated kinase, and the transcription factors PPARg coactivator-1 a/b (PGC-1) and Nrf-1/2 [32]. Each mitochondrion contains between 1 and 15 copies of the mtDNA [33], whereas each nucleoid is thought to consist from 1 to 3 mtDNA molecules [34].

The processes of fusion and fission are critical for correct mitochondrial function. Specifically, mitochondrial replication occurs via fission, which leads to the generation of new organelles during cell division, ensuring in this way that the number of mitochondria in the daughter cells remains the same as in the mother cell [35]. Additionally, fission facilitates the isolation of damaged or dysfunctional mitochondria. Autophagosomes target such organelles, and deliver them to lysosomes to be recycled (mitophagy). The process of fusion ensures the correct function of the mitochondria, and the distribution of mtDNA molecules in the entirety of the organelle [36]. It is also thought that fusion can rescue damaged mitochondria from undergoing mitophagy [37]. Fission and fusion are under the genetic regulation of the nuclear genome, through several factors, including mitofusin 1 and 2, and the GTPase dynamin-related protein [38].

Mitochondrial diseases

Studies assessing the rate of nucleotide substitutions seen in the mitochondrial genome of primate and human somatic tissues observed that it was evolving at a much higher rate compared to the nuclear genome [39–41]. These findings suggested that mutations are occurring much more frequently in the mitochondrial genome. A possible cause for the higher mtDNA mutation rate is ROS, due to the mtDNA's proximity to the ETC, in combination with its lack of histones and limited DNA repair capability. These mutations may have an effect on the ETC complexes' function, disrupting in this way the bioenergetics and leading to the generation of more ROS in a feedback loop [42]. mtDNA mutations are also caused due to errors taking place during replication via the polymerase gamma mechanism. It has been proposed that mistakes during replication are likely to be leading to mtDNA mutations more frequently, compared to those due to ROS (reviewed in Ref. [43]).

mtDNA mutations arising in oocytes are inherited, and depending on the number of affected molecules, may end up manifesting in children in the form of a mitochondrial disease. Wallace and colleagues [44] were the first to identify inherited mitochondrial diseases. Currently over 250 disease-causing mutations have been described, including point mutations and deletions [45].

Mitochondrial diseases are associated with several clinical symptoms most commonly affecting organs dependent on the generation of energy via OXPHOS, such as the brain, kidneys, heart, muscle, liver, and pancreas. The disease severity is affected by the type of mutation, and whether it is present in heteroplasmic or homoplasmic form, whereas their incidence is thought to be approximately one in every 200 newborns [46].

Mitochondrial diseases are incurable and can end up being debilitating or even lethal. The Mitochondrial Medicine Society has recently come up with some recommendations on certain therapies that could help individuals affected by mitochondrial disease. Specifically, certain supplements such as the reduced form CoQ10 (ubiquinol), alpha-lipoic acid, and riboflavin can be prescribed to mitochondrial disease patients. Others, such as L-carnitine or folinic acid can also be administered when patients are deficient [47].

Research has also focused on identifying ways of preventing the transmission of mitochondrial diseases from a carrier woman to her children, and several different approaches have been proposed. The safest is the use of oocyte donation. The issue with this approach is that the children conceived will be genetically related to the male partner, but not the female partner. Routine prenatal diagnosis is also feasible, but it is not advisable due to the inability to accurately predict the phenotype. The use of preimplantation genetic testing (PGT) to examine the presence and load of a mitochondrial mutation in the embryos generated by a carrier of this mutation has also been used, especially in cases of heteroplasmic mutations [48]. PGT has been clinically employed to identify several different mtDNA mutations, with blastomere and blastocyst biopsy both leading to accurate mutation detection and load prediction [49–53].

Two slightly different strategies have been proposed in order to enable carriers of homoplasmic mtDNA mutations or high-load heteroplasmic mtDNA mutations establish healthy pregnancies and the birth of unaffected children. Both involve transplanting the nuclear genome between oocytes before or after fertilization [45,54,55]. Transplantation of the nuclear genome from an oocyte affected by an mtDNA mutation to an enucleated oocyte provided by a healthy donor before fertilization has been defined as spindle transfer [45,54], while if this process takes place after fertilization, it is defined as pronuclear transfer [55]. The efficacy and safety of these strategies are still under evaluation, although spindle transfer has been employed clinically for the prevention of Leigh syndrome (caused by a heteroplasmic mtDNA 8993T > G mutation) and led to the birth of a healthy boy [56].

A summary of the different types of mitochondrial disease inheritance and associated symptoms is shown in Table 9.1.

Mitochondria in oocytes

An oocyte is deemed competent when it is able to complete maturation, become normally fertilized when it encounters sperm, resume and complete the second meiotic division, and support the embryo through its first few mitotic divisions, until it activates its own genome with its stored messenger RNA (mRNA) transcripts and proteins. Oocyte competence is a combination of many factors, including a correct chromosome number, as well as an adequate number of cytoplasmic organelles. The fact that, in their majority, chromosome errors observed in abnormal pregnancies and miscarriages arise during oogenesis is well known. The close relationship between advancing female age and an increase in chromosome malsegregation is also well established [57,58].

Oocyte competence acquisition is achieved during its growth in the follicle, and through the interaction with its surrounding cumulus and granulosa cells, and the follicular fluid [59]. The events leading to oocyte competence require energy in the form of ATP, which means that mitochondria are key influencers during this process [60,61]. The morphology of the mitochondria in the cytoplasm of a metaphase II oocyte is different compared to those found in somatic cells. Specifically, oocyte mitochondria are spherical with a 1 μM diameter, consisting of a few truncated cristae that surround a high-electron density matrix [6,62]. Despite their relatively immature morphology, oocyte mitochondria are functional and active in ATP generation through the OXPHOS reaction. This ATP will in turn provide the energy needed to take the embryo from fertilization to the blastocyst stage [6,63].

The number and distribution of mitochondria within the oocyte are believed to be critical determinants of its competence. It has been reported that good-quality oocytes have large

TABLE 9.1 The different inheritance types of mitochondrial diseases and associated symptoms.

Mitochondrial disease inheritance type	Mitochondrial disease symptoms
Autosomal recessive: The mutated gene is present in the nuclear genome. Both parents must be carriers of the mutated gene to transmit the mitochondrial disease to their offspring. There is a 25% risk for a child to be affected	*Muscular*: muscle weakness and pain, decreased muscular tone, and movement disorders
Autosomal dominant: The mutated gene is present in the nuclear genome. One of the two parents must be a carrier of the mutated gene to transmit the mitochondrial disease to their offspring. There is a 50% risk of a child being affected	*Gastrointestinal*: unexplained vomiting, difficulty in swallowing, diarrhea or constipation, reflux, and cramping
	Neurological: migraines, seizures, strokes, and dementia
	Heart, liver, and/or kidney disease
	Respiratory problems
	Thyroid problems
	Diabetes
	Lactic acidosis
	Vision and/or hearing impairment
Mitochondrial: The mutated gene is present in the mitochondrial genome and is transmitted exclusively from the mother to her offspring. The risk and severity of the mitochondrial disease will depend on whether the mutation is present in heteroplasmic or homoplasmic form in the maternal mitochondria	Poor growth
	Autism-like symptoms
	Learning difficulties and mental disabilities
	Increased risk of infection
De novo: The mutated gene is not present in either of the parents. The mutation arises spontaneously in the child	

numbers of evenly distributed mitochondria [59]. Considering that there is no mitochondria replication during preimplantation development, a large mitochondrial number and an even distribution in the oocyte's cytoplasm would ensure that the embryonic blastomeres will receive an adequate number of organelles [63,64]. Data on the number of mitochondria and their genome reported by different studies vary considerably. These investigations have suggested that a mature metaphase II oocyte contains ~100,000 mitochondria and between 50,000 and 550,000 copies of the mitochondrial genome [2,23,65].

Advancing female age has been shown to alter mitochondria and mtDNA copy number and morphology in animal and human oocytes. Older mice and hamster oocytes have been described as having structural differences in their mitochondria, compared to the oocytes of younger animals [66]. These differences included the presence of vacuoles, less well-defined cristae, and less electron-dense matrices in the oocytes of older animals. It should be noted that the fertility of the older animals was reduced, compared to the younger animals [66]. Some studies have also observed a decline in the mtDNA copy number of mouse, hamster, and cow oocytes [66–68], whereas such a decrease was not evident in others [69–71].

Data obtained during the analysis of human oocyte mitochondria and mtDNA copy number in relation to female age have also been contradictory. Specifically, some research groups have reported that mtDNA quantities are closely related to reproductive age, as calculated by follicle-stimulating hormone measurements, rather than chronological age [72], whereas others observed significant mtDNA quantity decreases in the oocytes of older women, compared to younger ones [22,73]. A significant decrease in oocyte/cumulus cell mtDNA quantity has also been observed in relation to endometriosis and reduced ovarian reserve [2,74]. Combination of the findings from these studies suggests that mitochondria and/or mtDNA dysfunction will adversely affect the competence of oocytes generated by reproductively older women.

Mitochondria are the main energy providers during both oocyte meiotic divisions with ATP levels increasing during polar body (PB) extrusion [75]. They can be found to aggregate around the first and second meiotic spindles, and move asymmetrically during extrusion of the first and second PBs, to ensure that most remain in the oocyte [60]. It is therefore likely that inadequate mitochondria numbers or defective organelles could be related to chromosome malsegregation and aneuploidy of female meiotic origin. Indeed, data suggest that specific mitochondrial haplogroups may predispose to the generation of chromosomally abnormal oocytes [12].

Considering the critical roles that mitochondria and their genome have during oogenesis, and the oocyte's ability to support the embryo during its first few developmental stages, some researchers have hypothesized that by supplementing the mitochondrial mass in oocytes of poor-prognosis patients, they could improve their clinical outcomes after in vitro fertilization (IVF) [76]. Cytoplasmic transfer from young donor oocytes to those generated by poorer prognosis and, in some cases, reproductively older women did indeed lead to embryos of better quality and increased implantation ability and the birth of children [77]. Some of these children, however, exhibited higher levels of mitochondrial heteroplasmy, with their cells containing two distinct mtDNA haplotypes, one coming from the donor, and the other from the recipient oocyte. Additionally, some of the children born were affected by autism or Turner's syndrome [77,78]. Combination of these findings led to the ooplasm transfer procedure being banned by the Food and Drug Administration.

Recently, the use of autologous mitochondria obtained from oocyte "precursor" cells has been proposed as an alternative supplementation approach to improve oocyte quality [79]. Autologous mitochondrial transfer would overcome ethical objections related to using genetically distinct mitochondria from an unrelated donor, and also circumvents theoretical clinical/biological issues potentially associated with heteroplasmy. This approach was the basis of a procedure called autologous germ line mitochondrial energy transfer, which was developed and offered clinically by a company called Ovascience. Initial application was associated with encouraging results [80,81], although a recently published randomized control trial did not demonstrate any actual benefit on the clinical outcomes of poorer prognosis patients [82].

Mitochondria in sperm

Contrary to oogenesis, which is characterized by an increase in mitochondrial numbers, sperm mitochondria and mtDNA go through a gradual decrease in quantity as sperm cells change shape from being round to elongated, during spermiogenesis [83,84]. The mitochondria that remain after this gradual depletion generate the energy required for the sperm cells to reach and fertilize the oocyte. Once fertilization is complete the sperm mitochondria are eliminated [85], via the process of ubiquitination and autophagy.

The reason for the gradual depletion of mitochondria and mtDNA during spermatogenesis is not clear. mtDNA lacks histones. It is therefore vulnerable to damage from ROS, and its elimination during spermiogenesis may occur to remove molecules carrying mutations [86]. Data obtained in studies examining the mitochondria and their genome in the male gamete suggest that mtDNA copy number and integrity could be indicative of sperm quality.

Wai and colleagues [15] assessed the effect that mtDNA copy number has on female and male fertility using two mouse models, one of which had lost one copy of Tfam, which is a critical part of the mitochondrial nucleoid. It was evident from their results that a threefold reduction of sperm mtDNA copy number is well tolerated in males, without affecting fertilization and live birth rates. They also observed that their mutant male mice preferentially transmitted the deleted Tfam allele to their offspring. The authors concluded that the mtDNA content of sperm cells and that of the reproductive tract is more than what is essential for male gametogenesis, and loss or dysfunction due to the presence of mutations occurs when the mutated mtDNA molecules are over a critical quantity threshold.

Another more recently published study provided evidence for a mechanism which could be involved in the gradual reduction of sperm mitochondria [87]. This investigation assessed the presence and levels of activity of proteins related to autophagy in human spermatozoa. It identified a total of eight such proteins in the sperm samples examined, including LC3, Atg5, Atg16, Beclin 1, p62, m-TOR, AMPKα, and PINK1. Activation of autophagy led to an increase in sperm motility, whereas its inhibition was associated with decreases in ATP, motility, viability, and intracellular calcium concentration. The authors also observed that mitochondrial protein expression was altered once autophagy was either activated or inhibited. They therefore concluded that autophagy (mitophagy) is likely to be regulating sperm motility and viability, and could also be involved in the depletion of mitochondria during male gametogenesis.

A higher mtDNA copy number and the presence of deletions have both been associated with abnormal sperm parameters [84,88–91]. Wu and colleagues [92] examined the mtDNA copy number and the presence of deletions in a total of 119 sperm samples obtained by men going through IVF procedures in a single infertility clinic. Their results very clearly showed that sperm samples with higher levels of mtDNA and/or deletions were associated with significantly lower fertilization rates ($P = .01$ and $P < .01$, respectively), and fewer good quality day-3 and day-5 embryos ($P = .02$ for both, $P = .01$ and $P = .09$). These findings are interesting as they illustrate the importance of mitochondrial depletion during spermatogenesis, and the adverse effect the failure of this process has on early embryogenesis.

Further work is necessary to obtain a better understanding of how mitochondria and their genome function during male gametogenesis, and their possible association with other sperm quality parameters, such as DNA fragmentation or aneuploidy. It is not possible currently to definitively determine sperm competence and ability to result in a live birth. The findings in some of the studies discussed above suggest that mitochondria and their genome may have the potential to objectively determine sperm quality.

Mitochondria in embryos

Once fertilization is complete, the resulting zygote initiates a series of mitotic cleavage divisions which lead to the formation of small cells known as blastomeres. During the first few cleavage divisions, the blastomeres are spherical and totipotent (genetically identical), with the overall size of the developing embryo remaining the same. The initial cleavage divisions take place under the control of the oocyte's stored mRNAs and proteins, with a transition to embryonic control occurring after embryonic genome activation at the four- to eight-cell stages [93]. As the embryo progresses through preimplantation development, it changes morphologically first into a morula (individual blastomeres no longer distinguished) and then into a blastocyst. The blastocyst stage is reached 5–6 days after fertilization and during this stage the embryo goes through the first cellular differentiation into two tissues, an external one known as TE, and an internal one known as ICM. Further TE differentiation will result in the formation of the placenta, whereas the ICM will develop into the embryo proper.

Little or no mitochondria and mtDNA replication is observed during the cleavage and morula stages of preimplantation development. Instead the oocyte's mitochondria are distributed into the newly formed blastomeres. Embryos start replicating their own mtDNA at some point after blastocyst differentiation, with replication being first observed in the TE part [3]. It has been estimated that each human TE cell contains ~150 mitochondria [94]. mtDNA replication is initiated later during development in the ICM. Mitochondrial organelle numbers are, therefore, lower in the ICM than in the TE [3,94].

Events taking place during the first few stages of preimplantation development such as metabolism, protein synthesis, cellular and chromosome divisions, and differentiation require significant amounts of energy. Such events are directly dependent on the correct function of mitochondria and their genome. Various investigations examining embryo culture have clearly demonstrated that suboptimal or adverse conditions, such as pH or calcium fluctuations, or the presence of glucose during the first few days of development, have a great impact on the metabolism of the embryo and the function of the mitochondria [95–98].

mtDNA and its quantity during preimplantation development have been the subjects of many recent investigations. Fragouli et al. [99] were the first to assess the quantity of mtDNA in cleavage and blastocyst stage embryos in relation to factors such as female age, embryo ploidy, and viability. It was evident from the obtained results that cleavage stage embryos generated by reproductively younger women (average age: 33.7 years) contained significantly more mtDNA ($P = .01$) compared to those generated by reproductively older women (average age: 39.2 years). These findings agreed with the notion that mtDNA replication does not start until the blastocyst stage, and suggested that the mtDNA of cleavage stage embryos has its origin in the oocyte. On the other hand, blastocysts generated by reproductively younger women (average age 34.8 years) had significantly lower mtDNA levels ($P = .003$), compared to those generated by reproductively older ones (average age: 39.8 years). These results suggested that an appreciable mtDNA replication amount had already taken place by the time that blastocyst differentiation was complete. A significant increase ($P = .025$) in mtDNA quantity was also observed in aneuploid blastocysts versus euploid ones. This investigation also reported the presence of a relationship between TE mtDNA quantity and the implantation ability of euploid blastocysts. Specifically, euploid blastocysts which failed to implant after transfer had mtDNA levels in their TE which were significantly higher ($P = .0066$) compared to those which led to ongoing pregnancies and live births. Thresholds of mtDNA quantity were established, above which implantation of euploid blastocysts was rarely observed [99].

These results were obtained in a blinded retrospective assessment of 89 embryos, 52.8% of which had not implanted after transfer. However, the failure rate seen in the subgroup of embryos with mtDNA levels above the set viability threshold was 100% (14 of 14), and this decrease in the ability to implant was independent of female age and embryo morphology

[99]. The reduction in embryo viability when mtDNA content was scored to be above established thresholds was further confirmed in a large blinded retrospective study of 1505 blastocysts, and a blinded prospective nonselective investigation of 199 embryos [100,101]. Data from both studies indicated that 5%–9% of all chromosomally normal good-quality blastocysts have elevated mtDNA levels, and are therefore likely to be of lower viability, compared to similar embryos with mtDNA levels below established thresholds. Both studies concluded that mtDNA quantification could potentially be used as an independent biomarker of embryo viability [100,101].

Several other research groups assessed mtDNA quantity in relation to various different parameters, including female age, embryo ploidy, morphology, and implantation ability [102–107]. Most of these studies agreed that chromosome abnormalities and suboptimal embryo morphology were associated with an increase in blastocyst mtDNA quantity [99,103–105,107–109]. The relationship between mtDNA quantity and embryo implantation ability proved to be more controversial. Of all investigations having taken place to date, those of Diez-Juan et al. [104] and Spinella et al. [106] agreed with the hypothesis that mtDNA quantities above set thresholds are associated with embryos of reduced viability, whereas those of Victor et al. [102], Treff et al. [107], and Klimczak et al. [105] did not observe such a relationship.

There are various explanations for the discrepancies seen among different studies. Methodological variation could be one of the main reasons causing some studies not to observe an association between mtDNA quantity and embryo implantation potential [102]. The optimization and validation of mtDNA quantification approaches, whether they are based in real-time PCR or next-generation sequencing, are critical in order for the obtained results to be accurate.

The discrepancies among published studies could also be attributed to an IVF clinic influence. The investigation carried out by Ravichandran and colleagues [101] was the only one to involve the assessment of mtDNA quantity in embryos generated in 35 different clinics. The obtained data demonstrated that certain clinics tended to frequently generate blastocysts with elevated (above established thresholds) mtDNA levels, whereas others did not generate any such embryos. The three studies [102,105,107] failing to see an association between mtDNA amounts and implantation ability examined embryos generated in a single IVF clinic. These studies were not able to determine "viability" thresholds of mtDNA quantity. Therefore it was difficult to determine whether any of the examined blastocysts fell into the "elevated mtDNA" group.

Blastocyst mtDNA quantities have been shown to be influenced by factors related to certain patient characteristics. Specifically, a recent investigation published by de los Santos and colleagues [103] examined the possible effect of several patient parameters, such as age, anti-Müllerian hormone, and body mass index (BMI) on embryo mtDNA quantities. What they observed was that an increased BMI was associated with a tendency to generate blastocysts with more mtDNA. It was also evident that an increase in serum progesterone was associated with a tendency to generate embryos with lower mtDNA quantities. These findings suggest that there could be several underlying reasons for the variable levels of mtDNA observed in blastocysts, and functional studies would be necessary in order to obtain a better understanding of this biological phenomenon.

One possibility is that embryos with elevated mtDNA levels carry functionally deficient mitochondria, unable to support their energetic requirements. An increase in the number of mitochondria could take place as a compensatory mechanism, but the newly formed organelles are also bound to be defective and

TABLE 9.2 Published studies assessing embryo mtDNA quantities in relation to different clinical parameters.

Study (reference)	No. of embryos included	mtDNA association with female age?	mtDNA association with embryo aneuploidy?	mtDNA association with embryo morphology?	mtDNA association with embryo implantation potential?
Fragouli et al. [99]	340	Yes	Yes	Not examined	Yes
Diez-Juan et al. [104]	65	No	Not examined	Yes	Yes
Victor et al. [102]	1396	No	No	Not examined	No
Treff et al. [107]	374	No	Not examined	Yes	No
Ravichandran et al. [101]	1505	Yes	Not examined	No	Yes
Fragouli et al. [100]	199	Yes	Not examined	Not examined	Yes
Tao et al. [109]	171/ mouse	Yes	Yes	Not examined	Not examined
Ho et al. [108]	57	Not examined	Yes	Yes	Not examined
Klimczak et al. [105]	1510	No	Not examined	Yes	No
de los Santos et al. [103]	1641	No	Yes	Yes	Not examined

incapable of correcting a possible ATP deficit, hence these embryos do not survive long term. Such increases in mitochondrial numbers have been shown to occur due to the presence of mutations in the mitochondrial genome [110]. Another possibility is that blastocysts with unusually high mtDNA quantities are experiencing some sort of stress, and as a response they have a more active metabolism, compared to normally developing embryos. A more active metabolism and its association with poorer viability have been described in the quiet embryo hypothesis which postulates that embryos with a quiet (i.e., less active) metabolism are more viable than those displaying elevated metabolic activity [97]. An increasingly active metabolism would require higher ATP levels to be generated, and therefore an increase in mitochondria numbers which could be reflected as a net gain in mtDNA. It should be noted that increasing ATP levels have been correlated with embryonic arrest in a mouse model [111].

Questions remain about the clinical value of mtDNA quantification. These questions can only be answered via well designed and appropriately carried out multicenter randomized control trials (RCTs). It is imperative, however, that any such RCTs employ well-validated technologies, in order to achieve accurate and meaningful mtDNA quantification.

All studies assessing embryo mtDNA quantities in relation to different clinical parameters are outlined in Table 9.2.

Conclusion

To summarize, the role of the mitochondria and their genome is critical during oogenesis, spermatogenesis, and early embryo development. Specifically, oocytes with reduced mtDNA levels and/or defective mitochondria are likely to be compromised and unable to adequately support the energy requirements of the developing embryo. Moreover, the gradual depletion of mitochondria is critical during spermatogenesis. At the blastocyst stage, thresholds or scores of mtDNA content have been established, above which implantation of a euploid embryo is extremely low. It is possible that elevated mtDNA amounts may be characteristic of embryos under some form of stress, although functional studies are needed to determine the factors leading to the increase in mtDNA levels. Data from published studies suggest that approximately 5%–10% of all blastocysts assessed tend to have elevated mtDNA levels, but these may represent approximately one-third of the nonimplanting embryos. It is therefore possible that the measurement of mtDNA quantities may give an indication of oocyte, sperm, and embryo quality and viability, although these findings need to be further confirmed in additional investigations, as well as in RCT settings.

References

[1] Wallace DC. A mitochondrial paradigm of metabolic and degenerative diseases, aging, and cancer: a dawn for evolutionary medicine. Annu Rev Genet 2005;39:359–407.

[2] May-Panloup P, Chrétien MF, Jacques C, Vasseur C, Malthièry Y, Reynier P. Low oocyte mitochondrial DNA content in ovarian insufficiency. Hum Reprod 2005;20(3):593–7.

[3] St John JC, Facucho-Oliveira J, Jiang Y, Kelly R, Salah R. Mitochondrial DNA transmission, replication and inheritance: a journey from the gamete through the embryo and into offspring and embryonic stem cells. Hum Reprod Update 2010;16(5):488–509.

[4] Wallace DC. Mitochondrial DNA in aging and disease. Sci Am 1997;277:40–7.

[5] Dumollard R, Carroll J, Duchen MR, Campbell K, Swann K. Mitochondria function and redox state in mammalian embryos. Semin Cell Dev Biol 2009;20(3):346–53.

[6] Van Blerkom J. Mitochondrial function in the human oocyte and embryo and their role in developmental competence. Mitochondrion 2011;11:797–813.

[7] Anderson S, Bankier AT, Barrell BG, et al. Sequence and organization of the human mitochondrial genome. Nature 1981;290(5806):457–65.

[8] Jansen RP. Germline passage of mitochondria: quantitative considerations and possible embryological sequelae. Hum Reprod 2000;15(Suppl. 2):112–28.

[9] Wallace DC, Brown MD, Lott MT. Mitochondrial DNA variation in human evolution and disease. Gene 1999;238:211–30.

[10] St John JC. The control of mtDNA replication during differentiation and development. Biochim Biophys Acta 2014;1840:1345–54.

[11] Ruiz-Pesini E, Lapena AC, Diez-Sanchez C, Perez-Martos A, Montoya J, Alvarez E, et al. Human mtDNA haplogroups associated with high or reduced spermatozoa motility. Am J Hum Genet 2000;67(3):682–96.

[12] Gianaroli L, Luiselli D, Crivello AM, et al. Mitochondrial DNA analysis and numerical chromosome condition in human oocytes and polar bodies. Mol Hum Reprod 2015;21(1):46–57.

[13] Giles RE, Blanc H, Cann HM, Wallace DC. Maternal inheritance of human mitochondrial DNA. Proc Natl Acad Sci USA 1980;77(1):6715–19.

[14] Marchington DR, Macaulay V, Hartshorne GM, Barlow D, Poulton J. Evidence from human oocytes for a genetic bottleneck in an mtDNA disease. Am J Hum Genet 1998;63(3):769–75.

[15] Wai T, Ao A, Zhang X, Cyr D, Dufort D, Shoubridge EA. The role of mitochondrial DNA copy number in mammalian fertility. Biol Reprod 2010;83(1):52–62.

[16] Hajjar C, Sampuda KM, Boyd L. Dual roles for ubiquitination in the processing of sperm organelles after fertilization. BMC Dev Biol 2014;15(14):6.

[17] Song WH, Ballard JW, Yi YJ, Sutovsky P. Regulation of mitochondrial genome inheritance by autophagy and ubiquitin-proteasome system: implications for health, fitness, and fertility. Biomed Res Int 2014;2014(2014):981867.

[18] Aitken RJ, Fisher HM, Fulton N, Gomez E, Knox W, Lewis B, et al. Reactive oxygen species generation by human spermatozoa is induced by exogenous NADPH and inhibited by the flavoprotein inhibitors diphenylene iodonium and quinacrine. Mol Reprod Dev 1997;47(4):468–82.

[19] Tilly JL, Sinclair DA. Germline energetics, aging and female infertility. Cell Metab 2013;17(6):838–50.

[20] Luo S, Valencia A, Zhang J, Lee N-C, Slone J, Gui B, et al. Biparental Inheritance of Mitochondrial DNA in Humans. Proc Natl Acad Sci USA 2018;115(51):13039–44.

[21] Larsson NG, Wang J, Wilhelmsson H, et al. Mitochondrial transcription factor A is necessary for mtDNA maintenance and embryogenesis in mice. Nat Genet 1998;18(3):231–6.

[22] Chan CC, Liu VW, Lau EY, Yeung WS, Ng EH, Ho PC. Mitochondrial DNA content and 4977 bp deletion in unfertilized oocytes. Mol Hum Reprod 2005;11(12):843–6.

[23] Reynier P, May-Panloup P, Chrétien MF, et al. Mitochondrial DNA content affects the fertilizability of human oocytes. Mol Hum Reprod 2001;7(5):425–9.

[24] Steuerwald N, Barritt JA, Adler R, et al. Quantification of mtDNA in single oocytes, polar bodies and subcellular components by real-time rapid cycle fluorescence monitored PCR. Zygote 2000;8(3):209–15.

[25] Pikó L, Taylor KD. Amounts of mitochondrial DNA and abundance of some mitochondrial gene transcripts in early mouse embryos. Dev Biol 1987;123 (2):364–74.

[26] Spikings EC, Alderson J, St John JC. Regulated mitochondrial DNA replication during oocyte maturation is essential for successful porcine embryonic development. Biol Reprod 2007;76(2):327–35.

[27] Thundathil J, Filion F, Smith LC. Molecular control of mitochondrial function in preimplantation mouse embryos. Mol Reprod Dev 2005;71(4):405–13.

[28] Tyynismaa H, Suomalainen A. Mouse models of mtDNA replication diseases. Methods 2010;51 (4):405–10.

[29] Korhonen JA, Gaspari M, Falkenberg M. TWINKLE Has 5′ -> 3′ DNA helicase activity and is specifically stimulated by mitochondrial single-stranded DNA-binding protein. J Biol Chem 2003;278(49):48627–32.

[30] Spelbrink JN, Li FY, Tiranti V, et al. Human mitochondrial DNA deletions associated with mutations in the gene encoding Twinkle, a phage T7 gene 4-like protein localized in mitochondria. Nat Genet 2001;28 (3):223–31.

[31] Bogenhagen DF, Rousseau D, Burke S. The layered structure of human mitochondrial DNA nucleoids. J Biol Chem 2008;283(6):3665–75.

[32] Seo AY, Joseph AM, Dutta D, Hwang JC, Aris JP, Leeuwenburgh C. New insights into the role ofmitochondria in aging: mitochondrial dynamics and more. J Cell Sci 2010;123(Pt 15):2533–42.

[33] Satoh M, Kuroiwa T. Organization of multiple nucleoids and DNA molecules in mitochondria of a human cell. Exp Cell Res 1991;196(1):137–40.

[34] Brown TA, Tkachuk AN, Shtengel G, et al. Super resolution fluorescence imaging of mitochondrial nucleoids reveals their spatial range, limits, and membrane interaction. Mol Cell Biol 2011;31 (24):4994–5010.

[35] Suárez-Rivero JM, Villanueva-Paz M, de la Cruz-Ojeda P, de la Mata M, Cotán D, Oropesa-Ávila M, et al. Mitochondrial dynamics in mitochondrial diseases. Diseases 2016;5(1) pii: E1.

[36] Chen H, Detmer SA, Ewald AJ, Griffin EE, Fraser SE, Chan DC. Mitofusins mfn1 and MFN2 coordinately regulate mitochondrial fusion and are essential for embryonic development. J Cell Biol 2003;160 (2):189–200.

[37] Twig G, Shirihai OS. The interplay between mitochondrial dynamics and mitophagy. Antioxid Redox Signal 2011;14(10):1939–51.

[38] Mears JA, Lackner LL, Fang S, Ingerman E, Nunnari J, Hinshaw JE. Conformational changes in dnm1 support a contractile mechanism for mitochondrial fission. Nat Struct Mol Biol 2011;18(1):20–6.

[39] Brown WM, George MJ, Wilson AC. Rapid evolution of animal mitochondrial DNA. Proc Natl Acad Sci USA 1979;76(4):1967–71.

[40] Brown WM, Prager EM, Wang A, Wilson AC. Mitochondrial DNA sequences of primates: tempo and mode of evolution. J Mol Evol 1982;18 (4):225–39.

[41] Tuppen HA, Blakely EL, Turnbull DM, Taylor RW. Mitochondrial DNA mutations and human disease. Biochim Biophys Acta 2010;1797(2):113–28.

[42] Kwong LK, Sohal RS. Age-related changes in activities of mitochondrial electron transport complexes in various tissues of the mouse. Arch Biochem Biophys 2000;373(1):16–22.

[43] DeBalsi KL, Hoff KE, William C, Copeland WC. Role of the mitochondrial DNA replication machinery in mitochondrial DNA mutagenesis, aging and age-related diseases. Ageing Res Rev 2017;33:89–104.

[44] Wallace DC, Singh G, et al. Mitochondrial DNA mutation associated with Leber's hereditary optic neuropathy. Science. 1988;242(4884):1427–30.

[45] Mitalipov S, Wolf D. Clinical and ethical implications of mitochondrial gene transfer. Trends Endocrinol Metab 2014;25(1):5–7.

[46] Elliott HR, Samuels DC, et al. Pathogenic mitochondrial DNA mutations are common in the general population. Am J Hum Genet 2008;83(2):254–60.

[47] Parikh S, Goldstein A, Koenig MK, Scaglia F, Enns GM, Saneto R, et al. Diagnosis and management of mitochondrial disease: a consensus statement from the Mitochondrial Medicine Society. Genet Med 2015;17 (9):689–701.

[48] Smeets HJM, Sallevelt SCEH, Dreesen JCFM, de Die-Smulders CEM, de Coo IFM. Preventing the transmission of mitochondrial DNA disorders using prenatal or preimplantation genetic diagnosis. Ann N Y Acad Sci 2015;1350:29–36.

[49] Gigarel N, Hesters L, Samuels DC, Monnot S, Burlet P, Kerbrat V, et al. Poor correlations in the levels of pathogenic mitochondrial DNA mutations in polar bodies versus oocytes and blastomeres in humans. Am J Hum Genet 2011;88(4):494–8.

[50] Monnot S, Gigarel N, Samuels DC, et al. Segregation of mtDNA throughout human embryofetal development: m.3243A > G as a model system. Hum Mutat 2011;32(1):116–25.

[51] Sallevelt SC, Dreesen JC, Drusedau M, et al. Preimplantation genetic diagnosis in mitochondrial DNA disorders: challenge and success. J Med Genet 2013;50(2):125–32.
[52] Steffann J, Frydman N, Gigarel N, et al. Analysis of mtDNA variant segregation during early human embryonic development: a tool for successful NARP preimplantation diagnosis. J Med Genet 2006;43(3):244–7.
[53] Thorburn DR, Wilton L, Stock-Myer S. Healthy baby girl born following pre-implantation genetic diagnosis for mitochondrial DNA m.8993T > G mutation. Mol Genet Metab 2009;98:5–6.
[54] Wolf DP, Hayama T, Mitalipov S. Mitochondrial genome inheritance and replacement in the human germline. EMBO J 2017;36(17):2659.
[55] Hyslop LA, Blakeley P, Craven L, Richardson J, Fogarty NME, Fragouli E, et al. Towards clinical application of pronuclear transfer to prevent mitochondrial DNA disease. Nature 2016;534(7607):383–6.
[56] Zhang J, Liu H, Luo S, Lu Z, Chávez-Badiola A, Liu Z, et al. Live birth derived from oocyte spindle transfer to prevent mitochondrial disease. Reprod Biomed Online 2017;34(4):361–8.
[57] Fragouli E, Alfarawati S, Spath K, et al. The origin and impact of embryonic aneuploidy. Hum Genet 2013;132(9):1001–13.
[58] Kuliev A, Cieslak J, Ilkevitch Y, Verlinsky Y. Chromosomal abnormalities in a series of 6,733 human oocytes in preimplantation diagnosis for age-related aneuploidies. Reprod Biomed Online 2003;6(1):54–9.
[59] Reader KL, Stanton J-AL, Juengel JL. The role of oocyte organelles in determining developmental competence. Biology 2017;6(3):35.
[60] Dalton CM, Carroll J. Biased inheritance of mitochondria during asymmetric cell division in the mouse oocyte. J Cell Sci 2013;126(Pt 13):2955–64.
[61] Jansen RP, de Boer K. The bottleneck: mitochondrial imperatives in oogenesis and ovarian follicular fate. Mol Cell Endocrinol 1998;145(1–2):81–8.
[62] Motta PM, Nottola SA, Makabe S, Heyn R. Mitochondrial morphology in human fetal and adult female germ cells. Hum Reprod 2000;15(Suppl. 2):129–47.
[63] Dumollard R, Duchen M, Carroll J. The role of mitochondrial function in the oocyte and embryo. Curr Top Dev Biol 2007;77:21–49.
[64] Van Blerkom J, Davis P, Alexander S. Differential mitochondrial distribution in human pronuclear embryos leads to disproportionate inheritance between blastomeres: relationship to microtubular organization, ATP content and competence. Hum Reprod 2000;15(12):2621–33.
[65] Cummins JM. Fertilization and elimination of the paternal mitochondrial genome. Hum Reprod 2000;15(Suppl. 2):92–101.
[66] Simsek-Duran F, Li F, Ford W, Swanson RJ, Jones Jr. HW, Castora FJ. Age-associated metabolic and morphologic changes in mitochondria of individual mouse and hamster oocytes. PLoS One 2013;8(5):e64955.
[67] Iwata H, Goto H, Tanaka H, Sakaguchi Y, Kimura K, Kuwayama T, et al. Effect of maternal age on mitochondrial DNA copy number, ATP content and IVF outcome of bovine oocytes. Reprod Fertil Dev 2011;23(3):424–32.
[68] Murakoshi Y, Sueoka K, Takahashi K, Sato S, Sakurai T, Tajima H, et al. Embryo developmental capability and pregnancy outcome are related to the mitochondrial DNA copy number and ooplasmic volume. J Assist Reprod Genet 2013;30(10):1367–75.
[69] Pawlak P, Cieslak A, Warzych E, Zejden Z, Szumacher-Strabel M, Molinska-Glura M, et al. No single way to explain cytoplasmic maturation of oocytes from prepubertal and cyclic gilts. Theriogenology 2012;78(9):2020–30.
[70] Pedersen HS, Lovendahl P, Larsen K, Madsen LB, Callesen H. Porcine oocyte mtDNA copy number is high or low depending on the donor. Zygote 2016;24(4):617–23.
[71] Reader KL, Cox NR, Stanton J-AL, Juengel JL. Mitochondria and vesicles differ between adult and prepubertal sheep oocytes during IVM. Reprod Fertil Dev 2015;27(3):513–22.
[72] Duran HE, Simsek-Duran F, Oehninger SC, Jones Jr HW, Castora FJ. The association of reproductive senescence with mitochondrial quantity, function, and DNA integrity in human oocytes at different stages of maturation. Fertil Steril 2011;96(2):384–8.
[73] Konstantinidis M, Alfarawati S, Hurd D, et al. Simultaneous assessment of aneuploidy, polymorphisms, and mitochondrial DNA content in human polar bodies and embryos with the use of a novel microarray platform. Fertil Steril 2014;102(5):1385–92.
[74] Hsu AL, Townsend PM, Oehninger S, Castora FJ. Endometriosis may be associated with mitochondrial dysfunction in cumulus cells from subjects undergoing in vitro fertilizationintracytoplasmic sperm injection, as reflected by decreased adenosine triphosphate production. Fertil Steril 2015;103(2):347–352.e1.
[75] Dalton CM, Szabadkai G, Carroll J. Measurement of ATP in single oocytes: impact of maturation and cumulus cells on levels and consumption. J Cell Physiol 2014;229:353–61.
[76] Cohen J, Scott R, Alikani M, Schimmel T, Munne S, Levron J, et al. Ooplasmic transfer in mature human oocytes. Mol Hum Reprod 1998;4(3):269–80.

[77] Barritt J, Willadsen S, Brenner C, Cohen J. Cytoplasmic transfer in assisted reproduction. Hum Reprod Update 2001;7(4):428–35.
[78] Barritt JA, Brenner CA, Malter HE, Cohen J. Mitochondria in human offspring derived from ooplasmic transplantation. Hum Reprod 2001;16:513–16.
[79] Chappel S. The role of mitochondria from mature oocyte to viable blastocyst. Obstet Gynecol Int 2013;183024.
[80] Fakih M, El Shmoury M, Szeptycki J, de la Cruz D, Lux C, Verjee S, et al. The AUGMENT treatment: physician reported outcomes of the initial global patient experience. JFIV Reprod Med Genet 2015;3 (3):154.
[81] Oktay K, Baltaci V, Sonmezer M, Turan V, Unsal E, Baltaci A, et al. Oogonial precursor cell-derived autologous mitochondria injection to improve outcomes in women with multiple IVF failures due to low oocyte quality: a clinical translation. Reprod Sci 2015;22(12):1612–17.
[82] Labarta E, de los Santos MJ, Herraiz S, Escriba MJ, Marzal A, Buigues A, et al. Autologous mitochondrial transfer as a complementary technique to intracytoplasmic sperm injection to improve embryo quality in patients undergoing in vitro fertilization—a randomized pilot study. Fertil Steril 2019;111 (1):86–96.
[83] Hecht NB, Liem H, Kleene KC, Distel RJ, Ho SM. Maternal inheritance of the mouse mitochondrial genome is not mediated by a loss or gross alteration of the paternal mitochondrial DNA or by methylation of the oocyte mitochondrial DNA. Dev Biol 1984;102 (2):452–61.
[84] May-Panloup P, Chretien MF, Savagner F, Vasseur C, Jean M, Malthiery Y, et al. Increased sperm mitochondrial DNA content in male infertility. Hum Reprod 2003;18(3):550–6.
[85] Sutovsky P, Van Leyen K, McCauley T, Day BN, Sutovsky M. Degradation of paternal mitochondria after fertilization: implications for heteroplasmy, assisted reproductive technologies and mtDNA inheritance. Reprod Biomed Online 2004;8(1):24–33.
[86] Tremellen K. Oxidative stress and male infertility—a clinical perspective. Hum Reprod Update 2008;14 (3):243–58.
[87] Aparicio IM, Espino J, Bejarano I, Gallardo-Soler A, Campo ML, Salido GM, et al. Autophagy-related proteins are functionally active in human spermatozoa and may be involved in the regulation of cell survival and motility. Sci Rep 2017;6:33647.
[88] Zhang G, Wang Z, Ling X, Zou P, Yang H, Chen Q, et al. Mitochondrial biomarkers reflect semen quality: results from the MARCHS Study in Chongqing, China. PLoS One 2016;11(12):e0168823.
[89] Bahrehmand Namaghi I, Vaziri H. Sperm mitochondrial DNA deletion in Iranian infertiles with asthenozoospermia. Andrologia 2017;49(3):e12627.
[90] Mughal IA, Irfan A, Jahan S, Hameed A. Male infertility is significantly associated with multiple deletions in an 8.7-kb segment of sperm mtDNA in Pakistan. Turk J Med Sci 2017;47(3):928–33.
[91] Talebi E, Karimian M, Nikzad H. Association of sperm mitochondrial DNA deletions with male infertility in an Iranian population. Mitochondrial DNA Part A DNA Mapp Seq Anal 2018;29 (4):615–23.
[92] Wu H, Whitcomb BW, Huffman A, Brandon N, Labrie S, Tougias E, et al. Associations of sperm mitochondrial DNA copy number and deletion rate with fertilization and embryo development in a clinical setting. Hum Reprod 2019;34(1):163–70.
[93] Braude P, Bolton V, Moore S. Human gene expression first occurs between the four- and eight-cell stages of preimplantation development. Nature 1988;332(6163):459–61.
[94] Van Blerkom J. Mitochondria as regulatory forces in oocytes, preimplantation embryos and stem cells. Reprod Biomed Online 2008;16(4):553–69.
[95] Barnett DK, Clayton MK, Kimura J, Bavister BD. Glucose and phosphate toxicity in hamster preimplantation embryos involves disruption of cellular organization, including distribution of active mitochondria. Mol Reprod Dev 1997;48(2):227–37.
[96] Lane M, Bavister BD. Calcium homeostasis in early hamster preimplantation embryos. Biol Reprod 1998;59(4):1000–7.
[97] Leese HJ. Quiet please, do not disturb: a hypothesis of embryo metabolism and viability. BioEssays 2002;24(9):845–9.
[98] Squirrell JM, Lane M, Bavister BD. Altering intracellular pH disrupts development and cellular organization in preimplantation hamster embryos. Biol Reprod 2001;64(6):1845–54.
[99] Fragouli E, Spath K, Alfarawati S, et al. Altered levels of mitochondrial DNA are associated with female age, aneuploidy, and provide an independent measure of embryonic implantation potential. PLoS Genet 2015;11(6):e1005241.
[100] Fragouli E, McCaffrey C, Ravichandran K, Spath K, Grifo J, Munne S, et al. Clinical implications of mitochondrial DNA quantification on pregnancy outcomes: a blinded prospective non-selection study. Hum Reprod 2017;32(11):2340–7.
[101] Ravichandran K, McCaffrey C, Grifo J, Morales A, Perloe M, Munne S, et al. Mitochondrial DNA quantification as a tool for embryo viability assessment: retrospective analysis of data from single euploid blastocyst transfers. Hum Reprod 2017;32 (6):1282–92.

[102] Victor AR, Brake AJ, Tyndall JC, Griffin DK, Zouves CG, Barnes FL, et al. Accurate quantitation of mitochondrial DNA reveals uniform levels in human blastocysts irrespective of ploidy, age, or implantation potential. Fertil Steril 2017;107(1):34–42.
[103] de Los Santos MJ, Diez Juan A, Mifsud A, Mercader A, Meseguer M, Rubio C, et al. Variables associated with mitochondrial copy number in human blastocysts: what can we learn from trophectoderm biopsies? Fertil Steril 2018;109(1):110–17.
[104] Diez-Juan A, Rubio C, Marin C, Martinez S, Al-Asmar N, Riboldi M, et al. Mitochondrial DNA content as a viability score in human euploid embryos: less is better. Fertil Steril 2015;104(3):534–41.
[105] Klimczak AM, Pacheco LE, Lewis KE, Massahi N, Richards JP, Kearns WG, et al. Embryonal mitochondrial DNA: relationship to embryo quality and transfer outcomes. J Assist Reprod Genet 2018;35(5):871–7.
[106] Spinella F, Cotroneo E, Bono S, Biricik A, Greco E, Minasi MG, et al. Quantification of mitochondrial DNA in preimplantation embryos: a tool to predict implantation potential of chromosomally normal embryos. Hum Reprod 2016;31:i26.
[107] Treff NR, Zhan Y, Tao X, Olcha M, Han M, Rajchel J, et al. Levels of trophectoderm mitochondrial DNA do not predict the reproductive potential of sibling embryos. Hum Reprod 2017;32(4):954–62.
[108] Ho JR, Arrach N, Rhodes-Long K, Salem W, McGinnis LK, Chung K, et al. Blastulation timing is associated with differential mitochondrial content in euploid embryos. J Assist Reprod Genet 2018;35 (4):711–20.
[109] Tao X, Landis JN, Krisher RL, Duncan FE, Silva E, Lonczak A, et al. Mitochondrial DNA content is associated with ploidy status, maternal age, and oocyte maturation methods in mouse blastocysts. J Assist Reprod Genet 2017;34(12):1587–94.
[110] Monnot S, Samuels DC, Hesters L, Frydman N, Gigarel N, Burlet P, et al. Mutation dependence of the mitochondrial DNA copy number in the first stages of human embryogenesis. Hum Mol Genet 2013;22(9):1867–72.
[111] Ginsberg L, Hillman N. ATP metabolism in tn/tn mouse embryos. J Embryol Exp Morphol 1975;33 (3):715–23.

CHAPTER

10

Endometrial receptivity and genetics

Nick Macklon[1,2]

[1]London Women's Clinic, London, United Kingdom [2]Zealand University Hospital, Koege, Denmark

Introduction

It can be reasonably stated that the first 40 years of in vitro fertilization (IVF) represented the golden age of embryo research. During this period, remarkable insights into early human development, the requirements of the preimplantation embryo, and markers of viability were gained. However, with embryo culture and selection technologies now reaching an advanced level of maturity, there is growing interest in the endometrial factor as the next frontier in the search to improve the management of subfertility and treatment outcomes. Given the relatively ready access that endometrial tissue affords to investigators, it is notable that our ability to interrogate endometrial function remains so limited, especially when compared with the large and still growing portfolio of techniques available to analyze embryo viability.

A number of reasons for the endometrium remaining the "Cinderella" of fertility research can be proposed. These include the prevailing view that the embryo is the dominant determinant of successful implantation, its exquisite sensitivity to its preimplantation environment and the commercial returns to be had from investing in developing culture media, incubator systems, and tests of quality.

However, another reason may lie in the language we use to describe endometrial function. The very term "receptivity" may be in part to blame. It implies a passivity of role, that is, further amplified by terms such as "embryo attachment" and "invasion," and belies the now emerging complex and active roles that the endometrium fulfills as a key and potentially modulatable determinant of successful human implantation. These new insights are encouraging the development of novel means of assessing endometrial function well beyond the limited concept of receptivity.

In this chapter, the contributions that genomics and transcriptomics have made to our understanding of the endometrial factor in implantation and its assessment are reviewed from a clinical perspective.

Genetic markers of endometrial function

The human endometrium is one of the most dynamic tissues in the body. Driven by ovarian estrogen and progesterone, it undergoes repeated cyclic growth, differentiation,

Human Reproductive Genetics
DOI: https://doi.org/10.1016/B978-0-12-816561-4.00010-7

desquamation, and regeneration [1]. Although the endometrium is nonreceptive to embryos for most of the menstrual cycle, it becomes receptive during a spatially and temporally restricted period in the secretory phase known as the "window of implantation" [2]. Gaining insight into the complex mechanisms controlling changes within the endometrium is crucial to understanding implantation.

From the first histologic dating methods [3] to the now established "omics" technologies, extensive efforts have been applied to understanding and characterizing receptive endometrium. Pioneering studies suggested that the application of high-throughput "omics" technologies held the key to endometrial biomarker research [4–8] and the following years witnessed an explosive growth in the number of "omics" studies involving the human endometrium.

Early studies investigated the specific patterns of gene expression that appeared to characterize the mid secretory phase. However, little consensus emerged, as the studies were small, employed different platforms, and often lacked controls. Further challenges arose from the examination of multicellular tissue and their inherent associated variation, and the biological differences between different subjects [9–12]. However, it became clear that gene array research was identifying the modulation of gene expression of proteins involved in the cell cycle, proliferation, and differentiation [9–11] of cytokines, chemokines and growth factors, and immune mediators [9,13], and attention increasingly turned to describing the dynamics of gene expression in the peri-implantation phase of the menstrual cycle.

The concept of the window of implantation that originated from studies of laboratory animals gained more credence as a feature of human reproduction with the classic studies of Wilcox et al. relating implantation outcome with its timing in relation to ovulation [14]. However, for many years the only means of assessing this was by histological examination of timed endometrial biopsies, and application of the "Noyes" criteria for dating endometrial maturation [3]. In the absence of any objective means of assessing endometrial receptivity, Noyes criteria became widely used, and the concept of endometrial dysfunction being rooted in the degree of secretory advancement gained currency. The emergence of genomics finally offered a more objective means of assessing endometrial maturity. Initially, Horcajadas et al. [15] defined a list of 25 target genes that were postulated to mark the implantation window. These included leukemia inhibitory factor, hyaluronan-binding protein 2, calpain, tissue factor pathway inhibitor 2, placental protein 14, and folate receptor. Subsequently, Diaz-Gimeno et al. identified a set of 238 genes that are differentially expressed in the transition from the prereceptive to the receptive state [8]. This finding paved the way to the creation of a diagnostic tool named the endometrial receptivity array (ERA). The accuracy and consistency of this molecular test for defining endometrial cycle phases appeared to be superior to classical histology methods [15,16]. The clinical potential of the ERA for detecting the personalized window of implantation in patients and thus guiding their personalized embryo transfer as a novel therapeutic strategy has been reported [16]. However, like the original Noyes criteria for the histological assessment of endometrial tissue which were originally designed only to enable the number of days of endometrial exposure to progesterone to be assessed [3], the ERA test is widely considered to represent a measure of endometrial receptivity in general. It can be argued that endometrial receptivity is determined by more factors than simply an appropriate maturation response to progesterone [17]. Moreover, the widespread and effective practice of transferring day 2 human embryos into the uterus, in the knowledge that they can "wait" for the endometrium to become receptive suggests a level of embryo tolerance of the nonreceptive endometrium. It can therefore be argued therefore that encountering perfectly synchronized endometrium is not mandatory for successful embryo implantation. However, it is likely that suboptimal embryo endometrial synchrony is a significant contributor to implantation failure in some women and merits investigation in certain clinical contexts. A recently completed large randomized clinical trial will help clarify the reliability and clinical value of ERA as a tool for synchronizing the timing of embryo transfer to endometrial maturity.

While asynchrony may be the cause in some [18], implantation failure may also arise as a result of other causes. The concept that transcriptomic profiles of the endometrium can be employed not just to assess maturity, but constitutive disorders of endometrial function is supported by studies that have shown other factors to impact on endometrial gene transcription. The presence of gynecological pathologies such as endometriosis or long-term presence of intrauterine contraceptive devices has been shown to be disruptive [19,20]. In recent years, a number of studies have appeared comparing transcriptomic profiles in endometrium from fertile women with those from women with a history of otherwise unexplained recurrent implantation failure (RIF) [21,22]. However, most of these studies have not been subjected to validation on an independent cohort. More recently, our group published a study that sought to address some of the methodological limitations of previous reports. The study design and approach adopted illustrate some of the issues that require consideration when investigating transcriptomic signatures in the endometrium for clinical purposes, and is therefore described here in some detail.

The aim of this study [22] was to determine whether an endometrial transcriptomic signature could be found in women with a history of RIF. In order to define a cohort of women in whom the presence of a significant endometrial factor underlying implantation failure was likely to be present, ovulatory women who had experienced RIF after undergoing three or more embryo transfer procedures or transfer of 10 or more high-quality embryos, despite a good ovarian response and in the absence of uterine pathology were identified. A control cohort included women who had readily conceived after intracytoplasmic sperm injection for male-factor fertility. RIF patients were screened for relevant inherited and acquired thrombophilias and abnormalities in glycosylated hemoglobin and thyroid-stimulating hormone levels, and those demonstrating abnormal results were excluded.

In this study, 43 patients with RIF and 72 control subjects were recruited, and each underwent an endometrial biopsy 7 days after an luteinizing hormone (LH) surge in their natural cycle. To identify a gene signature for RIF, a randomly selected subset of samples was created whereby the ratio of RIF patients to control subjects was kept similar to the full complement of samples. The remaining samples were assigned to the validation set in the same ratio of RIF patients to control subjects. Signature discovery consisted of 100 rounds of randomly selecting a training subset from the signature discovery set, which was subsequently used to rank genes based on their potential to differentiate RIF patients from control subjects. Samples were randomly assigned into a signature discovery set ($n = 81$) and an independent validation set ($n = 34$), keeping the ratio of RIF patients to control subjects similar. Iterative rounds of cross-validation were applied within the signature discovery set to find genes capable of distinguishing RIF patients from control subjects, because this reduces the risk of overfitting in the signature discovery set. Each iteration results in a separate gene set, and all genes were ranked according to how frequently they were present

TABLE 10.1 The accuracy of recurrent implantation failure (RIF) prediction with the use of a 303-gene classifier.

Metric	Signature discovery	Validation
NPV	94.0 (83.8–97.9)	81.5 (63.3–91.8)
PPV	90.3 (75.1–96.7)	100 (64.6–100)
Sensitivity	90.3 (75.1–96.7)	58.3 (32.0–80.7)
Specificity	94.0 (83.8–97.9)	100 (85.1–100)
Overall accuracy	92.6 (84.8–96.6)	85.3 (69.9–93.6)
P value	3.83×10^{-13}	

Notes: Values are presented as % (95% confidence interval). Sensitivity and specificity of *P* were calculated with the use of a Fisher exact test (two-sided). *NPV*, Negative predictive value; *PPV*, positive predictive value.
Source: *Reproduced with permission from Koot Y, van Hooff S, Boomsma C, van Leenen D, Groot Koerkamp M, Goddijn M, et al. An endometrial gene expression signature accurately predicts recurrent implantation failure after IVF. Sci Rep 2016;22:19411.*

in the separate gene sets. Selecting all genes with a frequency of ≥5% resulted in a 303-gene signature. To validate the gene signature, a classifier was built with the use of the full signature discovery set as input and the profile used to predict the class of the samples in the validation set, which, to ensure an independent validation, had not been used in any of the previous steps.

The positive predictive value (PPV) of the RIF prediction classifier was 90% with a sensitivity of 90% (Table 10.1). Most importantly, application to the independent validation set confirmed the signature's ability to distinguish RIF patients from control subjects (Fig. 10.1). All samples classified as RIF were indeed RIF patients (PPV 100%) with a sensitivity of 58%.

Besides classification of patients, an additional benefit of gene expression analyses is the potential to shed light on factors underlying a particular condition. A striking characteristic of the RIF signature genes is that there are many more genes with decreased expression (Fig. 10.2). This is consistent with an earlier study of RIF [23] that also reported enrichment for cell cycle-associated gene function within the set of downregulated genes. Gene ontology (GO) analysis revealed the various cellular processes and structures differentially affected in RIF patients versus controls. Most striking was the downregulation in RIF patients of genes involved in cell cycle regulation and cell division, indicative of a reduced rate of cellular proliferation. The RIF endometrium transcriptome also shows reduced expression of genes involved in cytoskeleton and cilia formation. The latter is of interest given the presence of ciliated cells during the implantation window in healthy women [24]. The number of enriched GO categories with increased expression was limited, but they were related to processes involved in extracellular organization and cell motility. Another feature of the RIF signature was the high proportion of transcription factors. The signature gene included established transcription factors such as the forkhead transcription factor FOXK2, family members of which have previously been implicated in ovary development and function [25,26].

Beyond endometrial receptivity

As stated in the introduction to this chapter, the term "endometrial receptivity" implies a passivity of function in implantation that recent discoveries have come to challenge. For many years, it has been understood that decidualization of the endometrium in the midluteal phase is necessary to ensure both receptivity to the implanting embryo and a supportive and nourishing environment after breach of the epithelium before the establishment of the early placenta. Recently, however, additional functions have been ascribed to the decidualized stromal compartment of the endometrium indicating that the decidua has a key role in

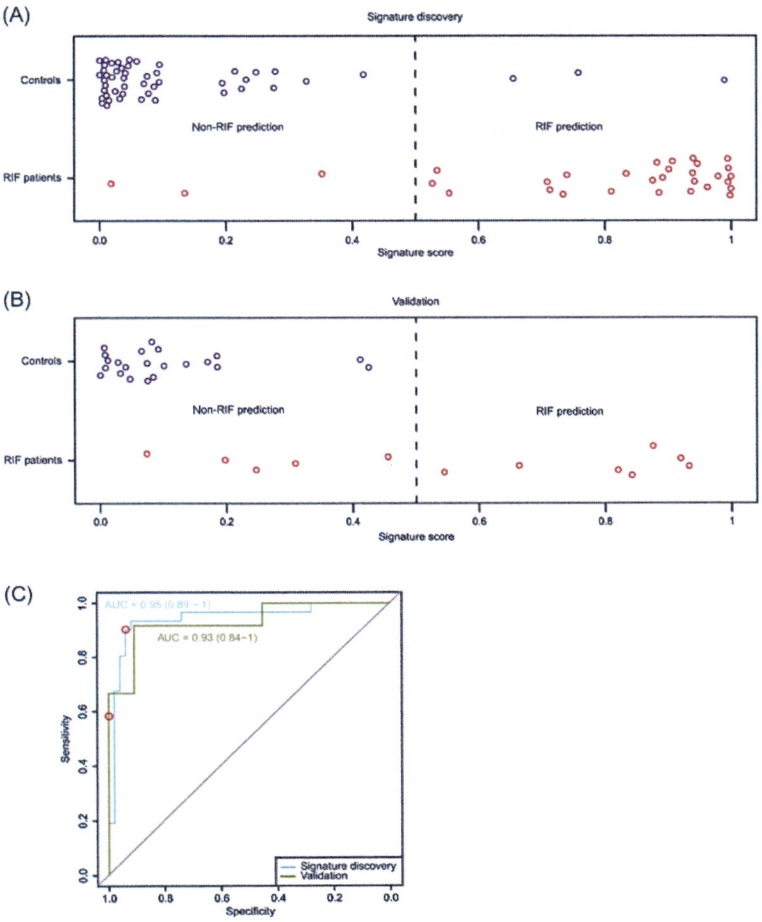

FIGURE 10.1 Support vector machine (SVM) classifier results on the (A) signature discovery and (B) validation sets of a 303-gene recurrent implantation failure (RIF) signature. (A) SVM classifier scores for the signature discovery set (RIF patients, *red*; control subjects, *blue*). Samples with a score of <0.5 are predicted to be control subjects, and those with a score of ≥0.5 are predicted to be RIF patients (the threshold is shown as a *dotted line*). (B) All samples from the validation set, scored based on the SVM classifier. (C) Receiver operating characteristic curves for the results shown in (A) (*blue line*) and (B) (*green line*). Areas under the receiver operating characteristic curve (AUC) with 95% confidence intervals are shown next to the curves. Source: *Reproduced with permission from Koot Y, van Hooff S, Boomsma C, van Leenen D, Groot Koerkamp M, Goddijn M, et al. An endometrial gene expression signature accurately predicts recurrent implantation failure after IVF. Sci Rep 2016;22:19411.*

directing the maternal response to the implanting embryo.

The need for such biosensor function becomes clear when one considers the challenge that the implanting embryo presents to the prospective mother. In contrast to other species, human embryos are characterized by their high rate of chromosomal abnormalities. Most of these will fail to establish an ongoing pregnancy, despite being invasive enough to initiate implantation. Although this may in part reflect incompetency, it has become evident that there is also an active maternal strategy to prevent investment in these invasive but poorly viable embryos [27].

If decidualization is suboptimal, then the biosensor function may be disrupted too. The consequence of this could be that rather than allowing early rejection of poor-quality embryos before the mother becomes aware that she may have conceived, the endometrium would allow poorly viable embryos to establish a clinical pregnancy, ultimately destined to fail, and present as a clinical miscarriage. Persistently impaired endometrial selectivity would result in recurrent early pregnancy loss in

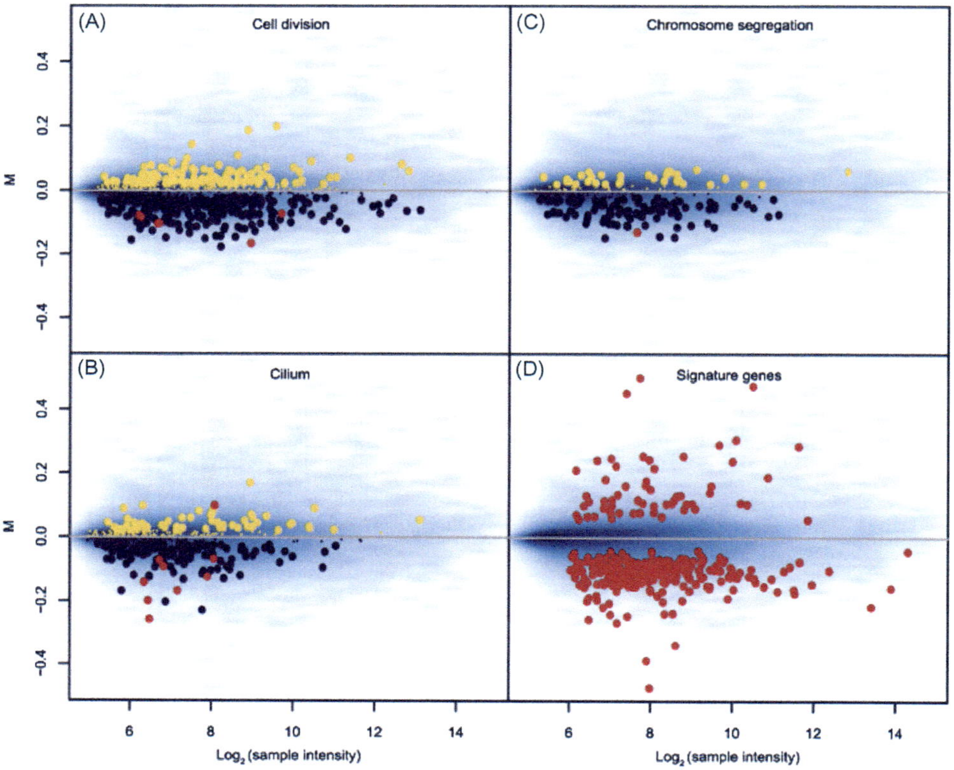

FIGURE 10.2 Gene expression of recurrent implantation failure (RIF) patients compared with control subjects ($\log_2$ fold change or *M* value) and the average expression across all samples ($\log_2$ sample intensity). (A–C) Each focus on an example of a gene ontology (GO) term which was found to be significant in gene set enrichment analysis. Genes in the GO term that are upregulated in RIF patients are shown in yellow, downregulated in blue. Shown in red are other genes that are part of the 303-gene signature. Genes that are not part of the GO term are shown as a blue density map, where darker blue indicates higher gene density. (D) All of the genes of the gene signature. Source: *Reproduced with permission from Koot Y, van Hooff S, Boomsma C, van Leenen D, Groot Koerkamp M, Goddijn M, et al. An endometrial gene expression signature accurately predicts recurrent implantation failure after IVF. Sci Rep 2016;22:19411.*

conjunction with paradoxic "superfertility." Conversely, an excessive decidual response would allow receptivity to dominate, reducing the incidence of miscarriage but increasing the likelihood of implantation delay or RIF after IVF (Fig. 10.3) [27]. Work by the Brosens group points to a possible plausible mechanism by which endometrial injury might increase stem cell numbers in the endometrium and encourage the removal of excessive senescent cells by stimulating natural killer cell activity [28]. Moreover, the differential constitutive disruption of endometrial gene expression in RIF and recurrent miscarriage has recently been demonstrated [29].

Evidence supporting the concept of active embryo selection at implantation in the human comes from a series of in vitro and in vivo studies which showed the response of the human endometrial stromal cells to be more profound in the presence of a developmentally incompetent than a competent human embryo.

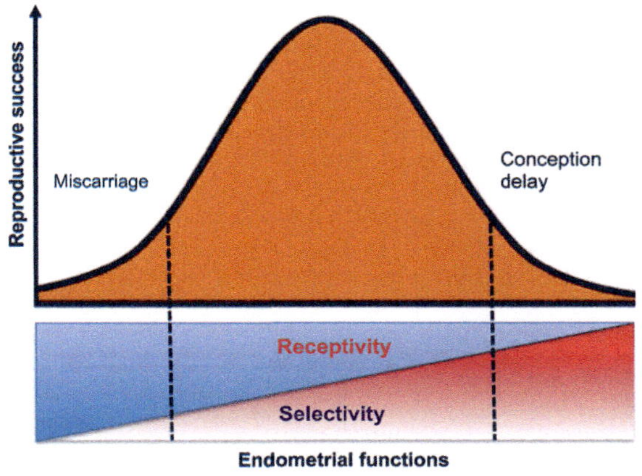

FIGURE 10.3 Schematic representation of the possible clinical consequences of dysbalance between the selective and receptive functions of the decidualized endometrium. Whereas excessive receptivity and poor selectivity may result in inappropriate implantation of poorly viable embryos, which may present as recurrent early pregnancy loss, poor-receptivity couples with excessive selectivity may present as recurrent implantation failure (RIF). Source: *Reproduced with permission from Macklon NS, Brosens JJ, The human endometrium as a sensor of embryo quality. Biol Reprod 2014;92:98.*

The pervasive embryo-centric paradigm predicts that developmentally competent embryos would signal their viability to the decidualized stromal cells, which would respond by upregulating production of proimplantation modulators. However, these studies demonstrated the reverse: embryos that showed morphological signs of developmental impairment elicited a strong response in decidualizing cells, characterized by selective inhibition of IL-1β, -6, -10, -17, -18, eotaxin (CCL11), and heparin-binding epidermal growth factor-like growth factor secretion. This apparent biosensor function was part of the decidual phenotype as human embryos did not trigger a response when cocultured with undifferentiated endometrial stromal cells [30].

The mechanisms underlying this novel concept of human embryo selectivity are beginning to emerge, and again transcriptomic studies have been key. In a study in which decidualizing cells were exposed for 12 hours to pooled medium conditioned from human embryos deemed insufficient for uterine transfer and high-quality embryos that resulted in an ongoing pregnancy after single embryo transfer, genome-wide expression profiling uncovered only 15 decidual genes responsive to soluble signals from competent human embryos [31]. In contrast, and consistent with the previously observed cytokine response [30], 449 maternal genes were deregulated in response to medium conditioned by poor-quality embryos. GO studies showed half of these genes to be associated with the broad biological process of transport, translation, and cell cycle regulation (Fig. 10.4) [31].

The most downregulated gene in the array analysis of exposed decidualized stromal cells was *HSPA8*, which encodes a protein involved in protein assembly and folding [32]. Knockdown of *HSPA8* in decidualizing cells has shown it to be a pivotal sensor molecule for embryonic signals by which soluble signals from developmentally impaired human embryos induce a proteotoxic stress response in decidualizing cells.

In vivo studies in which human embryo conditioned medium was injected into mouse uteri confirmed these findings, but also demonstrated a component consistent with the established paradigm of a competent embryo evoking a supportive intrauterine environment. A dual-phase response of the endometrium can therefore be proposed consisting of "recognition" and "selection." The ability of the luminal epithelium to "recognize" a high-quality embryo and modulate the decidual response it encounters on breaching the epithelium would aid subsequent nurturing and development in the postimplantation phase.

Once the embryo has successfully breached the luminal epithelium, it is thought to continue its journey into the endometrial stroma as the active party, "invading" through what

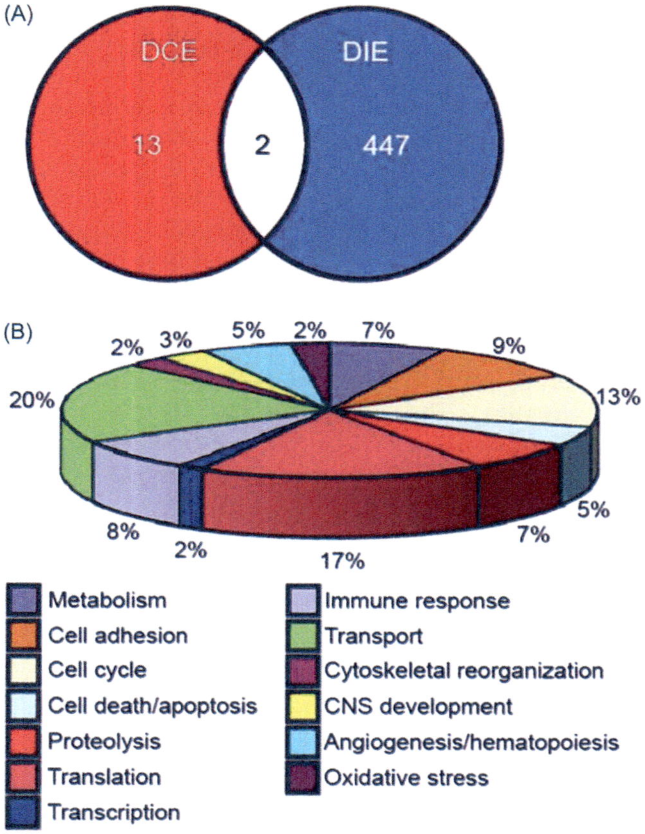

FIGURE 10.4 Venn diagram presenting the number of maternal genes significantly ($P < .01$) altered 24 h after exposure of mouse uterus to unconditioned embryo culture medium or medium conditioned by either developmentally competent or impaired human embryos (DCE and DIE, respectively). Source: *Reproduced with permission from Brosens JJ, Salker MS, Teklenburg G, Nautiyal J, Salter S, Lucas ES, et al. Uterine selection of human embryos at implantation. Sci Rep 2014;6:3894.*

has been considered a mechanically passive decidual matrix. However, recent studies indicate that active decidual cell migration and encapsulation of the conceptus are integral steps in the implantation process, and stromal cells move around the embryo to accommodate its expansion [33].

Further confirmation for this comes from imaging studies, which revealed that decidualizing endometrial stromal cells are programmed to migrate toward implantation-competent blastocysts (Fig. 10.5) [34]. This chemotactic and invasive migration of endometrial stromal cells is triggered by signals emanating from the trophoblast, especially platelet-derived growth factor-AA [35].

Time-lapse coculture studies showed that the propensity of decidual cells to migrate toward a conceptus was confined to high-quality human embryos and entirely inhibited in the presence of chromosomally abnormal tripronuclear embryos [34]. Taken together, these data indicate that decidual cells have the capacity to actively hinder invasion and outgrowth of abnormal human embryos that have breached the luminal epithelium.

A predictable consequence of a reduced ability to recognize embryonic signals would be increased frequency of implantation of impaired embryos that embark on a developmental trajectory destined to fail as a clinical miscarriage. If this supposition were correct,

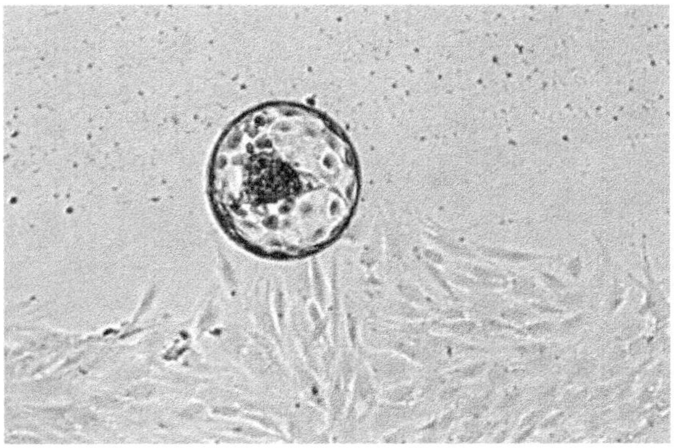

FIGURE 10.5 In an in vitro model, human decidualized stromal cells actively migrate to embrace the preimplantation blastocyst. Source: *Adapted from Weimar CH, Kavelaars A, Brosens JJ, Gellersen B, de Vreeden-Elbertse JM, et al. Endometrial stromal cells of women with recurrent miscarriage fail to discriminate between high- and low-quality human embryos. PLoS One 2012;7:e41424.*

persistently impaired endometrial selectivity would result in recurrent early pregnancy loss in conjunction with paradoxical "superfertility." This hypothesis is supported by two studies of the time-to-pregnancy intervals in women presenting with recurrent miscarriages [36,37]. In both studies, around 40% of women with recurrent pregnancy loss could be considered "superfertile" when defined by a mean time to pregnancy of 3 months or less.

Prolonged endometrial receptivity rather than impaired selectivity could also shorten the interpregnancy interval as well as the miscarriage rate by promoting out-of-phase implantation and again, clinical observations support this notion. In a study of the impact of timing of implantation following spontaneous conception on outcomes, 84% of conceptions were detected between 8 and 10 days after ovulation. Among the 102 pregnancies identified on day 9 after ovulation, 13% ended in an early pregnancy loss. This proportion rose to 26% with implantation on day 10, to 52% on day 11, and to 82% on day 12 and beyond [14].

Taken together, these clinical observations indicate that unrestrained endometrial receptivity and lack of embryo selection both contribute to subsequent pregnancy failure. This concept has been further supported by in vitro time-lapse assays in which the suppression of stromal cell migration observed in the presence of a developmentally incompetent embryo did not occur when the decidual cells had been obtained from women with recurrent miscarriage [34].

Emerging evidence indicates that an aberrant decidual response both prolongs the receptivity phenotype of the endometrium and impairs the ability of the endometrium to engage in embryo quality control.

Micro-RNAs as markers of endometrial function

Micro-RNAs (miRNAs) are small nonprotein-coding RNAs that function as posttranscriptional regulators of target mRNAs. Their effect is usually to silence the gene in question. These miRNAs are short, an average of 22 nucleotides long, and each one may repress 100 or more mRNAs, making them important for genetic regulation in many cell types [38].

A number of roles have been postulated for miRNAs in the endometrium. One role appears to be downregulating the expression of some cell cycle genes in the secretory-phase endometrial epithelium, thereby suppressing cell proliferation [39]. Another of the miRNAs, hsa-miR-222, has been shown to make stromal cells withdraw from the cell cycle, thus possibly influencing the differentiation process [40]. It has also been proposed that miRNA is responsible for the progesterone resistance seen in endometriosis [41].

Several miRNAs appear to be regulated by estrogen and progesterone in the endometrium. These in turn regulate estrogen receptor and progesterone receptors as well as paracrine factors, thereby being an important development toward receptivity [42].

miRNAs are emerging as potential biomarkers for human endometrial receptivity. Using a deep sequencing approach, miRNA expression profiles have been compared between a prereceptive (LH + 2) and a receptive (LH + 7) state in both natural and stimulated cycles [43]. In natural cycles, they found eight upregulated miRNAs and 12 downregulated miRNAs in LH + 7 compared to LH + 2. Bioinformatic analysis has revealed that these miRNAs target a set of genes that are characteristically expressed during the window of implantation. Four miRNAs have been identified that are specifically regulated in receptive endometrium at the time of implantation [44]. Another study has implicated miR-30d as a key miRNA regulating endometrial function, demonstrating that it is downregulated in decidualized stromal cells versus nondecidualized cells [40], and more recently that it is overexpressed during the window of implantation.

Extracellular miRNAs can be transported by both high- and low-density lipoproteins or bound to other proteins. However, recently it has been demonstrated that they may also be delivered in extracellular vesicles (EVs), which protect them from degradation and contribute to their stability within fluids [45]. EVs ranging in size from just 50 to 5000 nm in diameter can transport a wide range of selectively packaged components.

Recent research has focused on elucidating the role of maternally derived miRNAs loaded into exosomes in implantation. A novel cell-to-cell communication mechanism involving delivery of endometrial miRNAs from the maternal endometrium to preimplantation embryo trophectoderm cells has been described [46]. Vilella et al. observed that both EV-associated and free miR-30d could be observed in B6C3-derived mouse embryos, resulting in the overexpression of genes involved in adhesion processes, including Itgα7 and Cdh5 [46]. Moreover, it was shown that supplementation of murine embryos with miR-30d significantly improved embryo adhesion, suggesting that external miRNAs may play a functional role as transcriptomic modifiers in preimplantation embryos. Profiling miRNA expression in endometrial fluid has revealed that maternally derived miRNAs are present in EVs in the uterine microenvironment. While the mechanism(s) by which embryos take external miRNAs in remain unknown, the implications of this discovery are profound as it provides a mechanism by which the mother can program embryo development prior to its implantation. Moreover, it points to a deficiency in in vitro culture media that may underlie observed developmental differences between IVF and in vivo conceived offspring.

Conclusions and clinical implications

The introduction of molecular genetic analysis into the interrogation of endometrial function can be viewed as the first step in a revolution in clinical endometrial assessment. Prior to this, scrutiny of the endometrium has been limited to histological examination and ultrasound visualization, neither of which have provided the information required by clinicians to guide treatment or counseling. The knowledge gap that has grown between the embryo and the endometrium as determinants of successful implantation is beginning to be reduced, and with this comes the promise of novel therapeutic interventions that target specific endometrial causes of implantation failure.

Key to this revolution will be the realization that the endometrium is more than just "receptive." The reasons for which an embryo fails to implant once placed in the uterine cavity are many, and can intervene at any stage between arriving in the endometrial cavity and establishing pregnancy. It is clear that a new approach to diagnosing the endometrium is required if women are to benefit from personalized, effective treatments rather than the empirical therapies currently on offer [47]. Alongside transcriptomic analysis, the other "omics," including proteomic analysis of endometrial secretions, examination of the microbiome using next-generation sequencing techniques, and the development of clinical markers of decidual and endometrial biosensor function, will become part of an endometrial clinical "diagnostic toolbox" that will come to rival that enjoyed by embryologists in their scrutiny of embryo viability.

Implantation failure is no longer a clinical "black box" [48].

References

[1] Salamonsen LA, Nie G, Hannan NJ, Dimitriadis E. Society for Reproductive Biology Founders' Lecture 2009. Preparing fertile soil: the importance of endometrial receptivity. Reprod Fertil Dev 2009;21:923–34.

[2] Giudice LC. Potential biochemical markers of uterine receptivity. Hum Reprod 1999;14(Suppl. 2):3–16.

[3] Noyes RW, Hertig AT, Rock J. Dating the endometrial biopsy. Fertil Steril 1950;1:3–25.

[4] Boomsma CM, Kavelaars A, Eijkemans MJ, Amarouchi K, Teklenburg G, Gutknecht D, et al. Cytokine profiling in endometrial secretions: a non-invasive window on endometrial receptivity. Reprod Biomed Online 2009;18:85–94.

[5] Boomsma CM, Kavelaars A, Eijkemans MJ, Lentjes EG, Fauser BC, Heijnen CJ, et al. Endometrial secretion analysis identifies a cytokine profile predictive of pregnancy in IVF. Hum Reprod 2009;24:1427–35.

[6] Cheong Y, Boomsma C, Heijnen C, Macklon N. Uterine secretomics: a window on the maternal-embryo interface. Fertil Steril 2013;99:1093–9.

[7] Salamonsen LA, Edgell T, Rombauts LJ, Stephens AN, Robertson DM, Rainczuk A, et al. Proteomics of the human endometrium and uterine fluid: a pathway to biomarker discovery. Fertil Steril 2013;99:1086–92.

[8] Diaz-Gimeno P, Horcajadas JA, Martinez-Conejero JA, Esteban FJ, Alama P, Pellicer A, et al. A genomic diagnostic tool for human endometrial receptivity based on the transcriptomic signature. Fertil Steril 2011;95:50–60 60.e51-15.

[9] Talbi S, Hamilton AE, Vo KC, et al. Molecular phenotyping of human endometrium distinguishes menstrual cycle phases and underlying biological processes in normo-ovulatory women. Endocrinology. 2006;147(3):1097–121.

[10] Carson DD, Lagow E, Thathiah A, et al. Changes in gene expression during the early to mid-luteal (receptive phase) transition in human endometrium detected by high-density microarray screening. Mol Hum Reprod 2002;8(9):871–9.

[11] Riesewijk A, Martin J, van Os R, et al. Gene expression profiling of human endometrial receptivity on days LH + 2 versus LH + 7 by microarray technology. Mol Hum Reprod 2003;9(5):253–64.

[12] Macklon NS, van der Gaast MH, Hamilton A, Fauser BC, Giudice LC. The impact of ovarian stimulation with recombinant FSH in combination with GnRH antagonist on the endometrial transcriptome in the window of implantation. Reprod Sci 2008;15 (4):357–65.

[13] Ponnampalam AP, Weston GC, Trajstman AC, Susil B, Rogers PA. Molecular classification of human endometrial cycle stages by transcriptional profiling. Mol Hum Reprod 2004;10(12):879–93.

[14] Wilcox AJ, Baird DD, Weinberg CR. Time of implantation of the conceptus and loss of pregnancy. N Engl J Med 1999;340:1796–9.

[15] Horcajadas JA, Pellicer A, Simon C. Wide genomic analysis of human endometrial receptivity: new times, new opportunities. Hum Reprod Update 2007;13:77–86.

[16] Diaz-Gimeno P, Ruiz-Alonso M, Blesa D, Bosch N, Martinez-Conejero JA, Alama P, et al. The accuracy and reproducibility of the endometrial receptivity array is superior to histology as a diagnostic method for endometrial receptivity. Fertil Steril 2013;99:508–17.

[17] Macklon N. Recurrent implantation failure is a pathology with a specific transcriptomic signature. Fertil Steril 2017;108:9–14.

[18] Ruiz-Alonso M, Blesa D, Diaz-Gimeno P, Vilella F, Pellicer A, Simon C. The endometrial receptivity array as diagnosis and personalized embryo transfer as treatment for patients with receptive implantation failure. Fertil Steril 2013;100:818–24.

[19] Kao LC, Germeyer A, Tulac S, Lobo S, Yang JP, Taylor RN, et al. Expression profiling of endometrium from women with endometriosis reveals candidate genes for disease-based implantation failure and infertility. Endocrinology 2003;144:2870–81.

[20] Horcajadas JA, Sharkey AM, Catalano RD, Sherwin JR, Domínguez F, Burgos LA, et al. Effect of an intrauterine device on the gene expression profile of the endometrium. J Clin Endocrinol Metab 2006;91: 3199–207.
[21] Simon A, Laufer N. Assessment and treatment of repeated implantation failure (RIF). J Assist Reprod Genet 2012;29:1227–39.
[22] Koot Y, van Hooff S, Boomsma C, van Leenen D, Groot Koerkamp M, Goddijn M, et al. An endometrial gene expression signature accurately predicts recurrent implantation failure after IVF. Sci Rep 2016;22:19411.
[23] Koler M, Achache H, Tsafrir A, Smith Y, Revel A, Reich R. Disrupted gene pattern in patients with repeated in vitro fertilization (IVF) failure. Hum Reprod 2009;24(10):2541–8.
[24] Bartosch C, Lopes JM, Beires J, Sousa M. Human endometrium ultrastructure during the implantation window: a new perspective of the epithelium cell types. Reprod Sci 2011;18:525–39.
[25] Georges A, Auguste A, Bessière L, Vanet A, Todeschini AL, Veitia RA, et al. FOXL2: a central transcription factor of the ovary. J Mol Endocrinol 2014;52: R17–33.
[26] Richards JS, Pangas SA. The ovary: basic biology and clinical implications. J Clin Invest 2010;120:963–72.
[27] Macklon NS, Brosens JJ. The human endometrium as a sensor of embryo quality. Biol Reprod 2014;92:98.
[28] Lucas ES, Dyer NP, Murakami K, Lee YH, Chan YW, Grimaldi G, et al. Loss of endometrial plasticity in recurrent pregnancy loss. Stem Cell 2016;34:346–56.
[29] Huang J, Qin H, Chen X, Zhang J, Laird S, Wang C, et al. A comparison of transcriptomic profiles in endometrium during window of implantation between women with unexplained recurrent implantation failure and recurrent miscarriage. Reproduction 2017;153:749–58.
[30] Teklenburg G, Salker M, Molokhia M, Lavery S, Trew G, Aojanepong T, et al. Natural selection of human embryos: decidualizing endometrial stromal cells serve as sensors of embryo quality upon implantation. PLoS One 2010;5:e10258.
[31] Brosens JJ, Salker MS, Teklenburg G, Nautiyal J, Salter S, Lucas ES, et al. Uterine selection of human embryos at implantation. Sci Rep 2014;6:3894.
[32] Chen G, Bradford WD, Seidel CW, Li R. Hsp90 stress potentiates rapid cellular adaptation through induction of aeuploidy. Nature 2012;29(482):246–50.
[33] Weimar CH, Macklon NS, Post Uiterweer ED, Brosens JJ, Gellersen B. The motile and invasive capacity of human endometrial stromal cells: implications for normal and impaired reproductive function. Hum Reprod Update 2013;19:542–57.
[34] Weimar CH, Kavelaars A, Brosens JJ, Gellersen B, de Vreeden-Elbertse JM, Heijnen CJ, et al. Endometrial stromal cells of women with recurrent miscarriage fail to discriminate between high- and low-quality human embryos. PLoS One 2012;7:e41424.
[35] Schwenke M, Knöfler M, Velicky P, Weimar CH, Kruse M, Samalecos A, et al. Control of human endometrial stromal cell motility by PDGF-BB, HB-EGF and trophoblast-secreted factors. PLoS One 2013;8: e54336.
[36] Salker MS, Nautiyal J, Steel JH, Webster Z, Sućurović S, Nicou M, et al. Disordered IL-33/ST2 activation in decidualizing stromal cells prolongs uterine receptivity in women with recurrent pregnancy loss. PLoS One 2012;7:e52252.
[37] Orlando J, Coulam C. Is superfertility associated with recurrent pregnancy loss? Am J Reprod Immunol 2014;72:549–54.
[38] Williams AE. Functional aspects of animal microRNAs. Cell Mol Life Sci 2008;65(4):545–62.
[39] Kuokkanen S, Chen B, Ojalvo L, Benard L, Santoro N, Pollard JW. Genomic profiling of microRNAs and messenger RNAs reveals hormonal regulation in microRNA expression in human endometrium. Biol Reprod 2010;82(4):791–801.
[40] Qian K, Hu L, Chen H, et al. Hsa-miR-222 is involved in differentiation of endometrial stromal cells in vitro. Endocrinology 2009;150(10):4734–43.
[41] Filigheddu N, Gregnanin I, Porporato PE, et al. Differential expression of microRNAs between eutopic and ectopic endometrium in ovarian endometriosis. J Biomed Biotechnol 2010;2010:369549.
[42] Pan Q, Luo X, Toloubeydokhti T, Chegini N. The expression profile of micro-RNA in endometrium and endometriosis and the influence of ovarian steroids on their expression. Mol Hum Reprod 2007;13 (11):797–806.
[43] Sha AG, Liu JL, Jiang XM, Ren JZ, Ma CH, Lei W, et al. Genome-wide identification of micro-ribonucleic acids associated with human endometrial receptivity in natural and stimulated cycles by deep sequencing. Fertil Steril 2011;96(1):150–5.
[44] Altmäe S, Martinez-Conejero JA, Esteban FJ, Ruiz-Alonso M, Stavreus-Evers A, Horcajadas JA, et al. MicroRNAs miR-30b, miR-30d, and miR-494 regulate human endometrial receptivity. Reprod Sci 2013;20 (3):308–17.
[45] Pieters BC, Arntz OJ, Bennink MB, Broeren MG, van Caam AP, Koenders MI, et al. Commercial cow milk contains physically stable extracellular vesicles

expressing immunoregulatory TGF-β. PLoS One 2015;10(3):e0121123.
[46] Vilella F, Moreno-Moya JM, Balaguer N, Grasso A, Herrero M, Martínez S, et al. Hsa-miR-30d, secreted by the human endometrium, is taken up by the preimplantation embryo and might modify its transcriptome. Development 2015;142(18):3210–21.
[47] Hviid MM, Macklon N. Immune modulation treatments-where is the evidence? Fertil Steril 2017;107 (6):1284–93.
[48] Macklon NS, Geraedts JP, Fauser BC. Conception to ongoing pregnancy: the 'black box' of early pregnancy loss. Hum Reprod Update 2002;8 (4):333–43.

CHAPTER

11

Genetics of premature ovarian insufficiency

Jose Serna[1,2], *Elisa Varela*[2,3] *and Juan A. García-Velasco*[2,3,4]

[1]IVI RMA Zaragoza, Zaragoza, Spain [2]IVI Foundation, Madrid, Spain [3]IVI RMA Madrid, Madrid, Spain [4]Rey Juan Carlos University, Madrid, Spain

Introduction

Ovarian function, namely the production of mature oocytes and sexual hormones, spans from menarche to menopause and depends on follicular endowment and depletion, which are regulated by only partially understood mechanisms [1].

The human ovaries contain nearly 7 million germ cell at mid-gestation [2]. At birth there are 1–2 million primordial follicles (PFs) and they decline further, yielding an approximate number of 400,000 PFs at menarche. A progressive decline exists until menopause, when the number of PFs is around 1000 and ovulation ceases [2]. The mean age at natural menopause is 48.8 years, although this varies among countries and socioeconomical status and lifestyle [3].

Premature ovarian insufficiency (POI) is defined as the presence, before the age of 40, of amenorrhea for at least 4 months, low plasma estradiol levels, and FSH of more than 25 IU/mL on two occasions taken >4 weeks apart [4]. It was first described by Fuller Albright as "POI" [5]. The term was chosen to highlight the ovary as the primary source of dysfunction in order to differentiate it from secondary hypogonadotrophic hypogonadism. The terminology referring to this clinical picture is variable depending on the medical specialties or the part of the world [6]. Over time, this medical condition has received many different designations (e.g., gonadal dysgenesis, POI, premature ovarian failure, premature menopause, early menopause, hypergonadotrophic hypogonadism, POI, ovarian dysgenesis, primary ovarian failure, hypergonadotrophic amenorrhea, etc.). Although the ESHRE guideline developing group opted to use the term premature POI [4], it has not been extended in the literature (Table 11.1). "Insufficiency" is recommended in preference to "failure" because the former includes ovarian dysgenesis and hypergonadotrophic hypogonadism [7]. It should be called early menopause when it appears between the ages of 40 and 45 [4]. A clear distinction between POI and diminished ovarian reserve must be made [8]. The prevalence of POI has been estimated as 1% in the general population [9], and varies depending on ethnicity and lifestyle [10].

Human Reproductive Genetics
DOI: https://doi.org/10.1016/B978-0-12-816561-4.00011-9

TABLE 11.1 Terms utilized in the literature to refer to this clinical picture over time.

To January 2019[a]		From January 2014[b]		From January 2018[c]	
Gonadal dysgenesis	31%	Primary ovarian insufficiency	29%	Primary ovarian insufficiency	24%
Primary ovarian insufficiency	21%	Premature ovarian failure	20%	Premature ovarian failure	20%
Premature ovarian failure	18%	Gonadal dysgenesis	14%	Premature ovarian insufficiency	18%
Premature menopause	11%	Premature ovarian insufficiency	11%	Gonadal dysgenesis	13%
Early menopause	7%	Premature menopause	9%	Early menopause	11%
Hypergonadotropic hypogonadism	4%	Early menopause	9%	Premature menopause	7%
Premature ovarian insufficiency	3%	Hypergonadotropic hypogonadism	5%	Hypergonadotropic hypogonadism	6%
Ovarian dysgenesis	2%	Primary ovarian failure	1%	Primary ovarian failure	1%
Primary ovarian failure	1%	Ovarian dysgenesis	1%	Ovarian dysgenesis	<1%
Hypergonadotropic amenorrhea	<1%	Hypergonadotropic amenorrhea	<1%	Hypergonadotropic amenorrhea	<1%
Climacterium praecox	<1%	Climacterium praecox	<1%	Climacterium praecox	<1%
Menopause praecox	<1%	Menopause praecox	<1%	Menopause praecox	<1%

[a]*A PubMed search for each of the denominations was performed with no restricted publication date.*
[b]*Restricted from 2014 to date.*
[c]*Restricted from 2018 to early 2019.*
For each time period the denominations were sorted according to their relative frequency of appearance.

To date, there is no biochemical or clinical marker that predicts the age at menopause, although women with low ovarian reserve (OR) are prone to POI [11]. Due to the tendency in the Western world to increase mean maternal age [12], predicting the risk of POI is of paramount importance to preventing infertility. Furthermore, the cessation of ovarian hormone production leads to major symptoms and long-term side effects that must be addressed [13,14]. Moreover, some of the genetics influencing POI are also involved in metabolic, neurogenerative, and neoplastic diseases, therefore early diagnosis may improve the prognosis of such complications.

There are more than 50 genes whose mutations can be causative of POI and many other genes that may be implicated [15]. The genetics of POI is difficult to classify because there are many pathways and cellular functions that may be impaired, for example, gonadal development, DNA replication, DNA repair, meiosis, hormonal signaling, immune function, and metabolism. Some authors classify POI into isolated and syndromic POI, but for some genes that typically provoke syndromic POI, isolated POI may occasionally appear or be the initial presentation (i.e., *NBN*, *eIF2B*, genes in Perrault syndrome, *FOXL2*, *FMR1*, etc.).

Some of the genetic alterations producing POI are related to tumor predisposition or other complications later in life, highlighting the relevance of a genetic study and counseling in POI patients [16].

Premature ovarian insufficiency etiology

The potential causes of POI are shown in Table 11.2. There are well known genetic

TABLE 11.2 Potential causes of premature ovarian insufficiency (POI).

- Iatrogenic
  - Ovarian surgery
  - Chemotherapy
  - Radiotherapy
- Environmental factors
- Viral infections
- Metabolic diseases
- Autoimmune diseases
- Genetic alterations
- Idiopathic

causes of POI, but there is a high suspicion that idiopathic causes of POI bear a strong familial/genetic association [17], as occurs with the age at menopause [18]. The existence of animal models that match with mutations in suspected genes, and the association of chromosomal abnormalities, such as Turner syndrome (TS) (45,X), with POI support the strong suspicion that genetics is associated with many of the idiopathic cases of POI patients.

The possible genetic causes of POI may be related to:

1. Sex chromosomes;
   a. Aneuploidies
   b. X structural abnormalities
   c. Other sex chromosome abnormalities;
2. Specific genes on the X chromosome;
3. Mutations in autosomal genes;
4. Fragile X;
5. Noncoding RNAs.

Technical advances

Cytogenetic karyotyping has long been used for aneuploidies and structural chromosomal alterations. In terms of particular genes, the quest for candidate genes was hampered by Sanger's sequencing limitations. Next-generation sequencing (NGS) has revolutionized the genetics of POI. An important characteristic of NGS is the length of the genomic region to be covered. There are four main formats available:

1. *Target sequencing microarray (TSM)*: includes panels of particular selected genes/regions;
2. *Whole exome sequencing (WES)*: includes all the genome's coding region;
3. *Whole transcriptome sequencing or RNA-Seq*: includes coding plus noncoding RNA;
4. *Whole genome sequencing (WGS)*: adds all the intronic regions. As it includes vast sequences of unknown function, it is reserved for research purposes.

NGS data need bioinformatics to evaluate variants and their relevance base on multiple variables (type of genetic disease, amino acid conservation among species, tertiary structure predicted, etc.). Considerations on sequencing depth and coverage must be taken into account and variants found must be confirmed by Sanger's sequencing [19] Moreover, some genomic regions are not fully covered and variants in a heterozygous state might not be selected in the presence of a digenic/polygenic POI [20].

With the advent of NGS and lower cost, soon the workup in POI diagnosis will include target sequencing microarray/whole exome sequencing (TSM/WES) with ethical and relevant counseling for implications relative to familial and later-in-life possible complications.

Genetics of the ovarian reserve

Many genes are involved in the determination of the OR. The molecular mechanism associated with OR determination has been partially elucidated in recent years [15,21]. This insight can be carried out with the aid of animal models (e.g., mice and *Drosophila*) as it is a process highly conserved among species.

Primordial germ cells (PGCs) originate in the extraembryonic mesoderm and migrate to the genital ridge and after divisions and differentiations generate oogonias, which through aggregation end up forming the germ cell cyst that must break down to form the PF [22]. Commitment, migration, and proliferation of PGCs were subsequently driven by the following genes: bone morphogenetic proteins (BMPs) and Wnt3/β-catenin necessary to promote pluripotency and to inhibit differentiation, through Prdm1 and Prmd14, which mediate the expression of pluripotency genes (*Pou5F1*, *Nanog*, *Klf4*, and *Lin28a*) and germline-specific genes (*Nanos3*, *Kitlg*, *Tfapc2*, *Dppa3*; *Ddx4*, *Vasa*, *Mael*, and *Dazl*) [23]. From 12 weeks of pregnancy until birth, meiosis commences but stops in the diplotene stage of prophase I. Tab4b directly occupies the proximal promoter region of critical meiotic genes, including *Stra8*, *Dazl*, *Figla*, and *Nobox* [24]. *Dazl* expression is involved in meiosis activation, which induces responsiveness to retinoic acid, which in turn induces Stimulated by Retinoic Acid (Stra) 8 (Stra8)-dependent and -independent pathways. Finally, germ cell cysts break down via apoptosis and pregranulosa cells encapsulate a single oocyte and meiosis stops in prophase I. The number of follicles is reduce to one-third [22]. Factors driving these processes include: Gdf9, Bmp15, FoxL2, Nobox, Figla, Notch2, and Adam10 [23,25].

The synaptonemal complex (SC) is stabilized by cohesins. From this family of proteins, Stromal antigen 3 (STAG3), Recombination 8 (REC8), Structural Maintenance of Chromosomes 1 beta, and Radiation Sensitive 21-Like, are relevant in meiosis [26]. The last three have been proposed as candidates for POI but, to date, none has been described in humans [20]. However, by means of WES, a point-mutation in *STAG3*, whose transcript would either be not translated or result in a truncated unfunctional protein, has been described in a Middle Eastern family [27]. Inactivation of this protein in mice results in early oocyte death [28]. In another consanguineous family with Arabic origin, a mutation in the Synaptonemal Complex Central Element Protein 1, another member of the SC complex, was described in two sisters [29]. The inactivation of this protein in mice resulted in a lack of follicles in ovaries [30].

To ensure proper sister chromatid separation, the centromeric cohesion must be preserved during meiosis I. Shugoshin-like proteins, SGO1 and SGO2, are key proteins involved in this step. A combined pathogenic variant in *SGO2* and *CLDN14* (gene coding for Claudin14) has been describe in four members of a family with Perrault syndrome (PS) (see below) [31].

A critical point during meiosis is homologous recombination (HR). During DNA resection by the MRN complex (i.e., Mre11-Rad50-Nbs1), two helicases from the minichromosome maintenance (MCM) family assist in this step (i.e., MCM-8 and MCM-9) forming a complex [32]. In mutant mice for any of these genes there is an early loss of germ cells, and they were predisposed to cancer [33,34]. In some consanguineous families variants of *MCM8* and *MCM9* have been encountered causing genomic instability and POI [35,36].

The proteasome 26S subunit, ATPase, 3-interacting protein (PSMC3IP), crucial in HR, interacts DNA with recombinases RAD51 and DMC1 [37]. *PSMC3IP* homozygous mutations was found in five women with gonadal dysgenesis [38] and another mutation was found in six sisters with ovarian dysgenesis and a brother with azoospermia [39]. Two different mutations have been identified in women with POI in two different families [40,41].

ZMM proteins are responsible for crossover processing. These proteins include SYCP1, HFM1 helicase, the MSH4–MSH5 complex, and the MLH1–MLH3 heterodimer. HFM1 stabilized strand invasion catalyzed by RAD51 [42,43]. *Hfm1* knockout mice have ovaries with reduced size and a decreased number of follicles [43]. Two compound heterozygous mutations in *HFM1* were detected in two Chinese sisters with POI [44] and other mutations in some POI Chinese women [45]. A homozygous splice-site mutation in *MSH4* was detected in a Colombian family with POI-affected members [46]. In addition, *MSH5* mutations have been reported in several publications [47,48].

RecQ helicases have been proposed to be involved in HR. In one of these helicases, *REC8*, missense mutations have been described in patients with POI [20].

DNA repair proteins were also involved in POI. In a family with several members affected with POI, certain mutations in the Cockayne Syndrome B (*CSB*)-*PGBD3* gene have been described [49].

Nonhomologous end-joining is a secondary process involved in double-stranded break repair [50]. Two proteins involved in this process X-ray repair cross-complementing protein 4 (XRCC4) and Ligase 4 (LIG4). A homozygous variant in *XRCC4* was found in a female with a history of severe postnatal growth failure, microcephaly, primary gonadal failure, and early-onset metabolic syndrome. She developed a malignant gastrointestinal stromal tumor at age 28 [51]. Similarly, a mutation in *LIG4* was described in two patients with syndromic POI [52].

Finally, the Fanconi anemia DNA repair pathway, which repairs DNA interstrand cross-links, is also present in germinal cells. Several proteins are involved in this pathway and mutations in their genes have been associated with POI [53–55].

Follicular development

Folliculogenesis starts with initial recruitment to produce a cohort of follicles available for the cyclic recruitment. Several factors are implied in both recruitment and POI [56].

Loss-of-function mutation has been described in the *ESR1* gene. These patients present a plethora of peripheral symptoms, showing primary amenorrhea and multicystic anovulating ovaries [57,58]. By means of a candidate single-gene approach toward the *ESR2* gene, a mutation was described in a girl with primary amenorrhea but the contribution of other genes to the phenotype was not excluded [59]. In contrast, a girl with a defective mutation in the *ESR2* gene showed no ovaries visible by ultrasound and absence of markers of granulosa cells (such as anti-Müllerian hormone), suggesting the absence of follicles/streak gonads [60].

Mutations in the *FSHR* gene show varied phenotypes depending on the functionality of the protein they yield [61]. New mutations appear from time to time [62,63]. The first mutation described was in a Finnish family that showed a phenotype with absence of antral follicles [64] that later was characterized as a partial loss-of-function mutation [65]. A complete loss-of-function mutation was described in a patient whose ovarian histology showed that the receptor remained intracellularly, and the ovaries had an increase in the density of small follicles. There was a complete blockade of maturation after the primary stage [66].

With respect to the other gonadotrophin receptor, that is, *LHCGR*, a mutation was found in patients with oligoanovulation and recurrent cyst formation [67].

BMP15 and Growth and Differentiation Factor 9 (GDF9) are members of the TGF-β family with paramount relevance in controlling ovarian function. They are secreted by the ovary to act in granulosa cells (GCs) and drive proper oocyte maturation [68]. They may act alone or form a heterodimer, known as Cumulin [69]. *BMP15* mutations affect the ovary in several ways, for example, impaired early folliculogenesis, increased dizygotic twinning, ovarian hyperstimulation, and POI

[70–74]. The first mutation in *BMP15* identified in humans was a heterozygous POI patient with ovarian dysgenesis [75]. Thereafter, several mutations have been described in nonsyndromic POI patients [68]. Most of the variants were found in a heterozygous state, meaning that haploinsufficiency must be relevant, although in one publication, the mutation was only in a homozygous state with the progenitors being heterozygous for the mutations and with no phenotype [76]. It was proposed that variants of *BMP15* may affect POI patients in an oligogenic synergistic fashion [20] which was implicated in the POI phenotype related to TS [77]. Several variants of the *GDF9* also were related to POI [68].

Syndromic premature ovarian insufficiency

X chromosome defects

X chromosome changes in number and structure (i.e., monosomies, polysomies, Turner mosaicism, deletions, insertions, isochromosomes, and translocations) are associated with POI [78]. By means of cytogenetics in POI patients with balanced X-autosome translocations, a critical region on the long arm of the X chromosome was shown, that is, the Xq13.3–q27 interval [78]. Translocation may disrupt gene transcription due to the "position effect."

The 45,X is the typical karyotype associated with TS. Nevertheless, it has been proposed that surviving individuals are most likely 45, X/46,XX mosaicisms or have structural abnormalities of the X chromosome [79]. Although spontaneous puberty, menstruation, and pregnancies have been reported [80], the majority of TS women have primary amenorrhea due to complete oocyte depletion since the early stages of ovarian development [81,82]. The pathogenesis of TS phenotype is complex, but due to the fact that some X-linked genes escape the physiological inactivation, the most extended theory on this pathogenesis is the presence of only one single copy of these genes [83].

Moreover, the presence of unsynapsed regions might be recognized by meiotic checkpoints, leading to apoptosis and a decrease in the follicle number [84]. Epigenetics effects might also influence POI. It has been shown that X-linked genes in the critical region have a highly heterochromatic organization, downregulating the expression of critical genes in the oocyte [85].

Autoimmune polyendocrinopathy syndrome type I

Alterations in the Autoimmune Regulator (*AIRE*) gene may lead to multisystemic alterations: Addison's disease, hypoparathyroidism, alopecia, vitiligo, keratopathy, malabsorption, hepatitis, and mucocutaneous candidiasis [86]. *AIRE* is expressed in the thymus, where it regulates tolerance from T-cell attack [87]. It is an autosomal dominant disease with multiple mutations described [88]. Around 60% of females develop POI as a consequence of autoimmunity against steroidogenic enzymes [89]. Ovarian autoantibodies as detected by indirect immunofluorescence have poor specificity, as 30% of healthy women have positive test results [90].

Blepharophimosis, ptosis, epicanthus inversus syndrome

Blepharophimosis, ptosis, epicanthus inversus (BPES) syndrome is an autosomal dominant disease with a prevalence of 1:50,000 [2]. Depending on the presence or absence of POI, BPES syndrome has been divided into two categories, type I and type II. The functional alteration in forkhead box L2 transcription factor (FOXL2) is responsible for this syndrome. *FOXL2* was mapped on chromosome 2q23. To date, more than 270 *FOXL2* variants have been reported [91]. Depending on the functional alteration the mutation produces on the protein, the phenotype may vary [92,93]. Some mutations have been described producing POI without BPES syndrome [25,94,95].

Galactosemia and carbohydrate-deficient glycoprotein syndromes

Galactosemia is an autosomal dominant disease caused by deficiency of galactose-1-phosphatase uridyltransferase (GALT) enzyme, with an incidence of about 1:40,000–1:60,000 [96]. To date, more than 350 *GALT* variants have been described, with 277 known to be pathogenic and 16 mild or suspected pathogenic (arup.utah.edu/database/GALT/GALT_welcome.php). Despite dietary restrictions, long-term complications still occur. The majority of women with galactosemia will sooner or later develop POI [97–99]. Several hypotheses support the mechanism of POI in these women [99]: (1) direct toxicity of galactose to the oocytes and follicles, depleting the OR or compromising maturation, (2) impaired PGCs development [100], (3) alteration in glycosylation in gene pathways [101], hormones [102], and receptors [103], (4) effecting downregulation of the PI3K/Akt growth signaling pathway, targeting protein and gene expression, decreasing OR [104], and (5) oxidative stress [21]. POI may appear as primary or secondary amenorrhea and pregnancies have been described; the role of oocyte or ovarian cortex cryopreservation plays an important role in this pathology [105]. Medical treatment with salubridal may attenuate oocyte depletion [106].

Congenital disorders of glycosylation

Carbohydrate-deficient glycoprotein syndromes are a group of AR diseases related to mutations in the *PMM2* gene that encodes phosphomannomutase enzyme involved in the conversion of mannose-6-phosphate into mannose-1-phosphate. The clinical presentation shows a wide range of systemic disorders and early POI [21,107].

Pseudohypoparathyroidism type 1a

The *GNAS* gene encodes the α subunit of the guanine nucleotide-binding protein (G protein) implied in the process of signal transduction [108]. It is located on chromosome 20q13.32. Mutations and epigenetics modifications [109], due to its imprinting, result in diverse clinical syndromes, whose genetic mutations are sometimes difficult to study [110]. G proteins are downstream of hormone receptors, thus FSH and LH, among others, have impaired signaling [111].

Mitochondria

PS (sensorineural hearing loss and ovarian insufficiency) is a frequently clinically overlooked pathology mainly due to the variable expression and relationship between phenotype and genotype.

Polymerase DNA directed gamma (*POLG*) gene encodes mitochondrial DNA γ polymerase in charge of mitochondrial DNA replication and repair. *POLG* is located on chromosome 15q25. Mutations in this gene result in secondary accumulation of mtDNA deletions in patients' tissues and usually affect muscular and neurological systems [112]. Pathological variants provoke *progressive external ophthalmoplegia* (PEO), whose clinical picture includes proximal myopathy, sensory ataxia, POI, and Parkinsonism [112]. In a family with multiple members affected with PEO and POI, a compound heterozygosity was observed in three generations [113]. The pattern of inheritance is AR when mutations affect the polymerase domain, while it is AD when the exonuclease domain is affected [112,113]. There has been no POLG mutation described that produces isolated idiopathic POI [114].

Another gene involved in mtDNA maintenance that causes PEO and POI is *RNASEH1*, encoding ribonuclease H1 (RNase H1), which is physiologically located in the nucleus and mitochondria. Improper function of this RNase also provokes an accumulation of mtDNA mutations [115,116].

Twinkle mtDNA helicase gene or *C10ORF2* is a nuclear gene located in 10q24.31. *C10ORF2* codes for a helicase in charge of mtDNA unwinding during replication. Pathologic mutations are responsible for mtDNA depletion or deletions and POI with hearing loss, PEO, and PS [117,118].

During translation, aminoacyl transfer RNA (tRNA) synthases (aaRS) link amino acids with their cognate tRNAs. KARS and GARS are shared by the cytoplasmic and mitochondrial translation systems but the rest of the aaRS are specific for each system, that is, *-ARS* genes for cytoplasmic translation and *-ARS2* genes for the translation of the 13 mitochondrial genes. Diseases related with these synthases are leukodystrophies, peripheral neuropathies, and POI [119]. *HARS2*, *LARS2*, and *AARS2* encode mitochondrial histidyl-, leucyl-, and alanyl-tRNA synthetases 2, respectively. *HARS2* and *LARS2* mutations lead to PS with impaired hearing and POI [120,121]. When *AARS2* is mutated besides POI, adult-onset encephalopathy appears [122]. A compound heterozygous mutation in this gene has been encountered in a woman with POI and adult-onset leukodystrophy [123] In addition to this AR heritage, a compound heterozygous inheritance pattern may appear, as shown with *LARS2* and *KARS* (lysyl-tRNA synthetase) causing ovarioleukodystrophy [124]. Another gene involved in mitochondrial translation is *KIAA0391*, which encodes proteinaceous RNase P, a metallonuclease subunit of the mitochondrial RNase P complex, responsible for the 5′-end processing of mitochondrial precursor tRNAs. A missense variant has been detected in a consanguineous family with three members with PS being homozygous for this mutation [125].

CLPP encodes mitochondrial ATP-dependent chambered protease, a component of a mitochondrial ATP-dependent proteolytic complex, involved in the degradation of unfolded or misfolded proteins, that when mutated is associated with PS [126–128].

Other recently described genes encoding mitochondrial-acting proteins related with PS are *ERAL1* and *KIAA0391*. ERAL1 protein binds to the mitochondrial 12S rRNA and is involved in the assembly of the small mitochondrial ribosomal subunit. A single homozygous mutation in *ERAL1* has been described in three unrelated women with PS [129].

17β-Hydroxysteroid dehydrogenase type 4 (HSD17B4), also known as D-bifunctional protein, is a multifunctional peroxisomal enzyme involved in fatty acid β-oxidation and steroid metabolism. Homozygous mutations in the *HSD17B4* gene leading to DBP deficiency provoke an autosomal-recessive disorder of peroxisomal fatty acid β-oxidation that is generally fatal within the first 2 years of life. Nevertheless, a compound heterozygous mutation has been described in different families with members affected with PS [130,131]. It has been hypothesized that peroxisome dysfunction leads to (among other molecular and metabolic changes within the cell) impaired mitochondrial function [132]. Recently, a homozygous *HSD17B4* mutation causing PS has been described, suggesting that depending on how this enzyme is impaired the phenotype may vary [133].

Complex V of mitochondrial ATP synthase defects impairs mitochondrial energy production. Mutations of *MT-ATP6/8* encoding two subunits of this complex are related with syndromes including cerebellar ataxia, peripheral neuropathy, diabetes mellitus, and POI [134].

Ovarioleukodystrophy

Ovarioleukodystrophy is a leukoencephalopathy with vanishing white matter of the central nervous system associated with POI. Eukaryotic initiation factor 2B (eIF2B) is a nucleotide-exchange factor that plays a key regulatory role in the translation initiation phase of protein synthesis and is required to prevent the synthesis of denatured proteins under cellular stress [135]. Pathologic variants of three of its units (i.e., *EIF2B2*, *EIF2B4*, and *EIF2B5*) have been related with POI associated or not with neurological symptomatology [136]. POI may be diagnosed before the neurological symptoms appear [137,138]. The reason for the degree of the phenotype remains unclear. *EIF2B* gene should be considered a potential candidate for patients with isolated POI [15]. In addition, some *AARS2*, *LARS2*, and *KARS* mutations are also implicated in leukoencephalopathies and POI [122,124].

Ataxia telangiectasia

The Ataxia Telangiectasia Mutated (*ATM*) gene encodes for a protein kinase implicated in cell cycle control, detecting DNA damage known to result in a chromosome breakage disorder. Pathologic mutations in *ATM* result in ataxia telangiectasia, an AR disease showing cerebellar degeneration, oculomotor dysfunction, immunodeficiency, cancer susceptibility, increased radiation sensitivity, and chromosomal instability, as well as POI [139].

Demirhan syndrome

Bone morphogenetic protein receptor 1B (BMPR1B) is a receptor for Growth and Differentiation Factor 5 (GDF5). Mutations in *BMPR1B* have been found to cause a skeletal syndrome with absent or hypoplastic ovaries [140].

Premature aging syndromes

Several syndromes characterized by symptoms of premature aging are associated with POI. *Bloom syndrome* is an AR disease related with mutations in the gene which encodes the DNA helicase BLM. The main symptoms of Bloom syndrome include short stature, typical skin rashes on sun-exposed areas, moderate immunodeficiency, increased cancer risk due to chromosome instability, and hypogonadism [141]. *WRN* codes for another DNA helicase that, when mutated, provokes *Werner syndrome*, an adult progeria with increased cancer risk and atrophic gonads [142].

Another POI-related syndromic premature aging is *GAPO* caused by recessive mutations in *ANTXR1* gene, whose protein is involved in cell adhesion and migration. Ovaries show premature follicular depletion [143].

Fragile X syndrome

Fragile X syndrome (FXS) is member of a large group of neurological conditions known as the repeat expansion diseases. It was first described in 1943 by Martin and Bell as a familial syndrome of intellectual disability with dysmorphic features and macroorchidism affecting men [144]. It was named after the fragility showed in X chromosome cytogenetics in Xq27.3, as FXS [145]. *FMR1* enclosed in the 5′ untranslated region of exon 1, a highly polymorphic CGG repeat, and a CpG island 250 bp in the previous noncoding region [146].

Based on the CGG repeat sequence four alleles has been differentiated, that is, (1) normal, (2) intermediate or gray zone,

TABLE 11.3 *FMR1* CGG triplet expansion, modifiers, simplified molecular effects, and clinical picture.

Allele size	Number of triplets	Modifiers[a]	Produces	Clinical picture
Normal	6–44 CGGs	–	Normal mRNA	Normal
			Normal FMRP	
Intermediate allele (gray zone)	45–54 CGGs	–	Normal mRNA	Normal
			Normal FMRP	
		+	Excess mRNA	FXTAS/FXPOI[b]
			Normal or slightly decreased FMRP	
Premutation	55–200 CGGs	–	Excess mRNA	FXTAS/FXPOI[b]
			Normal or slightly decreased FMRP	
		+	No FMRP	FXS
Mutation	> 200	CpG islands and repeats methylated	No FMRP	FXS
		Unmethylated	Excess mRNA	FXTAS/FXPOI[a]

[a]*Mainly methylation.*
[b]*Other disorders. The effect of intermediate allele, premutation, and mutation categories may change depending on the degree of methylation, AGG interspersion, and maybe other modifiers.*
FMRP, Fragile X mental retardation protein; *FXTAS*, fragile X-associated tremor/ataxia syndrome; *FXPOI*, fragile X-associated premature ovarian; *FXS*, fragile X syndrome.

(3) premutation (PM), and (4) mutation. The mutation process is by expansion in each generation depending on several factors (gender, CGG repeat number, the presence of AGG interspersion, external agents, and possibly others) [147–151]. The level of triplet expansion modifies the methylation pattern that, combined, produces changes in *FMR1*-mRNA size and changes in their translation properties (Table 11.3) [147]. *FMR1* gene physiologically escapes from X chromosome methylation, but in the full mutated allele it is methylated and *FMR1* expression is silenced [152]. This picture is further complicated by the presence of mosaicism, both in length and methylation, blurring the boundaries between the phenotypes of the PM and the full mutation [153,154]. The prevalence of the different alleles change depending on the population studied [155,156].

A mother will transmit the affected allele to 50% of her sons or daughters, while a father will pass it on to all his daughters and none of his sons. In the presence of PM alleles and in some cases of intermediate alleles, in 20% of women and 50% of older men, fragile X-associated premature ovarian (FXPOI) and fragile X-associated tremor/ataxia syndrome (FXTAS) appear (Table 11.4).

Fragile X-associated premature ovarian insufficiency

The *FMR1* PM is the most common genetic cause of POI [157]. Women carrying *FMR1* PM and intermediate alleles are at risk of developing POI. Alternatively, having the full mutation alleles carries the same POI risk as the general population [158]. Around 20% of women carrying the PM develop POI but full mutation

TABLE 11.4 Clinical involvement associated with the premutation.

	Prevalence (permutation carriers vs general population)			
Phenotype	Male carriers	Female carriers	Male noncarriers	Female noncarriers
FXTAS	40%	16%	N/A	N/A
Fragile X-associated primary ovarian insufficiency	N/A	16%–20%	N/A	~1% (primary ovarian insufficiency)
Hypertension	57%	22%	~30%	~30%
Migraine	27%	54%	~12%	~20%
Neuropathy	62%	17%	<5%	<5%
Sleep apnea	32% with FXTAS	32% with FXTAS	~15%	~5%
Psychiatric problems	~50%	~50%	~3.6% (>45 years old)	~10.3% (>45 years old)

19,20,23–28.
FXTAS, Fragile X-associated tremor ataxia syndrome; *N/A*, not applicable.
Creative common license. Based on Rajaratnam A, Shergill J, Salcedo-Arellano M, Saldarriaga W, Duan X, Hagerman R. Fragile X syndrome and fragile X-associated disorders. F1000Research [Internet]. 2017;6:2112. Available from: https://f1000research.com/articles/6-2112/v1.

carriers will not [159,160]. Those with PM in the range of 80–100 repeats have the highest risk for POI [161]. *FMR1* gene is the cause of approximately 6% of POI cases [159]. Among women with sporadic or familial POI, the PM carrier was present in 3.2% and 11.5%, respectively [162]. *FMR1* PM can be detected in about 11% of familial POI and 3% of sporadic POI [163–165]. The prevalence of PM alleles among the general population is estimated to be of 1:150–300 in females and 1:400–850 in males [166,167]. Nevertheless, due to both founder effects and racial differences in haplotypes, the frequency of expanded *FMR1* alleles is highly variable around the world, with the highest prevalence in Colombia and the lowest in Ireland and Asia [168,169].

Triplet expansion must be tested in (1) individuals with intellectual disability, developmental delay, or autism, (2) individuals who have a family history of FXS, (3) women with a family history of FMR1-associated disorders (POI or early menopause, individuals with late-onset tremor or cerebellar ataxia), and (4) gamete donors [147].

Protein expression and function

In human fetal ovaries fragile X mental retardation protein (FMRP) is expressed in germ cells surrounded by FMRP-negative pregranulosa and interstitial cells [170]. FMRP expression in these germ cells coincides with the loss of expression of the pluripotency-associated protein [171]. In contrast, in adult women it is expressed in granulosa cells of mature follicles [172].

FMRP acts as a posttranscriptional factor binding to different RNAs and modifying translational activity. One-third of all RNAs encoding pre- and postsynaptic proteins are targets of FMRP. This role as a posttranscription factor may explain the phenotypic complexity of the FXS and its variable expression [147].

Molecular mechanism

The precise mechanism of developing FXPOI remains elusive. It may be related to an initial decrease in the OR, altered recruitment of follicles, increased atresia, or altered hypothalamic–pituitary–gonadal axis. At least in mice, the establishment of a PF pool is normal and there is an increased loss of follicles [173,174], suggesting that depletion occurs by follicle loss later in life [175].

Several hypotheses related to oocyte loss have been postulated. The most supported is the increased levels of *FMR1*-mRNA in PM and in intermediate carriers, leading to an RNA gain-of function toxicity. Interestingly there is no increased translation into FMRP. Elevated levels of *FMR1*-mRNA form aggregates with RNA-binding proteins, that might impair cellular functions, at least in FXTAS [176]. Granulosa cells of PM women have increased level of *FMR1*-mRNA [172]. Signaling mechanisms necessary for the maintenance of the survival and activation of the PF, as well as oocyte maturation, are downregulated in FXPOI women [177]. Another proposed mechanism is repeat-associated non-ATG (RAN) translation. Repetitive RNA motifs can cause the initiation of translation in the absence of an AUG start codon. Translation of CGG repeats results in polyglycine-containing protein causing cellular toxicity in FXTAS [178]. Similarly, FMRpolyG were found in ubiquitin-positive inclusions in ovarian stromal cells of PM women [179,180]. Moreover, 49 alternative-spliced isoforms from the 17 exons of *FMR1* are described with tissue-specific differential expression. In PM carriers, the distribution pattern and expression levels of this isoforms were different in asymptomatics compared with patients with FXTAS [181]. Whether this also happens in FXPOI is unknown. Moreover, several long noncoding RNAs are generated from *FMR1* [147]. Specifically, one of these is *FMR6*, which has been detected with the highest levels in granulosa cells of PM women in the range of 80–120 repeats [182].

Other nontranscriptional processes might cause cell death and POI. R-loops (stable RNA–DNA hybrids) are formed during transcription through the expanded CGG repeat track in FXTAS. These loops might activate a cellular DNA-damage response [183]. Furthermore, FAN1 is a nuclease that has both 5′–3′ exonuclease and 5′ flap endonuclease activities. Mutations in *FAN1* may contribute to tissue-specific triplet expansion via a replication-independent process [150]. External agents may worsen the expansion and thus the clinical picture [151]. However, no effect of the loss of FAN1 was apparent for germ-line expansions [150]. Finally, women carrying a PM have shorter telomeres and, hence, are "biologically older" than women carrying the normal-size allele, as the telomere length is not associated with the repeat length but with the diagnosis of FXPOI [184].

FMR2 (*AFF2*) is a gene mapped to Xq28 that behaves similar to *FMR1*. It bears a (GCC)n triplet repeat in exon 1 and has been found to be mutated in 1.5% of POI women studied [185].

Noncoding RNAs

MicroRNAs posttranscriptionally regulate gene expression and are widely expressed in mammalian ovaries [186]. Their expression pattern and levels differentially shift during ovarian development and folliculogenesis [187]. The mRNA expression levels of *FOXO3*, *FOXL2*, and *CCND2* change in transfected granulosa cells with mutated miRNAs, suggesting a role in POI [188]. MiRNA polymorphisms have been described in Asiatic families with POI, suggesting a role of this epigenetic modification in cell survival [189,190].

Role of telomeres in premature ovarian insufficiency

There are several molecular pathways implicated in organismal aging but the telomere pathway, whose function is to safeguard chromosome stability, is a critical one because it is betrothed to and affects other pathways implicated in aging [191].

Telomere history

The existence of telomeres (from Greek "telos" end, and "meros" part) was first proposed by Herman Muller (Nobel Prize 1946) and Barbara McClintock (Nobel Price 1983), who observed that chromosome ends (in *Drosophila melanogaster* and *Zea mays*) were protected from fusions, while chromosome breaks were repaired (fused back together) to maintain their integrity [192–194]. In 1978, Elisabeth Blackburn and Joseph Gall found that telomeres of the protozoan *Tetrahymena* consisted of tandem repeats of the sequence "TTGGGG" and were able to demonstrate that telomeres protect chromosomes from degradation [195,196]. Independent studies by Leonard Hayflick had shown that cells grown in culture could only undergo a limited number of divisions. This was called the replicative senescence phenomenon [197], which was explained on the basis of the unidirectional nature of the chromosome replication machinery, which cannot copy the very ends of chromosomes [198–200]. Therefore on every round of cell division a fragment of telomeric DNA sequence is lost during replication. However, Blackburn and colleagues observed telomere length variations in *Tetrahymena* [195] and hypothesized that a terminal-transferase activity could add repeats onto telomere ends during replication, and that this transferase might be responsible for those variations in telomere length. In 1985, the presence of a terminal-transferase activity was demonstrated in *Tetrahymena* cell-free extracts [201]. Later, it was purified and shown to be composed of both an RNA and a protein component, that were required for activity. This new transferase was called telomerase [202]. Telomerase, a reverse transcriptase able to add DNA using an RNA template, is the main mechanism for telomere elongation and is conserved in higher eukaryotes.

Telomere structure and function

The protective ends of linear chromosomes consist of several kilobases of repeats of the hexameric sequence "TTAGGG," ending in a G-rich 3′ overhang of approximately 300–450 nucleotides [203]. The 3′ overhang can invade the double-stranded telomere DNA sequence to generate a loop structure called the T-loop (telomere loop) [204], which is the first mechanism to hide the telomere end. The telomere sequence and the T-loop are bound by a complex of proteins that protect chromosome ends from degradation and repair activities [205]. This complex is called shelterin and comprises six proteins (TRF1, TRF2, RAP1, TIN2, TPP1, and POT1), which, in addition to telomere protection, control telomere length [206,207]. Telomere and subtelomere regions contain heterochromatic marks which protect telomeres from unscheduled recombination [208] and control telomere length [209]. Moreover, telomeres are further protected by especially long noncoding RNAs which contain telomeric repeats, called TERRAS [210,211], which stabilize telomeres and control telomere length [210,212].

Telomeres and aging

Cell division is required to maintain tissue homeostasis and organ function during the life span of individuals, but after many divisions, telomeres can be reduced to a critically short length. When this happens, shelterins cannot bind and protect telomeres and the T-loop structure cannot be sustained [213], leaving telomeres more accessible to repair and degradation activities. If most telomeres had a critically short length, cells would enter crisis [214], leading to chromosome instability, which is a hallmark of cancer. If only a few telomeres (just five) were critically short, then the DDR pathways would be activated, leading to cell senescence (cells cannot divide further, but they can carry out their function) or apoptosis [215,216]. Accumulation of senescent cells leads to aged tissue and organ dysfunction. Furthermore, if adult stem cells have critically short telomeres and cannot further divide, tissue homeostasis would be compromised. Therefore a certain telomere length is needed to sustain life. Each species has a genetically determined telomere length from birth. Adult mice of the *Mus musculus* species have a mean telomeric length of 40–50 kb, while humans have about 10–15 kb. However, the rate of telomere shortening, and not absolute telomere length, is related to organismal life span [217]. In mice telomeres shorten approximately 7000 bases per year while in humans, telomere attrition is about 100 times slower [217].

Telomerase, which is activated during the blastocyst stage [218,219] can counteract telomere shortening by adding de novo repeats to telomeres, but this activity is undetectable in most cells of the organism, except for embryonic and adult stem cells, the germ line, and cancer cells [220]. Although the lack of telomerase activity may be seen as a disadvantage, it is a mechanism for cancer protection [221].

Attempts to dissect the function of telomerase in aging led to the generation of telomerase-deficient mice [197,222,223] which had short telomeres, decreased regenerative capacity, and a shorter life span [197,222,223], but were cancer resistant. In a very elegant experiment, Jaskelioff and coworkers demonstrated that telomerase reactivation in the fourth generation of mice lacking telomerase reversed tissue degeneration [224]. Telomerase was overexpressed to study its effects on life span and fitness. Indeed, better tissue regeneration was found, but also, a decreased in survival due to spontaneous cancer incidence at young ages [225]. When telomerase was overexpressed in cancer-resistant mice, the regenerative capacity of tissues was higher and the life span was significantly increased [226]. Similar results were observed when telomerase was overexpressed in wild-type mice during adulthood, 1- and 2-year-old mice [227], with an increase in life span and normal incidence of spontaneous cancer. These results are critical to design possible telomerase treatments in humans without increasing the risk of cancer. In humans, accelerated telomere attrition caused bay mutations in genes related to telomere maintenance and telomerase, increasing the risk of suffering aging-associated diseases [228].

Telomeres in female reproduction

Ovaries are atypical because they age at a faster pace than the rest of the organs. Even the uterus can play its role at advanced ages. Apart from the environmental insults that organs can be exposed to, undoubtedly, genetic factors affect ovarian function. The question is whether the telomere pathway can impact on ovarian function. In wild-type mice, telomeres are longer in immature oocytes, and their length shortens as they become mature. After zygote formation, the telomere length increases up to the blastocyst stage [229,230]. The longest telomeres localize at the inner cell mass of the blastocyst [218,219]. Regarding telomerase activity, in immature oocytes more telomerase activity is detected. The activity decreases as oocytes mature, until the morula stage, and then increases with the highest peak at the blastocyst stage, where telomere length is thought to be reset in the organism [231,232]. An increase in telomerase activity after zygote formation has been observed in other species, such as bovine and humans [200,231,233,234]. The implication of telomerase in fertility was clearly observed in telomerase-deficient mouse models. In mice of the sixth generation without telomerase, fertility was greatly reduced. The size of the ovaries was diminished compared to controls, and the uterine horns had aberrant shapes with reduced thickness of the myometrium [223]. The percentage of oocytes retrieved after stimulation was lower than controls, and most of the fertilized eggs did not reached the blastocyst stage [223]. Liu and coworkers found that oocytes from the fourth generation had spindle aberrations and chromosome misalignments [230].

The tendency of parents to delay childbearing turns to a disadvantage due to the loss of oocyte quantity and/or quality with age, leading to a decrease in spontaneous pregnancies and an increase in aneuploidy [235,236]. Indeed, telomeres in oocytes shorten after fetal development, possibly due to toxic compounds that reach the ovaries and the accumulation of reactive oxygen species [237]. Short telomeres have been associated with endometrial pathologies [238], miscarriage, and failure in IVF cycles [239]. Furthermore, shorter telomeres have been found in GCs obtained from patients suffering premature ovarian insufficiency, and telomerase activity was low or undetectable in GCs from these patients [233,240]. In patients with premature ovarian failure, exposure to estrogens is lower [240], and this could affect telomerase enzyme, which is activated by sexual hormones [241,242]. More studies are necessary to understand in depth how the telomere pathway affects fertility in order to both minimize the disadvantages for fertility caused by telomeric attrition and maximize the health of women at late ages.

Future diagnosis and treatment

Targeted therapy for genetic causes of POI currently remains elusive. Nevertheless, basic research gives insights into future treatment. For instance, epigenetic changes blocking transcription in *FMR1* are potentially reversible. Moreover, CRISPR/Cas9 genome editing has been used to shorten expansions in the gene in cell lines.

Nevertheless, assisted reproductive technologies may, at least, allow oocytes or ovarian cortex be preserved to prevent POI, highlighting the paramount relevance of early diagnosis and prevention.

Actually, most of the laboratory workup of POI women consists of karyotype and FMR1 gene testing. Based on the recent increase in knowledge of the POI genetic background and the association with major health issues, knowledge of specific gene panels directed toward POI will accelerate in clinical practice.

References

[1] Pelosi E, Simonsick E, Forabosco A, Garcia-Ortiz JE, Schlessinger D. Dynamics of the ovarian reserve and impact of genetic and epidemiological factors on age of menopause. Biol Reprod [Internet] 2015;92(5):130. Available from: <http://www.ncbi.nlm.nih.gov/pubmed/25904009>.

[2] Baker TG. A quantitative and cytological study of germ cells in human ovaries. Proc R Soc Lond B Biol Sci 1964;158:417–33.

[3] Schoenaker DA, Jackson CA, Rowlands JV, Mishra GD. Socioeconomic position, lifestyle factors and age at natural menopause: a systematic review and meta-analyses of studies across six continents. Int J Epidemiol [Internet] 2014;43(5):1542–62. Available from: <https://academic.oup.com/ije/article-lookup/doi/10.1093/ije/dyu094>.

[4] Webber L, Davies M, Anderson R, Bartlett J, Braat D, Cartwright B, et al. ESHRE guideline: management of women with premature ovarian insufficiency. Hum Reprod [Internet] 2016;31(5):926–37. Available from: <http://humrep.oxfordjournals.org/lookup/doi/10.1093/humrep/dew027%5Cn>, <http://www.ncbi.nlm.nih.gov/pubmed/27008889>.

[5] Albright F, Smith PH, Fraser R. A syndrome characterized by primary ovarian insufficiency and decreased stature: report of 11 cases with a digression on hormonal control of axillary and pubic hair. Am J Med Sci 1942;204:625–48.
[6] Cooper AR, Baker VL, Sterling EW, Ryan ME, Woodruff TK, Nelson LM. The time is now for a new approach to primary ovarian insufficiency. Fertil Steril [Internet] 2011;95(6):1890–7. Available from: <http://www.ncbi.nlm.nih.gov/pubmed/20188353>.
[7] Welt CK. Primary ovarian insufficiency: a more accurate term for premature ovarian failure. Clin Endocrinol (Oxf) [Internet] 2008;68(4):499–509. Available from: <http://doi.wiley.com/10.1111/j.1365-2265.2007.03073.x>.
[8] Pastore LM, Christianson MS, Stelling J, Kearns WG, Segars JH. Reproductive ovarian testing and the alphabet soup of diagnoses: DOR, POI, POF, POR, and FOR. J Assist Reprod Genet [Internet] 2018;35(1):17–23. Available from: <http://link.springer.com/10.1007/s10815-017-1058-4>.
[9] Coulam CB, Adamson SC, Annegers JF. Incidence of premature ovarian failure. Obstet Gynecol [Internet] 1986;67(4):604–6 Apr [cited 2019 Feb 5]; Available from: <http://www.ncbi.nlm.nih.gov/pubmed/3960433>.
[10] Luborsky JL, Meyer P, Sowers MF, Gold EB, Santoro N. Premature menopause in a multi-ethnic population study of the menopause transition. Hum Reprod 2003;18(1):199–206.
[11] Kim C, Slaughter JC, Wang ET, Appiah D, Schreiner P, Leader B, et al. Anti-Müllerian hormone, follicle stimulating hormone, antral follicle count, and risk of menopause within 5 years. Maturitas [Internet] 2017;102(20):18–25. Available from: <http://www.ncbi.nlm.nih.gov/pubmed/25986448>.
[12] Mathews TJ, Hamilton BE. Mean age of mothers is on the rise: United States, 2000-2014. NCHS Data Brief [Internet] 2016;232:1–8. Available from: <http://www.ncbi.nlm.nih.gov/pubmed/26828319>.
[13] Nicoloro-SantaBarbara JM, Lobel M, Bocca S, Stelling JR, Pastore LM. Psychological and emotional concomitants of infertility diagnosis in women with diminished ovarian reserve or anatomical cause of infertility. Fertil Steril 2017;108(1):161–7.
[14] Kanj RV, Ofei-Tenkorang NA, Altaye M, Gordon CM. Evaluation and management of primary ovarian insufficiency in adolescents and young adults. J Pediatr Adolesc Gynecol 2018;31(1):13–18.
[15] Tucker EJ, Grover SR, Bachelot A, Touraine P, Sinclair AH. Premature ovarian insufficiency: new perspectives on genetic cause and phenotypic spectrum. Endocr Rev 2016;37(6):609–35.
[16] Katari S, Aarabi M, Kintigh A, Mann S, Yatsenko SA, Sanfilippo JS, et al. Chromosomal instability in women with primary ovarian insufficiency. Hum Reprod [Internet] 2018;33(3):531–8. Available from: <https://academic.oup.com/humrep/article/33/3/531/4841816>.
[17] Vegetti W, Grazia Tibiletti M, Testa G, de Lauretis Y, Alagna F, Castoldi E, et al. Inheritance in idiopathic premature ovarian failure: analysis of 71 cases. Hum Reprod [Internet] 1998;13(7):1796–800. Available from: <http://www.ncbi.nlm.nih.gov/pubmed/9740426>.
[18] Torgerson DJ, Thomas RE, Reid DM. Mothers and daughters menopausal ages: is there a link? Eur J Obstet Gynecol Reprod Biol [Internet] 1997;74(1):63–6. Available from: <http://linkinghub.elsevier.com/retrieve/pii/S0301211597000857>.
[19] Sims D, Sudbery I, Ilott NE, Heger A, Ponting CP. Sequencing depth and coverage: key considerations in genomic analyses. Nat Rev Genet [Internet] 2014;15(2):121–32. Available from: https://doi.org/10.1038/nrg3642.
[20] Bouilly J, Beau I, Barraud S, Bernard V, Azibi K, Fagart J, et al. Identification of multiple gene mutations accounts for a new genetic architecture of primary ovarian insufficiency. J Clin Endocrinol Metab [Internet] 2016;101(12):4541–50. Available from: <https://academic.oup.com/jcem/article-lookup/doi/10.1210/jc.2016-2152>.
[21] Huhtaniemi I, Hovatta O, La Marca A, Livera G, Monniaux D, Persani L, et al. Advances in the molecular pathophysiology, genetics, and treatment of primary ovarian insufficiency. Trends Endocrinol Metab [Internet] 2018;29(6):400–19. Available from: https://doi.org/10.1016/j.tem.2018.03.010.
[22] Sun Y-C, Sun X-F, Dyce PW, Shen W, Chen H. The role of germ cell loss during primordial follicle assembly: a review of current advances. Int J Biol Sci [Internet] 2017;13(4):449–57. Available from: <http://www.ijbs.com/v13p0449.htm>.
[23] Wear HM, McPike MJ, Watanabe KH. From primordial germ cells to primordial follicles: a review and visual representation of early ovarian development in mice. J Ovarian Res [Internet] 2016;9(1):36. Available from: https://doi.org/10.1186/s13048-016-0246-7.
[24] Grive KJ, Gustafson EA, Seymour KA, Baddoo M, Schorl C, Golnoski K, et al. TAF4b regulates oocyte-specific genes essential for meiosis. PLOS Genet [Internet] 2016;12(6):e1006128 Barsh GS, editor. Available from: <https://dx.plos.org/10.1371/journal.pgen.1006128>.
[25] Pannetier M, Chassot A-A, Chaboissier M-C, Pailhoux E. Involvement of ***FOXL2*** and ***RSPO1*** in ovarian determination, development, and maintenance in

mammals. Sex Dev [Internet] 2016;10(4):167–84. Available from: <https://www.karger.com/Article/FullText/448667>.

[26] Ishiguro K. The cohesin complex in mammalian meiosis. Genes Cell [Internet] 2019;24(1):6–30. Available from: <http://doi.wiley.com/10.1111/gtc.12652>.

[27] Caburet S, Arboleda VA, Llano E, Overbeek PA, Barbero JL, Oka K, et al. Mutant cohesin in premature ovarian failure. N Engl J Med 2014;370(10):943–9.

[28] Winters T, McNicoll F, Jessberger R. Meiotic cohesin STAG3 is required for chromosome axis formation and sister chromatid cohesion. EMBO J [Internet] 2014;33(11):1256–70. Available from: <http://emboj.embopress.org/cgi/doi/10.1002/embj.201387330ovari>.

[29] de Vries L, Behar DM, Smirin-Yosef P, Lagovsky I, Tzur S, Basel-Vanagaite L. Exome sequencing reveals SYCE1 mutation associated with autosomal recessive primary ovarian insufficiency. J Clin Endocrinol Metab [Internet] 2014;99(10):E2129–32. Available from: <https://academic.oup.com/jcem/article-lookup/doi/10.1210/jc.2014-1268>.

[30] Bolcun-Filas E, Speed R, Taggart M, Grey C, de Massy B, Benavente R, et al. Mutation of the mouse syce1 gene disrupts synapsis and suggests a link between synaptonemal complex structural components and DNA repair. PLoS Genet [Internet] 2009;5(2):e1000393 Lichten M, editor. Available from: <https://dx.plos.org/10.1371/journal.pgen.1000393>.

[31] Faridi R, Rehman AU, Morell RJ, Friedman PL, Demain L, Zahra S, et al. Mutations of SGO2 and CLDN14 collectively cause coincidental Perrault syndrome. Clin Genet [Internet] 2017;91(2):328–32. Available from: <http://doi.wiley.com/10.1111/cge.12867>.

[32] Lamarche BJ, Orazio NI, Weitzman MD. The MRN complex in double-strand break repair and telomere maintenance. FEBS Lett 2010;584(17):3682–95.

[33] Hartford SA, Luo Y, Southard TL, Min IM, Lis JT, Schimenti JC. Minichromosome maintenance helicase paralog MCM9 is dispensible for DNA replication but functions in germ-line stem cells and tumor suppression. Proc Natl Acad Sci USA [Internet] 2011;108(43):17702–7. Available from: <http://www.pnas.org/cgi/doi/10.1073/pnas.1113524108>.

[34] Lutzmann M, Grey C, Traver S, Ganier O, Maya-Mendoza A, Ranisavljevic N, et al. MCM8- and MCM9-deficient mice reveal gametogenesis defects and genome instability due to impaired homologous recombination. Mol Cell [Internet] 2012;47(4):523–34. Available from: <https://linkinghub.elsevier.com/retrieve/pii/S1097276512004947>.

[35] Rossetti R, Ferrari I, Bonomi M, Persani L. Genetics of primary ovarian insufficiency. Clin Genet [Internet]. 2017;91(2):183–98. Available from: <http://doi.wiley.com/10.1111/cge.12921>.

[36] Dondik Y, Lei Z, Gaskins J, Pagidas K. Minichromosome maintenance complex component 8 and 9 gene expression in the menstrual cycle and unexplained primary ovarian insufficiency. J Assist Reprod Genet 2019;36(1):57–64.

[37] Zhao W, Sung P. Significance of ligand interactions involving Hop2-Mnd1 and the RAD51 and DMC1 recombinases in homologous DNA repair and XX ovarian dysgenesis. Nucleic Acids Res 2015;43(8):4055–66.

[38] Zangen D, Kaufman Y, Zeligson S, Perlberg S, Fridman H, Kanaan M, et al. XX ovarian dysgenesis is caused by a PSMC3IP/HOP2 mutation that abolishes coactivation of estrogen-driven transcription. Am J Hum Genet [Internet] 2011;89(4):572–9. Available from: https://doi.org/10.1016/j.ajhg.2011.09.006.

[39] Al-Agha AE, Ahmed IA, Nuebel E, Moriwaki M, Moore B, Peacock KA, et al. Primary ovarian insufficiency and azoospermia in carriers of a homozygous PSMC3IP stop gain mutation. J Clin Endocrinol Metab [Internet] 2018;103(2):555–63. Available from: <https://academic.oup.com/jcem/article/103/2/555/4731742>.

[40] Mandon-Pépin B, Touraine P, Kuttenn F, Derbois C, Rouxel A, Matsuda F, et al. Genetic investigation of four meiotic genes in women with premature ovarian failure. Eur J Endocrinol [Internet] 2008;158(1):107–15. Available from: <https://eje.bioscientifica.com/view/journals/eje/158/1/107.xml>.

[41] He W-B, Tu C-F, Liu Q, Meng L-L, Yuan S-M, Luo A-X, et al. DMC1 mutation that causes human non-obstructive azoospermia and premature ovarian insufficiency identified by whole-exome sequencing. J Med Genet [Internet] 2018;55(3):198–204 [cited 2019 Feb 6]; jmedgenet-2017-104992. Available from: <http://jmg.bmj.com/lookup/doi/10.1136/jmedgenet-2017-104992>.

[42] Mazina OM, Mazin AV, Nakagawa T, Kolodner RD, Kowalczykowski SC. Saccharomyces cerevisiae Mer3 helicase stimulates 3′–5′ heteroduplex extension by Rad51. Cell [Internet] 2004;117(1):47–56. Available from: <https://linkinghub.elsevier.com/retrieve/pii/S0092867404002946>.

[43] Guiraldelli MF, Eyster C, Wilkerson JL, Dresser ME, Pezza RJ. Mouse HFM1/Mer3 is required for crossover formation and complete synapsis of homologous chromosomes during meiosis. PLoS Genet [Internet] 2013;9(3):e1003383 Hawley RS, editor. Available from: <http://dx.plos.org/10.1371/journal.pgen.1003383>.

[44] Wang J, Zhang W, Jiang H, Wu B-L. Mutations in HFM1 in recessive primary ovarian insufficiency. N Engl J Med [Internet] 2014;370(10):972–4. Available from: <http://www.nejm.org/doi/10.1056/NEJMc1310150>.

[45] Pu D, Wang C, Cao J, Shen Y, Jiang H, Liu J, et al. Association analysis between HFM1 variation and primary ovarian insufficiency in Chinese women. Clin Genet [Internet] 2016;89(5):597–602. Available from: <http://www.ncbi.nlm.nih.gov/pubmed/26679638>.

[46] Carlosama C, Elzaiat M, Patiño LC, Mateus HE, Veitia RA, Laissue P. A homozygous donor splice-site mutation in the meiotic gene MSH4 causes primary ovarian insufficiency. Hum Mol Genet [Internet] 2017;26(16):3161–6. Available from: <https://academic.oup.com/hmg/article-lookup/doi/10.1093/hmg/ddx199>.

[47] Guo T, Zhao S, Zhao S, Chen M, Li G, Jiao X, et al. Mutations in MSH5 in primary ovarian insufficiency. Hum Mol Genet 2017;26(8):1452–7.

[48] Moyses-Oliveira M, Mancini TI, Takeno SS, Rodrigues ADS, Bachega TASS, Bertola D, et al. Congenital adrenal hyperplasia, ovarian failure and Ehlers-Danlos syndrome due to a 6p deletion. Sex Dev 2014;8(4):139–45.

[49] Qin Y, Guo T, Li G, Tang T-S, Zhao S, Jiao X, et al. CSB-PGBD3 mutations cause premature ovarian failure. PLOS Genet [Internet] 2015;11(7):e1005419 Ford JM, editor. Available from: <https://dx.plos.org/10.1371/journal.pgen.1005419>.

[50] Davis AJ, Chen DJ. DNA double strand break repair via non-homologous end-joining. Transl Cancer Res [Internet] 2013;2(3):130–43. Available from: <http://www.ncbi.nlm.nih.gov/pubmed/24000320>.

[51] de Bruin C, Mericq V, Andrew SF, van Duyvenvoorde HA, Verkaik NS, Losekoot M, et al. An XRCC4 splice mutation associated with severe short stature, gonadal failure, and early-onset metabolic syndrome. J Clin Endocrinol Metab [Internet] 2015;100(5):E789–98. Available from: <https://academic.oup.com/jcem/article-lookup/doi/10.1210/jc.2015-1098>.

[52] Murray JE, Bicknell LS, Yigit G, Duker AL, van Kogelenberg M, Haghayegh S, et al. Extreme growth failure is a common presentation of ligase IV deficiency. Hum Mutat [Internet] 2014;35(1):76–85. Available from: <http://doi.wiley.com/10.1002/humu.22461>.

[53] Fu C, Begum K, Overbeek PA. Primary ovarian insufficiency induced by fanconi anemia E mutation in a mouse model. PLoS One 2016;11(3):e0144285.

[54] Pyun J-A, Kim S, Cha DH, Kwack K. Polymorphisms within the FANCA gene associate with premature ovarian failure in Korean women. Menopause. 2014;21(5):530–3.

[55] Fouquet B, Pawlikowska P, Caburet S, Guigon C, Makinen M, Tanner L, et al. A homozygous FANCM mutation underlies a familial case of non-syndromic primary ovarian insufficiency. Elife. 2017;6:e30490.

[56] Hsueh AJW, Kawamura K, Cheng Y, Fauser BC. Intraovarian control of early folliculogenesis. Endocr Rev 2015;36(1):1–24.

[57] Quaynor SD, Stradtman EW, Kim H-G, Shen Y, Chorich LP, Schreihofer DA, et al. Delayed puberty and estrogen resistance in a woman with estrogen receptor α variant. N Engl J Med [Internet] 2013;369(2):164–71. Available from: <http://www.nejm.org/doi/10.1056/NEJMoa1303611>.

[58] Bernard V, Kherra S, Francou B, Fagart J, Viengchareun S, Guéchot J, et al. Familial multiplicity of estrogen insensitivity associated with a loss-of-function ESR1 mutation. J Clin Endocrinol Metab [Internet] 2016;102(1):93–9. Available from: <https://academic.oup.com/jcem/article-lookup/doi/10.1210/jc.2016-2749>.

[59] Asadi M, Ghafouri-Fard S, Zare-Abdollahi D, Ebrahim-Habibi A, Matin N. Estrogen receptor mutation in a girl with primary amenorrhea. Clin Genet [Internet] 2013;83(5):497–8. Available from: <http://doi.wiley.com/10.1111/cge.12083>.

[60] Lang-Muritano M, Sproll P, Wyss S, Kolly A, Hürlimann R, Konrad D, et al. Early-onset complete ovarian failure and lack of puberty in a woman with mutated estrogen receptor β (ESR2). J Clin Endocrinol Metab [Internet] 2018;103(10):3748–56. Available from: <https://academic.oup.com/jcem/article/103/10/3748/5063510>.

[61] Meduri G, Bachelot A, Cocca MP, Vasseur C, Rodien P, Kuttenn F, et al. Molecular pathology of the FSH receptor: new insights into FSH physiology. Mol Cell Endocrinol [Internet] 2008;282(1–2):130–42. Available from: <https://linkinghub.elsevier.com/retrieve/pii/S0303720707004212>.

[62] Katari S, Wood-Trageser MA, Jiang H, Kalynchuk E, Muzumdar R, Yatsenko SA, et al. Novel inactivating mutation of the FSH receptor in two siblings of Indian origin with premature ovarian failure. J Clin Endocrinol Metab [Internet] 2015;100(6):2154–7. Available from: <https://academic.oup.com/jcem/article-lookup/doi/10.1210/jc.2015-1401>.

[63] França MM, Lerario AM, Funari MFA, Nishi MY, Narcizo AM, de Mello MP, et al. A novel homozygous missense FSHR variant associated with hypergonadotropic hypogonadism in two siblings from a Brazilian family. Sex Dev [Internet] 2017;11(3):137–42. Available from: <https://www.karger.com/Article/FullText/477193>.

[64] Aittomäki K, Lucena JL, Pakarinen P, Sistonen P, Tapanainen J, Gromoll J, et al. Mutation in the follicle-stimulating hormone receptor gene causes hereditary hypergonadotropic ovarian failure. Cell [Internet] 1995;82(6):959–68. Available from: <http://www.ncbi.nlm.nih.gov/pubmed/7553856>.

[65] Rannikko A, Pakarinen P, Manna PR, Beau I, Misrahi M, Aittomäki K, et al. Functional characterization of the human FSH receptor with an inactivating Ala189Val mutation. Mol Hum Reprod [Internet] 2002;8(4):311–17. Available from: <http://www.ncbi.nlm.nih.gov/pubmed/11912278>.

[66] Meduri G, Touraine P, Beau I, Lahuna O, Desroches A, Vacher-Lavenu MC, et al. Delayed puberty and primary amenorrhea associated with a novel mutation of the human follicle-stimulating hormone receptor: clinical, histological, and molecular studies. J Clin Endocrinol Metab [Internet] 2003;88(8):3491–8. Available from: <https://academic.oup.com/jcem/article-lookup/doi/10.1210/jc.2003-030217>.

[67] Bentov Y, Kenigsberg S, Casper RF. A novel luteinizing hormone/chorionic gonadotropin receptor mutation associated with amenorrhea, low oocyte yield, and recurrent pregnancy loss. Fertil Steril [Internet] 2012;97(5):1165–8. Available from: https://doi.org/10.1016/j.fertnstert.2012.02.002.

[68] Belli M, Shimasaki S. Molecular aspects and clinical relevance of GDF9 and BMP15 in ovarian function. Vitam Horm [Internet] 2018;107:317–48 [cited 2019 Feb 6]; Available from: <https://linkinghub.elsevier.com/retrieve/pii/S0083672917300596>.

[69] Mottershead DG, Sugimura S, Al-Musawi SL, Li J-J, Richani D, White MA, et al. Cumulin, an oocyte-secreted heterodimer of the transforming growth factor-β family, is a potent activator of granulosa cells and improves oocyte quality. J Biol Chem [Internet] 2015;290(39):24007–20. Available from: <http://www.jbc.org/lookup/doi/10.1074/jbc.M115.671487>.

[70] Abir R, Fisch B. Invited commentary: A single nucleotide polymorphism in BMP15 is associated with high response to controlled ovarian hyperstimulation. Reprod Biomed Online [Internet] 2011;23(1):77–80. Available from: https://doi.org/10.1016/j.rbmo.2011.03.025.

[71] Hanevik HI, Hilmarsen HT, Skjelbred CF, Tanbo T, Kahn JA. A single nucleotide polymorphism in BMP15 is associated with high response to ovarian stimulation. Reprod Biomed Online [Internet] 2011;23(1):97–104. Available from: https://doi.org/10.1016/j.rbmo.2011.02.015.

[72] Margulis S, Abir R, Felz C, Nitke S, Krissi H, Fisch B. Bone morphogenetic protein 15 expression in human ovaries from fetuses, girls, and women. Fertil Steril [Internet] 2009;92(5):1666–73. Available from: https://doi.org/10.1016/j.fertnstert.2008.08.119.

[73] Morón FJ, de Castro F, Royo JL, Montoro L, Mira E, Sáez ME, et al. Bone morphogenetic protein 15 (BMP15) alleles predict over-response to recombinant follicle stimulation hormone and iatrogenic ovarian hyperstimulation syndrome (OHSS). Pharmacogenet Genomics [Internet] 2006;16(7):485–95. Available from: <https://insights.ovid.com/crossref?an = 01213011-200607000-00004>.

[74] Shimasaki S, Moore RK, Otsuka F, Erickson GF. The bone morphogenetic protein system in mammalian reproduction. Endocr Rev [Internet] 2004;25(1):72–101. Available from: <https://academic.oup.com/edrv/article-lookup/doi/10.1210/er.2003-0007>.

[75] Di Pasquale E, Beck-Peccoz P, Persani L. Hypergonadotropic ovarian failure associated with an inherited mutation of human bone morphogenetic protein-15 (BMP15) gene. Am J Hum Genet [Internet] 2004;75(1):106–11. Available from: <https://linkinghub.elsevier.com/retrieve/pii/S0002929707619995>.

[76] Mayer A, Fouquet B, Pugeat M, Misrahi M. BMP15 "knockout-like" effect in familial premature ovarian insufficiency with persistent ovarian reserve. Clin Genet 2017;92(2):208–12.

[77] Castronovo C, Rossetti R, Rusconi D, Recalcati MP, Cacciatore C, Beccaria E, et al. Gene dosage as a relevant mechanism contributing to the determination of ovarian function in Turner syndrome. Hum Reprod [Internet] 2014;29(2):368–79. Available from: <https://academic.oup.com/humrep/article-lookup/doi/10.1093/humrep/det436>.

[78] Toniolo D. X-linked premature ovarian failure: a complex disease. Curr Opin Genet Dev [Internet] 2006;16(3):293–300. Available from: <https://linkinghub.elsevier.com/retrieve/pii/S0959437X06000669>.

[79] Hook EB, Warburton D. Turner syndrome revisited: review of new data supports the hypothesis that all viable 45,X cases are cryptic mosaics with a rescue cell line, implying an origin by mitotic loss. Hum Genet [Internet] 2014;133(4):417–24. Available from: <http://link.springer.com/10.1007/s00439-014-1420-x>.

[80] Bouchlariotou S, Tsikouras P, Dimitraki M, Athanasiadis A, Papoulidis I, Maroulis G, et al. Turner's syndrome and pregnancy: has the 45,X/47,XXX mosaicism a different prognosis? Own clinical experience and literature review. J Matern Neonatal Med [Internet] 2011;24(5):668–72. Available from: <http://www.tandfonline.com/doi/full/10.3109/14767058.2010.520769>.

[81] Reynaud K, Cortvrindt R, Verlinde F, De Schepper J, Bourgain C, Smitz J. Number of ovarian follicles in human fetuses with the 45,x karyotype. Fertil

Steril [Internet] 2004;81(4):1112–19. Available from: <https://linkinghub.elsevier.com/retrieve/pii/S0015028203032023>.

[82] Fechner PY, Davenport ML, Qualy RL, Ross JL, Gunther DF, Eugster EA, et al. Differences in follicle-stimulating hormone secretion between 45,X monosomy Turner syndrome and 45,X/46,XX mosaicism are evident at an early age. J Clin Endocrinol Metab [Internet]. 2006;91(12):4896–902 [cited 2019 Feb 5]; Available from: <https://academic.oup.com/jcem/article-lookup/doi/10.1210/jc.2006-1157>.

[83] Zinn AR, Ross JL. Turner syndrome and haploinsufficiency. Curr Opin Genet Dev [Internet] 1998;8(3):322–7. Available from: <http://linkinghub.elsevier.com/retrieve/pii/S0959437X98800890>.

[84] Turner JMA, Mahadevaiah SK, Fernandez-Capetillo O, Nussenzweig A, Xu X, Deng CX, et al. Silencing of unsynapsed meiotic chromosomes in the mouse. Nat Genet 2005;37(1):41–7.

[85] Rizzolio F, Pramparo T, Sala C, Zuffardi O, De Santis L, Rabellotti E, et al. Epigenetic analysis of the critical region I for premature ovarian failure: demonstration of a highly heterochromatic domain on the long arm of the mammalian X chromosome. J Med Genet 2009;46(9):585–92.

[86] Fierabracci A, Bizzarri C, Palma A, Milillo A, Bellacchio E, Cappa M. A novel heterozygous mutation of the AIRE gene in a patient with autoimmune polyendocrinopathy-candidiasis-ectodermal dystrophy syndrome (APECED). Gene. 2012;511(1):113–17.

[87] Eisenbarth GS, editor. Immunoendocrinology: scientific and clinical aspects [Internet]. Totowa, NJ: Humana Press; 2011. Available from: <http://link.springer.com/10.1007/978-1-60327-478-4>.

[88] Oftedal BE, Hellesen A, Erichsen MM, Bratland E, Vardi A, Perheentupa J, et al. Dominant mutations in the autoimmune regulator AIRE are associated with common organ-specific autoimmune diseases. Immunity 2015;42(6):1185–96.

[89] Söderbergh A, Myhre AG, Ekwall O, Gebre-Medhin G, Hedstrand H, Landgren E, et al. Prevalence and clinical associations of 10 defined autoantibodies in autoimmune polyendocrine syndrome type I. J Clin Endocrinol Metab 2004;.

[90] Novosad JA, Kalantaridou SN, Tong Z-B, Nelson LM. Ovarian antibodies as detected by indirect immunofluorescence are unreliable in the diagnosis of autoimmune premature ovarian failure: a controlled evaluation. BMC Womens Health [Internet] 2003;3(1):2. Available from: <http://bmcwomenshealth.biomedcentral.com/articles/10.1186/1472-6874-3-2>.

[91] Chai P, Li F, Fan J, Jia R, Zhang H, Fan X. Functional analysis of a Novel FOXL2 indel mutation in Chinese families with blepharophimosis-ptosis-epicanthus inversus syndrome type I. Int J Biol Sci [Internet] 2017;13(8):1019–28. Available from: <http://www.ijbs.com/v13p1019.htm>.

[92] Nallathambi J, Laissue P, Batista F, Benayoun BA, Lesaffre C, Moumné L, et al. Differential functional effects of novel mutations of the transcription factor FOXL2 in BPES patients. Hum Mutat [Internet] 2008;29(8):E123–31. Available from: <http://doi.wiley.com/10.1002/humu.20809>.

[93] Todeschini A-L, Dipietromaria A, L'Hôte D, Boucham FZ, Georges AB, Pandaranayaka PJE, et al. Mutational probing of the forkhead domain of the transcription factor FOXL2 provides insights into the pathogenicity of naturally occurring mutations. Hum Mol Genet [Internet] 2011;20(17):3376–85. Available from: <https://academic.oup.com/hmg/article-lookup/doi/10.1093/hmg/ddr244>.

[94] Elzaiat M, Todeschini AL, Caburet S, Veitia RA. The genetic make-up of ovarian development and function: the focus on the transcription factor FOXL2. Clin Genet 2017;91(2):173–82.

[95] Harris SE. Identification of novel mutations in FOXL2 associated with premature ovarian failure. Mol Hum Reprod 2002;8(8):729–33.

[96] Thakur M, Feldman G, Puscheck EE. Primary ovarian insufficiency in classic galactosemia: current understanding and future research opportunities. J Assist Reprod Genet [Internet] 2018;35(1):3–16 [cited 2019 Feb 6]; Available from: <http://link.springer.com/10.1007/s10815-017-1039-7>.

[97] Berry GT. Galactosemia and amenorrhea in the adolescent. Ann N Y Acad Sci [Internet]. 2008;1135(1):112–1137. Available from: <http://doi.wiley.com/10.1196/annals.1429.038>.

[98] Fridovich-Keil JL, Gubbels CS, Spencer JB, Sanders RD, Land JA, Rubio-Gozalbo E. Ovarian function in girls and women with GALT-deficiency galactosemia. J Inherit Metab Dis [Internet] 2011;34(2):357–66. Available from: <http://doi.wiley.com/10.1007/s10545-010-9221-4>.

[99] Rubio-Gozalbo ME, Gubbels CS, Bakker JA, Menheere PPCA, Wodzig WKWH, Land JA. Gonadal function in male and female patients with classic galactosemia. Hum Reprod Update [Internet] 2010;16(2):177–88. Available from: <https://academic.oup.com/humupd/article-lookup/doi/10.1093/humupd/dmp038>.

[100] Bandyopadhyay S. Prenatal exposure to high galactose adversely affects initial gonadal pool of germ cells in rats. Hum Reprod [Internet] 2003;18

(2):276–82. Available from: <https://academic.oup.com/humrep/article-lookup/doi/10.1093/humrep/deg058>.

[101] Coss KP, Treacy EP, Cotter EJ, Knerr I, Murray DW, Shin YS, et al. Systemic gene dysregulation in classical galactosaemia: is there a central mechanism? Mol Genet Metab [Internet] 2014;113(3):177–87. Available from: <https://linkinghub.elsevier.com/retrieve/pii/S1096719214002583>.

[102] Knerr I, Coss KP, Doran PP, Hughes J, Wareham N, Burling K, et al. Leptin levels in children and adults with classic galactosaemia. JIMD Rep [Internet] 2012;125–31. Available from: <http://link.springer.com/10.1007/8904_2012_191>.

[103] Gubbels CS, Land JA, Evers JLH, Bierau J, Menheere PPCA, Robben SGF, et al. Primary ovarian insufficiency in classic galactosemia: role of FSH dysfunction and timing of the lesion. J Inherit Metab Dis [Internet] 2013;36(1):29–34. Available from: <http://doi.wiley.com/10.1007/s10545-012-9497-7>.

[104] Balakrishnan B, Chen W, Tang M, Huang X, Cakici DD, Siddiqi A, et al. Galactose-1 phosphate uridylyltransferase (GalT) gene: a novel positive regulator of the PI3K/Akt signaling pathway in mouse fibroblasts. Biochem Biophys Res Commun [Internet] 2016;470(1):205–12. Available from: https://doi.org/10.1016/j.bbrc.2016.01.036.

[105] van Erven B, Berry GT, Cassiman D, Connolly G, Forga M, Gautschi M, et al. Fertility in adult women with classic galactosemia and primary ovarian insufficiency. Fertil Steril [Internet] 2017;108(1):168–74. Available from: <https://linkinghub.elsevier.com/retrieve/pii/S0015028217303709>.

[106] Balakrishnan B, Nicholas C, Siddiqi A, Chen W, Bales E, Feng M, et al. Reversal of aberrant PI3K/Akt signaling by Salubrinal in a GalT-deficient mouse model. Biochim Biophys Acta Mol Basis Dis [Internet] 2017;1863(12):3286–93. Available from: <https://linkinghub.elsevier.com/retrieve/pii/S0925443917303058>.

[107] Matthijs G, Schollen E, Pardon E, Veiga-Da-Cunha M, Jaeken J, Cassiman J-J, et al. Mutations in PMM2, a phosphomannomutase gene on chromosome 16p13 in carbohydrate-deficient glycoprotein type I syndrome (Jaeken syndrome). Nat Genet [Internet] 1997;16(1):88–92. Available from: <http://www.nature.com/articles/ng0597-88>.

[108] Plagge A, Kelsey G, Germain-Lee EL. Physiological functions of the imprinted Gnas locus and its protein variants Gαs and XLαs in human and mouse. J Endocrinol [Internet] 2008;196(2):193–214. Available from: <https://joe.bioscientifica.com/view/journals/joe/196/2/193.xml>.

[109] Weinstein LS, Chen M, Liu J. Gs α mutations and imprinting defects in human disease. Ann N Y Acad Sci [Internet] 2002;968(1):173–97. Available from: <http://doi.wiley.com/10.1111/j.1749-6632.2002.tb04335.x>.

[110] Lo F-S, Chen T-L, Chiou C-C. Detection of rare somatic GNAS mutation in McCune-Albright syndrome using a novel peptide nucleic acid probe in a single tube. Molecules [Internet] 2017;22(11):1874. Available from: <http://www.mdpi.com/1420-3049/22/11/1874>.

[111] Mantovani G, Spada A. Mutations in the Gs alpha gene causing hormone resistance. Best Pract Res Clin Endocrinol Metab [Internet] 2006;20(4):501–13. Available from: <https://linkinghub.elsevier.com/retrieve/pii/S1521690X06000728>.

[112] Luoma P, Melberg A, Rinne JO, Kaukonen JA, Nupponen NN, Chalmers RM, et al. Parkinsonism, premature menopause, and mitochondrial DNA polymerase γ mutations: clinical and molecular genetic study. Lancet [Internet] 2004;364(9437):875–82. Available from: <https://linkinghub.elsevier.com/retrieve/pii/S0140673604169833>.

[113] Pagnamenta AT, Taanman J-W, Wilson CJ, Anderson NE, Marotta R, Duncan AJ, et al. Dominant inheritance of premature ovarian failure associated with mutant mitochondrial DNA polymerase gamma. Hum Reprod [Internet] 2006;21(10):2467–73. Available from: <https://academic.oup.com/humrep/article-lookup/doi/10.1093/humrep/del076>.

[114] Qin Y, Jiao X, Simpson JL, Chen ZJ. Genetics of primary ovarian insufficiency: new developments and opportunities. Hum Reprod Update 2015;21(6):787–808.

[115] Reyes A, Melchionda L, Nasca A, Carrara F, Lamantea E, Zanolini A, et al. RNASEH1 mutations impair mtDNA replication and cause adult-onset mitochondrial encephalomyopathy. Am J Hum Genet [Internet] 2015;97(1):186–93. Available from: <https://linkinghub.elsevier.com/retrieve/pii/S0002929715001998>.

[116] Young MJ, Copeland WC. Human mitochondrial DNA replication machinery and disease. Curr Opin Genet Dev 2016;38:52–62.

[117] Morino H, Pierce SB, Matsuda Y, Walsh T, Ohsawa R, Newby M, et al. Mutations in Twinkle primase-helicase cause Perrault syndrome with neurologic features. Neurology [Internet] 2014;83(22):2054–61. Available from: <http://www.neurology.org/cgi/doi/10.1212/WNL.0000000000001036>.

[118] Ołdak M, Oziębło D, Pollak A, Stępniak I, Lazniewski M, Lechowicz U, et al. Novel neuro-audiological findings and further evidence for TWNK involvement in Perrault syndrome. J Transl

Med [Internet] 2017;15(1):25. Available from: <http://translational-medicine.biomedcentral.com/articles/10.1186/s12967-017-1129-4>.

[119] Yao P, Fox PL. Aminoacyl-tRNA synthetases in medicine and disease. EMBO Mol Med [Internet] 2013;5 (3):332–43. Available from: <http://embomolmed.embopress.org/cgi/doi/10.1002/emmm.201100626>.

[120] Pierce SB, Gersak K, Michaelson-Cohen R, Walsh T, Lee MK, Malach D, et al. Mutations in LARS2, encoding mitochondrial leucyl-tRNA synthetase, lead to premature ovarian failure and hearing loss in Perrault syndrome. Am J Hum Genet [Internet] 2013;92(4):614–20. Available from: https://doi.org/10.1016/j.ajhg.2013.03.007.

[121] Pierce SB, Chisholm KM, Lynch ED, Lee MK, Walsh T, Opitz JM, et al. Mutations in mitochondrial histidyl tRNA synthetase HARS2 cause ovarian dysgenesis and sensorineural hearing loss of Perrault syndrome. Proc Natl Acad Sci USA [Internet] 2011;108(16):6543–8. Available from: <http://www.pnas.org/cgi/doi/10.1073/pnas.1103471108>.

[122] Dallabona C, Diodato D, Kevelam SH, Haack TB, Wong L-J, Salomons GS, et al. Novel (ovario) leukodystrophy related to AARS2 mutations. Neurology [Internet] 2014;82(23):2063–71. Available from: <http://www.neurology.org/cgi/doi/10.1212/WNL.0000000000000497>.

[123] Hamatani M, Jingami N, Tsurusaki Y, Shimada S, Shimojima K, Asada-Utsugi M, et al. The first Japanese case of leukodystrophy with ovarian failure arising from novel compound heterozygous AARS2 mutations. J Hum Genet 2016;61(10):899–902.

[124] van der Knaap MS, Bugiani M, Mendes MI, Riley LG, Smith DEC, Rudinger-Thirion J, et al. Biallelic variants in LARS2 and KARS cause deafness and (ovario)leukodystrophy. Neurology [Internet] 2019;92(11):e1225–37. Available from: https://doi.org/10.1212/WNL.0000000000007098. Available from: <http://www.neurology.org/lookup/doi/10.1212/WNL.0000000000007098>.

[125] Hochberg I, Demain LAM, Urquhart JE, Amberger A, Deutschmann AJ, Demetz S, et al. A homozygous variant in mitochondrial RNase P subunit PRORP is associated with Perrault syndrome characterized by hearing loss and primary ovarian insufficiency. bioRxiv 2017;. Available from: https://doi.org/10.1101/168252.

[126] Jenkinson EM, Rehman AU, Walsh T, Clayton-Smith J, Lee K, Morell RJ, et al. Perrault syndrome is caused by recessive mutations in CLPP, encoding a mitochondrial ATP-dependent chambered protease. Am J Hum Genet 2013;92(4):605–13.

[127] Ahmed S, Jelani M, Alrayes N, Mohamoud HSA, Almramhi MM, Anshasi W, et al. Exome analysis identified a novel missense mutation in the CLPP gene in a consanguineous Saudi family expanding the clinical spectrum of Perrault syndrome type-3. J Neurol Sci [Internet] 2015;353(1–2):149–54. Available from: <https://linkinghub.elsevier.com/retrieve/pii/S0022510X15002488>.

[128] Dursun F, Mohamoud HSA, Karim N, Naeem M, Jelani M, Kırmızıbekmez H. A novel missense mutation in the CLPP gene causing Perrault syndrome type 3 in a Turkish family. J Clin Res Pediatr Endocrinol [Internet] 2016;8(4):472–7. Available from: <http://cms.galenos.com.tr/Uploads/Article_1710/JCRPE-8-472.pdf>.

[129] Chatzispyrou IA, Alders M, Guerrero-Castillo S, Zapata Perez R, Haagmans MA, Mouchiroud L, et al. A homozygous missense mutation in ERAL1, encoding a mitochondrial rRNA chaperone, causes Perrault syndrome. Hum Mol Genet [Internet] 2017;26(13):2541–50. Available from: <https://academic.oup.com/hmg/article/26/13/2541/3755423>.

[130] Pierce SB, Walsh T, Chisholm KM, Lee MK, Thornton AM, Fiumara A, et al. Mutations in the DBP-deficiency protein HSD17B4 cause ovarian dysgenesis, hearing loss, and ataxia of Perrault syndrome. Am J Hum Genet [Internet] 2010;87(2):282–8. Available from: <https://linkinghub.elsevier.com/retrieve/pii/S0002929710003630>.

[131] Amor DJ, Marsh APL, Storey E, Tankard R, Gillies G, Delatycki MB, et al. Heterozygous mutations in HSD17B4 cause juvenile peroxisomal D-bifunctional protein deficiency. Neurol Genet [Internet] 2016;2(6): e114. Available from: <http://ng.neurology.org/lookup/doi/10.1212/NXG.0000000000000114>.

[132] Crane DI. Revisiting the neuropathogenesis of Zellweger syndrome. Neurochem Int [Internet] 2014;69:1–8. Available from: <https://linkinghub.elsevier.com/retrieve/pii/S0197018614000370>.

[133] Chen K, Yang K, Luo S-S, Chen C, Wang Y-XY, Wang Y-XY, et al. A homozygous missense variant in HSD17B4 identified in a consanguineous Chinese Han family with type II Perrault syndrome. BMC Med Genet [Internet] 2017;18(1):91. Available from: <http://bmcmedgenet.biomedcentral.com/articles/10.1186/s12881-017-0453-0>.

[134] Kytövuori L, Lipponen J, Rusanen H, Komulainen T, Martikainen MH, Majamaa K. A novel mutation m.8561C>G in MT-ATP6/8 causing a mitochondrial syndrome with ataxia, peripheral neuropathy, diabetes mellitus, and hypergonadotropic hypogonadism. J Neurology [Internet] 2016;263(11):2188–95.

Available from: <http://link.springer.com/10.1007/s00415-016-8249-2>.

[135] Fogli A, Boespflug-Tanguy O. The large spectrum of eIF2B-related diseases. Biochem Soc Trans [Internet] 2006;34(1):22. Available from: <http://www.biochemsoctrans.org/bst/034/bst0340022.htm>.

[136] Lynch DS, Rodrigues Brandão de Paiva A, Zhang WJ, Bugiardini E, Freua F, Tavares Lucato L, et al. Clinical and genetic characterization of leukoencephalopathies in adults. Brain [Internet] 2017;140(5):1204–11. Available from: <https://academic.oup.com/brain/article/140/5/1204/3060041>.

[137] Fogli A, Schiffmann R, Bertini E, Ughetto S, Combes P, Eymard-Pierre E, et al. The effect of genotype on the natural history of eIF2B-related leukodystrophies. Neurology [Internet] 2004;62(9):1509–17. Available from: <http://www.neurology.org/lookup/doi/10.1212/01.WNL.0000123259.67815.DB>.

[138] Humayun M, Khan A. Case Report: Cerebral leukodystrophy and the gonadal endocrinopathy: a rare but real association. F1000Research 2018;7:158.

[139] Miller ME, Chatten J. Ovarian changes in ataxia telangiectasia. Acta Paediatr [Internet] 1967;56(5):559–61. Available from: <http://doi.wiley.com/10.1111/j.1651-2227.1967.tb15424.x>.

[140] Demirhan O. A homozygous BMPR1B mutation causes a new subtype of acromesomelic chondrodysplasia with genital anomalies. J Med Genet [Internet] 2005;42(4):314–17. Available from: <http://jmg.bmj.com/cgi/doi/10.1136/jmg.2004.023564>.

[141] Arora H, Chacon AH, Choudhary S, Mcleod MP, Meshkov L, Nouri K, et al. Bloom syndrome. Int J Dermatol 2014;53(7):798–802.

[142] Oshima J, Sidorova JM, Monnat RJ. Werner syndrome: clinical features, pathogenesis and potential therapeutic interventions. Ageing Res Rev [Internet] 2017;33:105–14. Available from: <https://linkinghub.elsevier.com/retrieve/pii/S1568163716300265>.

[143] Benetti-Pinto CL, Ferreira V, Andrade L, Yela DA, De Mello MP. GAPO syndrome: a new syndromic cause of premature ovarian insufficiency. Climacteric 2016;19(6):594–8.

[144] Martin JP, Bell J. A pedigree of mental defect showing sex-linkage. J Neurol Neurosurg Psychiatry [Internet] 1943;6(3–4):154–7. Available from: <http://jnnp.bmj.com/cgi/doi/10.1136/jnnp.6.3-4.154>.

[145] Lubs HA. A marker X chromosome. Am J Hum Genet 1969;21(3):231–44.

[146] Naumann A, Hochstein N, Weber S, Fanning E, Doerfler W. A distinct DNA-methylation boundary in the 5′- upstream sequence of the FMR1 promoter binds nuclear proteins and is lost in fragile X syndrome. Am J Hum Genet 2009;85(5):606–16.

[147] Mila M, Alvarez-Mora MI, Madrigal I, Rodriguez-Revenga L. Fragile X syndrome: an overview and update of the FMR1 gene. Clin Genet [Internet] 2018;93(2):197–205. Available from: <http://doi.wiley.com/10.1111/cge.13075>.

[148] Nolin SL, Sah S, Glicksman A, Sherman SL, Allen E, Berry-Kravis E, et al. Fragile X AGG analysis provides new risk predictions for 45-69 repeat alleles. Am J Med Genet Part A [Internet] 2013;161(4):771–8. Available from: <http://doi.wiley.com/10.1002/ajmg.a.35833>.

[149] Zeesman S, Zwaigenbaum L, Whelan DT, Hagerman RJ, Tassone F, Taylor SAM. Paternal transmission of fragile X syndrome. Am J Med Genet [Internet] 2004;129A(2):184–9. Available from: <http://doi.wiley.com/10.1002/ajmg.a.30191>.

[150] Zhao X-N, Usdin K. FAN1 protects against repeat expansions in a Fragile X mouse model. DNA Repair (Amst) [Internet] 2018;69:1–5. Available from: <https://linkinghub.elsevier.com/retrieve/pii/S1568786418301113>.

[151] Saldarriaga W, Salcedo-Arellano MJ, Rodriguez-Guerrero T, Rios M, Fandino-Losada A, Ramirez-Cheyne J, et al. Increased severity of fragile X spectrum disorders in the agricultural community of Ricaurte, Colombia. Int J Dev Neurosci 2019;72:1–5.

[152] Warren ST. The epigenetics of fragile X syndrome. Cell Stem Cell [Internet] 2007;1(5):488–9. Available from: <https://linkinghub.elsevier.com/retrieve/pii/S1934590907002342>.

[153] Loesch DZ, Huggins RM, Hagerman RJ. Phenotypic variation and FMRP levels in fragile X. Ment Retard Dev Disabil Res Rev [Internet] 2004;10(1):31–41. Available from: <http://doi.wiley.com/10.1002/mrdd.20006>.

[154] Pretto D, Yrigollen CM, Tang HT, Williamson J, Espinal G, Iwahashi CK, et al. Clinical and molecular implications of mosaicism in FMR1 full mutations. Front Genet 2014;5:318.

[155] Pastore LM, Manichaikul A, Wang XQ, Finkelstein JS. FMR1 CGG repeats. Reprod Sci [Internet] 2016;23(9):1225–33. Available from: <http://journals.sagepub.com/doi/10.1177/1933719116632927>.

[156] Tosh D, Rao KL, Rani HS, Deenadayal DA, Murty USN, Grover P. Association between fragile X premutation and premature ovarian failure: a case–control study and meta-analysis. Arch Gynecol Obstet [Internet] 2014;289(6):1255–62. Available from: <http://link.springer.com/10.1007/s00404-014-3145-4>.

[157] Fortuño C, Labarta E. Genetics of primary ovarian insufficiency: a review. J Assist Reprod Genet 2014;31(12):1573–85.

[158] Avraham S, Almog B, Reches A, Zakar L, Malcov M, Sokolov A, et al. The ovarian response in fragile X patients and premutation carriers undergoing IVF–PGD: reappraisal. Hum Reprod [Internet] 2017;32 (7):1508–11. Available from: <http://academic.oup.com/humrep/article/32/7/1508/3791675/The-ovarian-response-in-fragile-X-patients-and>.

[159] Barasoain M, Barrenetxea G, Huerta I, Télez M, Criado B, Arrieta I. Study of the genetic etiology of primary ovarian insufficiency: FMR1 gene. Genes (Basel) [Internet] 2016;7(12):1–18. Available from: <http://www.ncbi.nlm.nih.gov/pubmed/27983607>.

[160] Pastore LM, Johnson J. The FMR1 gene, infertility, and reproductive decision-making: a review. Front Genet [Internet] 2014;5:195. Available from: <http://journal.frontiersin.org/article/10.3389/fgene.2014.00195/abstract>.

[161] Sullivan AK, Marcus M, Epstein MP, Allen EG, Anido AE, Paquin JJ, et al. Association of FMR1 repeat size with ovarian dysfunction. Hum Reprod 2005;20(2):402–12.

[162] De Caro JJ, Dominguez C, Sherman SL. Reproductive health of adolescent girls who carry the FMR1 premutation. Ann N Y Acad Sci [Internet] 2008;1135 (1):99–111. Available from: <http://doi.wiley.com/10.1196/annals.1429.029>.

[163] Bussani C, Papi L, Sestini R, Baldinotti F, Bucciantini S, Bruni V, et al. Premature ovarian failure and fragile X premutation: a study on 45 women. Eur J Obstet Gynecol Reprod Biol [Internet] 2004;112(2):189–91. Available from: <https://linkinghub.elsevier.com/retrieve/pii/S0301211503004196>.

[164] Murray A, Ennis S, MacSwiney F, Webb J, Morton NE. Reproductive and menstrual history of females with fragile X expansions. Eur J Hum Genet [Internet] 2000;8(4):247–52. Available from: <http://www.nature.com/articles/5200451>.

[165] Marozzi A, Vegetti W, Manfredini E, Tibiletti MG, Testa G, Crosignani PG, et al. Association between idiopathic premature ovarian failure and fragile X premutation. Hum Reprod [Internet] 2000;15 (1):197–202. Available from: <https://academic.oup.com/humrep/article-lookup/doi/10.1093/humrep/15.1.197>.

[166] Tassone F, Iong K, Tong T-H, Lo J, Gane LW, Berry-Kravis E, et al. FMR1 CGG allele size and prevalence ascertained through newborn screening in the United States. Genome Med [Internet] 2012;4(12):100. Available from: <http://genomemedicine.biomedcentral.com/articles/10.1186/gm401>.

[167] Hunter J, Rivero-Arias O, Angelov A, Kim E, Fotheringham I, Leal J. Epidemiology of fragile X syndrome: a systematic review and meta-analysis. Am J Med Genet Part A [Internet] 2014;164 (7):1648–58. Available from: <http://doi.wiley.com/10.1002/ajmg.a.36511>.

[168] O'Byrne JJ, Sweeney M, Donnelly DE, Lambert DM, Beattie ED, Gervin CM, et al. Incidence of Fragile X syndrome in Ireland. Am J Med Genet Part A [Internet] 2017;173(3):678–83. Available from: <http://doi.wiley.com/10.1002/ajmg.a.38081>.

[169] Saldarriaga W, Forero-Forero JV, González-Teshima LY, Fandiño-Losada A, Isaza C, Tovar-Cuevas JR, et al. Genetic cluster of fragile X syndrome in a Colombian district. J Hum Genet 2018;63:509–16.

[170] Rifé M, Nadal A, Milà M, Willemsen R. Immunohistochemical FMRP studies in a full mutated female fetus. Am J Med Genet Part A [Internet] 2004;124A(2):129–32. Available from: <http://doi.wiley.com/10.1002/ajmg.a.20342>.

[171] Rosario R, Filis P, Tessyman V, Kinnell H, Childs AJ, Gray NK, et al. FMRP associates with cytoplasmic granules at the onset of meiosis in the human oocyte. PLoS One 2016;11(10):e0163987.

[172] Elizur SE, Lebovitz O, Derech-Haim S, Dratviman-Storobinsky O, Feldman B, Dor J, et al. Elevated levels of FMR1 mRNA in granulosa cells are associated with low ovarian reserve in FMR1 premutation carriers. PLoS One [Internet] 2014;9(8):e105121 Bardoni B, editor. Available from: <https://dx.plos.org/10.1371/journal.pone.0105121>.

[173] Hoffman GE, Le WW, Entezam A, Otsuka N, Tong Z-B, Nelson L, et al. Ovarian abnormalities in a mouse model of fragile X primary ovarian insufficiency. J Histochem Cytochem [Internet] 2012;60 (6):439–56. Available from: <http://journals.sagepub.com/doi/10.1369/0022155412441002>.

[174] Sherman SL, Curnow EC, Easley CA, Jin P, Hukema RK, Tejada MI, et al. Use of model systems to understand the etiology of fragile X-associated primary ovarian insufficiency (FXPOI). J Neurodev Disord 2014;6(1):26.

[175] Pastore LM, McMurry TL, Williams CD, Baker VL, Young SL. AMH in women with diminished ovarian reserve: potential differences by FMR1 CGG repeat level. J Assist Reprod Genet [Internet] 2014;31 (10):1295–301. Available from: <http://link.springer.com/10.1007/s10815-014-0276-2>.

[176] Galloway JN, Nelson DL. Evidence for RNA-mediated toxicity in the fragile X-associated tremor/ataxia syndrome. Future Neurol [Internet] 2009;4 (6):785–98. Available from: <https://www.futuremedicine.com/doi/10.2217/fnl.09.44>.

[177] Alvarez-Mora MI, Rodriguez-Revenga L, Madrigal I, Garcia-Garcia F, Duran M, Dopazo J, et al. Deregulation of key signaling pathways involved in

oocyte maturation in FMR1 premutation carriers with Fragile X-associated primary ovarian insufficiency. Gene [Internet] 2015;571(1):52–7. Available from: <https://linkinghub.elsevier.com/retrieve/pii/S0378111915007489>.

[178] Sellier C, Buijsen RAM, He F, Natla S, Jung L, Tropel P, et al. Translation of expanded CGG repeats into FMRpolyG is pathogenic and may contribute to fragile X tremor ataxia syndrome. Neuron [Internet] 2017;93(2):331–47. Available from: <https://linkinghub.elsevier.com/retrieve/pii/S0896627316309588>.

[179] Buijsen RAM, Visser JAA, Kramer P, Severijnen EAWFM, Gearing M, Charlet-Berguerand N, et al. Presence of inclusions positive for polyglycine containing protein, FMRpolyG, indicates that repeat-associated non-AUG translation plays a role in fragile X-associated primary ovarian insufficiency. Hum Reprod [Internet] 2016;31(1):158–68. Available from: <https://academic.oup.com/humrep/article-lookup/doi/10.1093/humrep/dev280>.

[180] Man L, Lekovich J, Rosenwaks Z, Gerhardt J. Fragile X-associated diminished ovarian reserve and primary ovarian insufficiency from molecular mechanisms to clinical manifestations. Front Mol Neurosci [Internet] 2017;10:290 [cited 2019 Feb 6]; Available from: <http://journal.frontiersin.org/article/10.3389/fnmol.2017.00290/full>.

[181] Tseng E, Tang H-T, AlOlaby RR, Hickey L, Tassone F. Altered expression of the FMR1 splicing variants landscape in premutation carriers. Biochim Biophys Acta Gene Regul Mech [Internet] 2017;1860(11):1117–26. Available from: <https://linkinghub.elsevier.com/retrieve/pii/S1874939917301761>.

[182] Elizur SE, Dratviman-Storobinsky O, Derech-Haim S, Lebovitz O, Dor J, Orvieto R, et al. FMR6 may play a role in the pathogenesis of fragile X-associated premature ovarian insufficiency. Gynecol Endocrinol 2016;32(4):334–7.

[183] Loomis EW, Sanz LA, Chédin F, Hagerman PJ. Transcription-associated R-loop formation across the human FMR1 CGG-repeat region. PLoS Genet [Internet] 2014;10(4):e1004294 Aguilera A, editor. Available from: <http://dx.plos.org/10.1371/journal.pgen.1004294>.

[184] Albizua I, Rambo-Martin BL, Allen EG, He W, Amin AS, Sherman SL. Women who carry a fragile X premutation are biologically older than noncarriers as measured by telomere length. Am J Med Genet Part A [Internet] 2017;173(11):2985–94. Available from: <http://doi.wiley.com/10.1002/ajmg.a.38476>.

[185] Murray A, Webb J, Dennis N, Conway G, Morton N. Microdeletions in FMR2 may be a significant cause of premature ovarian failure. J Med Genet [Internet]. 1999;36(10):767–70. Available from: <http://jmg.bmj.com/cgi/doi/10.1136/jmg.36.10.767>.

[186] Ahn HW, Morin RD, Zhao H, Harris RA, Coarfa C, Chen Z-J, et al. MicroRNA transcriptome in the newborn mouse ovaries determined by massive parallel sequencing. MHR Basic Sci Reprod Med [Internet] 2010;16(7):463–71. Available from: <https://academic.oup.com/molehr/article-lookup/doi/10.1093/molehr/gaq017>.

[187] Veiga-Lopez A, Luense LJ, Christenson LK, Padmanabhan V. Developmental programming: gestational bisphenol-A treatment alters trajectory of fetal ovarian gene expression. Endocrinology [Internet] 2013;154(5):1873–84. Available from: <https://academic.oup.com/endo/article-lookup/doi/10.1210/en.2012-2129>.

[188] Cho SH, An HJ, Kim KA, Ko JJ, Kim JH, Kim YR, et al. Single nucleotide polymorphisms at miR-146a/196a2 and their primary ovarian insufficiency-related target gene regulation in granulosa cells. PLoS One [Internet] 2017;12(8):e0183479 Yang BB, editor. Available from: <https://dx.plos.org/10.1371/journal.pone.0183479>.

[189] Rah H, Jeon YJ, Shim SH, Cha SH, Choi DH, Kwon H, et al. Association of miR-146aC > G, miR-196a2T > C, and miR-499A > G polymorphisms with risk of premature ovarian failure in Korean women. Reprod Sci [Internet] 2013;20(1):60–8. Available from: <http://journals.sagepub.com/doi/10.1177/1933719112450341>.

[190] Dang Y, Zhao S, Qin Y, Han T, Li W, Chen Z-J. MicroRNA-22-3p is down-regulated in the plasma of Han Chinese patients with premature ovarian failure. Fertil Steril [Internet] 2015;103(3):802–807.e1. Available from: https://doi.org/10.1016/j.fertnstert.2014.12.106.

[191] López-Otín C, Blasco MA, Partridge L, Serrano M, Kroemer G. The hallmarks of aging. Cell 2013;153:1194–217.

[192] McClintock B. The stability of broken ends of chromosomes in Zea Mays. Genetics 1941;28:234–82.

[193] McClintock B. The behavior in successive nuclear divisions of a chromosome broken at meiosis. Proc Natl Acad Sci USA 1939;25:405–16.

[194] Müller HJ. Bar duplication. Collecting Net (Woods Hole) 1938;13:181–98.

[195] Blackburn EH, Gall JG. A tandemly repeated sequence at the termini of the extrachromosomal ribosomal RNA genes in Tetrahymena. J. Mol. Biol. 1978;120:33–53.

[196] Szostak JW, Blackburn EH. Clonig yeast telomeres on linear plasmid vectors. Cell 1982;29:245–55.

[197] Herrera E, Samper E, Martín-Caballero J, Flores JM, Lee HW, Blasco MA. Disease states associated with

telomerase deficiency appear earlier in mice with short telomeres. EMBO J 1999;18:2950–60.
[198] Olovnikov AM. A theory of marginotomy. The incomplete copying of template margin in enzymic synthesis of polynucleotides and biological significance of the phenomenon. J Theor Biol 1973;41:181–90.
[199] Olovnikov AM. Principle of marginotomy in template synthesis of polynucleotides. Dokl Akad Nauk SSSR 1971;201:1496–9.
[200] Watson JD. Origin of concatemeric T7 DNA. Nat New Biol 1972;239:197–201.
[201] Greider CW, Blackburn EH. Identification of a specific telomere terminal transferase activity in Tetrahymena extracts. Cell 1985;43:405–13.
[202] Greider Cw, Blackburn EH. The telomere transferase of Tetrahymena is a ribonucleoprotein enzyme with two kinds of primer specificity. Cell 1987;51:887–98.
[203] Blasco MA. Telomeres and human disease: ageing, cancer and beyond. Nat Rev Genet 2005;6:611–22.
[204] de Lange T. A loopy view of telomere evolution. Front Genet 2015;6:321.
[205] Palm W, de Lange T. How shelterin protects mammalian telomeres. Annu Rev Genet 2008;42:301–34.
[206] Schmutz I, de Lange T. Shelterin. Curr Biol 2016;26 (10):397–9.
[207] de Lange T. Shelterin: the protein complex that shapes and safeguards human telomeres. Genes Dev. 2005;19:2100–10.
[208] Shoeftner S, Blasco MA. A higher order of telomere regulation: telomere heterochromatin and telomeric RNAs. EMBO J 2009;28:2323–36.
[209] Gonzalo S, Jaco I, Fraga MF, Chen T, Li E, Esteller M, et al. DNA methyltransferases control telomere length and telomere recombination in mammalian cells. Nat Cell Biol 2006;8:416–24.
[210] Schoeftner S, Blasco MA. Developmentally regulated transcription of mammalian telomeres by DNA-dependent RNA polymerase II. Nat Cell Biol 2008;10:228236.
[211] Azzalin CM, Reichenbach P, Khoriauli L, Giulotto E, Lingner J. Telomeric repeat containing RNA and RNA surveillance factors at mammalian chromosome ends. Science 2007;318:798–801.
[212] Chu HP, Cifuentes-Rojas C, Kesner B, Aeby E, Lee HG, Wei C, et al. TERRA RNA antagonizes ATRX and protects telomeres. Cell 2017;170:86–101.
[213] Doksani Y, Wu JY, de Lange T, Zhuang X. Super-resolution fluorescence imaging of telomeres reveals TRF2-dependent T-loop formation. Cell 2013;155:345–56.
[214] Maciejowski J, Li Y, Bosco N, Campbell PJ, de Lange T. Chromothripsis and kataegis induced by telomere crisis. Cell 2015;163:1641–54.
[215] Martínez P, Blasco MA. Telomere-driven diseases and telomere-targeting therapies. J Cell Biol 2017;216:875–87.
[216] Collado M, Blasco MA, Serrano M. Cellular senescence in cancer and aging. Cell 2007;130:223–33.
[217] Vera E, Bernardes de Jesus B, Foronda M, Flores JM, Blasco MA. The rate of increase of short telomeres predicts longevity in mammals. Cell Rep 2012;2:732–7.
[218] Varela E, Muñoz-Lorente MA, Tejera AM, Ortega S, Blasco MA. Generation of mice with longer and better preserved telomeres in the absence of genetic manipulations. Nat Commun 2016;7:11739–55.
[219] Varela E, Schneider RP, Ortega S, Blasco MA. Different telomere-length dynamics at the inner cell mass versus established embryonic stem (ES) cells. Proc Natl Acad Sci USA 2011;108(37):15207–12.
[220] Bernardes de Jesus B, Blasco MA. Telomerase at the intersection of cancer and aging. Trends Genet 2013;29:513–20.
[221] Maciejowski J, de Lange T. Telomeres in cancer: tumour suppression and genome instability. Nat Rev Mol Cell Biol 2017;18:175–86.
[222] Blasco MA, Lee HW, Hande MP, Samper E, Lansdorp PM, dePinho RA, et al. Telomere shortening and tumor formation by mouse cells lacking telomerase RNA. Cell 1997;9:25–34.
[223] Lee HW, Blasco MA, Gottlieb GJ, et al. Essential role of mouse telomerase in highly proliferative organs. Nature 1998;392:569–74.
[224] Jaskelioff M, Muller FL, Paik JH, Thomas E, Jiang S, Adams AC, et al. Telomerase reactivation reverses tissue degeneration in aged telomerase-deficient mice. Nature 2011;469(7328):102–6.
[225] González-Suárez E, Samper E, Flores JM, Blasco MA. Telomerase-deficient mice with short telomeres are resistant to skin tumorigenesis. Nat Genet 2000;26:114–17.
[226] Tomás-Loba A, Flores I, Fernández-Marcos PJ, Cayuela ML, Maraver A, Tejera A, et al. Telomerase reverse transcriptase delays aging in cancer-resistant mice. Cell 2008;135:609–22.
[227] Bernardes de Jesus B, Vera E, Schneeberger K, Tejera AM, Ayuso E, Bosch F, et al. Telomerase gene therapy in adult and old mice delays aging and increases longevity without increasing cancer. EMBO Mol Med 2012;4:691–704.
[228] Armanios MY, et al. Telomerase mutations in families with idiopathic pulmonary fibrosis. N Engl J Med 2007;356:1317–26.
[229] Turner S, Wong HP, Rai J, Hartshorne GM. Telomere lengths in human oocytes, cleavage stage embryos and blastocysts. Mol Hum Reprod 2010;16:685–94.

[230] Liu L, Blasco MA, Keefe DL. Requirement of functional telomeres for metaphase chromosome alignments and integrity of meiotic spindles. EMBO Rep 2002;3(3):230–4.
[231] Wright WE, Piatyszek MA, Rainey WE, Byrd W, Shay JW. Telomerase activity in human germline and embryonic tissues and cells. Dev Genet 1996;18:173–9.
[232] Schaetzlein S, Lucas-Hahn A, Lemme E, Kues WA, Dorsch M, Manns MP, et al. Telomere length is reset during early mammalian embryogenesis. Proc Natl Acad Sci USA 2004;101:8034–8.
[233] Betts DH, King WA. Telomerase activity and telomere detection during early bovine development. Dev Genet 1999;25:397–403.
[234] Xu J, Yang X. Telomerase activity in bovine embryos during early development. Biol Reprod 2000;63:1124–8.
[235] Franasiak J, Forman E, Hong K, Werner M, Upham K, Treff N, et al. The nature of aneuploidy with increasing age of the female partner: a review of 15,169 consecutive trophectoderm biopsies evaluated with comprehensive chromosomal screening. Fertil Steril 2014;101:656–63.
[236] Treff NR, Su J, Taylor D, Scott Jr. RT. Telomere DNA deficiency is associated with development of human embryonic aneuploidy. PLoS Genet 2011;7:1–19.
[237] Keefe DL. Telomeres, reproductive aging, and genomic instability during early development. Reprod Sci 2016;23:1612–15.
[238] Hapangama DK, Kamal A, Saretzki G. Implications of telomeres and telomerase in endometrial pathology. Hum Reprod Update 2017;23:166–87.
[239] Keefe DL, Franco S, Liu L, Trimarchi J, Cao B, Weitzen S, et al. Telomere length predicts embryo fragmentation after in vitro fertilization in women—toward a telomere theory of reproductive aging in women. Am J Obstet Gynecol 2005;192:1256–60.
[240] Xu X, Chen X, Zhang X, Liu Y, Wang Z, Wang P, et al. Impaired telomere length and telomerase activity in peripheral blood leukocytes and granulosa cells in patients with biochemical primary ovarian insufficiency. Hum Reprod 2017;32:201–7.
[241] Calado RT, et al. Sex hormones, acting on the *TERT* gene, increase telomerase activity in human primary hematopoietic cells. Blood 2016;114:2236–43.
[242] Guo C, et al. In vivo regulation of hTERT expression and telomerase activity by androgen. J Urol 2003;170:615–18.

Further reading

Iqbal K, Kues WA, Baulain U, Garrels W, Herrmann D, Niemann H. Species-specific telomere length differences between blastocyst cell compartments and ectopic telomere extension in early bovine embryos by human telomerase reverse transcriptase. Biol Reprod 2011;84:723–33.

CHAPTER

12

Prenatal testing

Joshua A. Copel, Katherine Kohari and Audrey A. Merriam

Department of Obstetrics, Gynecology, and Reproductive Sciences, Section of Maternal-Fetal Medicine, Yale School of Medicine, New Haven, CT, United States

Prenatal testing is a rapidly evolving field in genetics and obstetrics. This field encompasses specialists in obstetrics and gynecology, maternal–fetal medicine, reproductive endocrinology and infertility, and medical genetics. As early as 1909 an association was reported between maternal age and Down syndrome [1]. For years this stood as the only method of "screening." Today highly sensitive and specific noninvasive screening methods plus diagnostic methods of testing that have progressed beyond karyotype alone exist to inform families about their pregnancies. This chapter describes the commonly used screening modalities and the different methods and tests available through diagnostic testing procedures in pregnancy.

Aneuploidy screening tests

Nuchal translucency

Background

The nuchal translucency (NT) is an ultrasound measurement defined as the collection of fluid under the skin behind the neck of the fetus obtained between 10 and 14 weeks' gestation (crown–rump length between 38–45 and 84 mm) (Fig. 12.1). While some fluid is present in the nuchal space of all fetuses, regardless of chromosomal status, it tends to increase among aneuploid fetuses, as well as those with other congenital anomalies. This measurement was introduced as the first screening method to detect fetal trisomy 21 in the first trimester [2]. While the mechanism leading to the increased NT measurement is not fully known, it is thought to be multifactorial and linked to abnormalities in lymphatic drainage, fetal cardiovascular abnormalities, and abnormalities in the extracellular matrix [3,4].

The fetal NT increases with gestational age/crown–rump length. Due to this the NT measurement may considered abnormal when it is above 3.0 mm, or above the 99th percentile for the gestational age. In pooled data from 30 studies, NT screening alone has a sensitivity for trisomy 21 of 77% with a 6% false-positive rate. The cutoff used to determine an abnormal NT varied in these studies between gestational-age cut-offs for the 95th percentile and 3.0 mm [5]. The cutoff picked for an abnormal NT screen will affect the test statistics, which explains the variation in detection rate for trisomy 21 in the literature.

Human Reproductive Genetics
DOI: https://doi.org/10.1016/B978-0-12-816561-4.00012-0

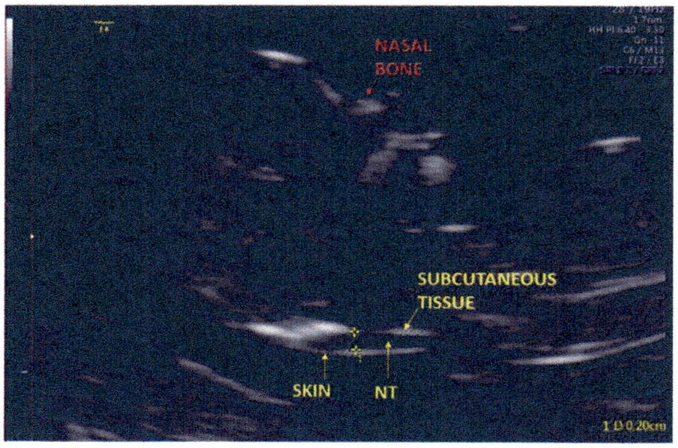

FIGURE 12.1 Transabdominal ultrasound image of an nuchal translucency (NT) measurement. The calipers are placed perpendicularly between the skin and the subcutaneous tissue, with the fetus in a neutral position. The amnion is clearly seen below the skin. Nasal bone is also present in this image.

TABLE 12.1 The criteria needed to obtain a proper nuchal translucency (NT) measurement [6,7].

- The crown–rump length must be between 45 and 84 mm, which typically falls between 10 0/7 and 13 6/7 weeks' gestation.
- Transabdominal or transvaginal scanning may be used but transabdominal imaging is successful in about 95% of patients.
- The fetus must be midline sagittal.
- The fetus should occupy three-fourths of the image.
- The calipers for measurement should be set to 0.1 mm increments to insure accuracy.
- The amnion must be distinguishable from the fetal skin and can be accomplished by waiting for fetal movement away from the membrane or by asking the mother to cough, which may move the fetus.
- The NT measurement should be obtained behind the cervical spine.
- The fetal head should be in a neutral position. If it is flexed or extended the measurement will not be correct.
- The maximum thickness of the space between the skin and the soft tissue over the cervical spine should be measured. The calipers should be placed perpendicular to the fetal body on the inner edge of the skin and the inner edge of the soft tissue.
- The maximum measurement of at least three NT measurements obtained should be used to calculate risk.

Limitations

There is an extensive list of criteria needed to obtain a satisfactory image (Table 12.1), so it is not surprising that obtaining consistent, reliable measurements may be difficult. Studies have shown interoperator differences of up to 0.5–0.6 mm and is largely attributable to caliper placement [8,9]. Given these difficulties, quality review programs for NT measurement have been developed. The Fetal Medicine Foundation in London and the Nuchal Translucency Quality Review program in the United States are two examples of these programs, which teach proper image capture and measurement, perform image review and perform ongoing epidemiologic feedback to the sonographers and physicians performing and reading the ultrasounds.

Maternal obesity also impacts the ability to obtain a quality NT image. The rising obesity rates, particularly in developed countries, have negatively impacted the ability to obtain an image, with failure rates as high as 23% in patients with class III obesity. The failure rates decrease with repeated attempts and bringing patients back for repeat ultrasounds, but remain almost four times higher for morbidly obese patients [10].

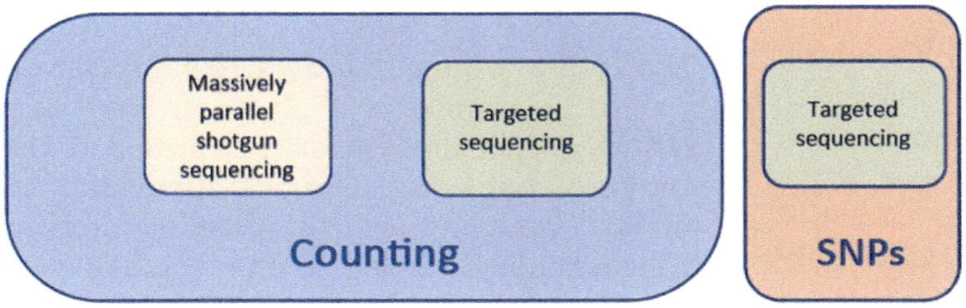

FIGURE 12.2 Differentiating cell-free fetal DNA technologies.

Other ultrasound markers

There are other ultrasound markers that can be used in the first trimester to assess risk for aneuploidy; the primary one is the presence or absence of a nasal bone. This can be identified in the same image used for the NT measurement (Fig. 12.1) and is seen as an equal sign (=), with the nasal bone ossification and overlying skin. A third echogenic line should be seen slightly distally and is the skin over the tip of the nose. One large literature review found a sensitivity of 65% with nasal bone alone, which is less than that of NT alone [11]. There are multiple issues with nasal bone measurement that make it less than ideal for use as a screening test, for example, it is more likely to be visualized with advancing gestational ages [12] and it is more commonly absent in women of African ethnicity, without an increase in the risk of trisomy 21 [13].

Doppler measurements showing tricuspid regurgitation and pulsation in the ductus venosus have also been associated with increased risk of trisomy 21 in the first trimester; however, these are technically challenging measurements to obtain and have not been widely used in the United States.

Biochemical screening

Serum analytes

Specific maternal serum analytes are also available for first-trimester screening for aneuploidy. Alterations in the levels of maternal serum pregnancy-associated plasma protein A (PAPP-A) and the free β subunit of human chorionic gonadotropin (hCG) have been found to be associated with the common trisomies 21, 13, and 18. In trisomy 21 pregnancies the level of PAPP-A is decreased and free β-hCG is elevated. In trisomy 12, 13, and 18 pregnancies both analytes are decreased compared to normal pregnancies [14]. The combination of serum analytes alone identifies 68.2% of pregnancies with trisomy 21 with a 5% false-positive rate [15].

First trimester screen

The combination of NT and first-trimester serum analyte screening is conventionally known as the first-trimester screen (FTS). The combination improves detection rates for trisomy 21 ranging from 79% to93% [16–19]. In women over 35 the detection rate reaches 92% [16,17], with a 5% screen-positive rate (Fig. 12.2). The timing for the FTS correlates with the optimal gestational age for obtaining the NT and is typically performed between 11 and 14 weeks' gestation. Although the presence or absence of the nasal bone may be reported on the FTS report, it is not used in the risk calculation.

Maternal serum alpha-fetoprotein

Screening for aneuploidy, outside of maternal age, originally began in the second trimester with the use of a maternal serum analyte. Maternal serum alpha-fetoprotein (MSAFP) was noted to be low in women with a pregnancy with trisomy 21 [20,21]. Alpha-fetoprotein (AFP) is one of the most abundant proteins in the fetus in the first trimester. Levels decrease during the second trimester in normal pregnancies. Although the physiologic reason for low levels in pregnancies with trisomy 21 is unclear, elevated levels are found in cases of fetal anomalies where the fetus is lacking a skin barrier in some capacity (i.e., open neural tube defect, anencephaly, gastroschisis). The "leaking" of AFP from the fetus into the amniotic fluid then crosses the maternal–placental interface causing elevated levels in the maternal serum (Table 12.2).

Quadruple screen

The quadruple screen or quad screen is another serum analyte test that is performed only in the second trimester, making it an attractive option for women who present late to care. This test uses four maternal serum analytes to provide a risk for trisomy 21 and trisomy 18, and can also provide a risk assessment for the pregnancy being affected by an open neural tube or ventral wall defect. The four proteins used are MSAFP, hCG, inhibin A, and unconjugated estriol (Table 12.3).

Unconjugated estriol and hCG were the first two analytes to be added to MSAFP to produce the triple screen. Low levels of unconjugated estriol and elevated levels of hCG were found together in women with pregnancies carrying trisomy 21 fetuses. The triple screen is no longer in use as a screening test alone since the discovery of elevated inhibin A levels in trisomy 21 pregnancies.

The combination of these four analytes can provide a risk assessment for aneuploidy from 15 to 22 weeks' gestation. The detection rate in women less than 35 years old is 75%, but jumps to 92% in women older than 35 years old at delivery, with a false-positive rate of 5% and 13%, respectively [17].

Combination screening

The results of aneuploidy screening can be improved by combining the various screening tests above, since the tests are performed at different gestational ages. The two approaches to combined screening are the integrated screen and the combined screen.

Integrated screening

The primary method of this screening uses two parts of the FTS (NT measurement and PAPP-A) combined with the quad screen in the second trimester. The free β-hCG is not used since hCG is part of the second-trimester screen. The patient does not get a result for the screening until all parts are completed in the second trimester. This method has a detection rate for trisomy 21 of 95% with a 5% false-positive rate [18,22].

A second method of integrated screening involves serum analytes only (PAPP-A in the first trimester and the quad screen in the second trimester). This is an attractive option for women who are in an area without access to first-trimester NT measurement capabilities, or if maternal obesity precludes adequate image acquisition. The detection rate using serum analytes alone is around 86% with a 5% false-positive rate [18,22].

The disadvantages of these methods include lack of any test result until the second trimester, resulting in later diagnostic testing and potentially later pregnancy termination. Second, up to 25% of patients may not return for their quad screen, leaving them without any aneuploidy screening results for the pregnancy [23].

Sequential screen

The sequential screening method eliminates the issue with quad screen nonadherence and return of aneuploidy screen results until the second trimester. This screening method allows for results to be released in the first trimester after the FTS and is then used to guide management for second-trimester screening.

TABLE 12.2 FTS screening [combination of nuchal translucency (NT), pregnancy-associated plasma protein A (PAPP-A), and free β subunit of human chorionic gonadotropin (β-hCG)] results in four of the largest studies.

Source	Pregnancies screened	All ages detection rate for trisomy 21 (%)	All ages false-positive rate for trisomy 21 (%)	All ages detection rate for trisomy 18 (%)	All ages false-positive rate for trisomy 18 (%)	Pregnancies screened	≥35 years old detection rate for trisomy 21 (%)	≥35 years old false-positive rate for trisomy 21 (%)	≥35 years old detection rate for trisomy 18 (%)	≥35 years old false-positive rate for trisomy 18 (%)
Wapner et al. (2003) (BUN study) [16]	8216	79	5	91	2	4120	78	5	100	2.6
Malone et al. (2005) (FASTER trial) [17]	38,033	86	5	–	–	8199	95	22	–	–
Wald et al. (2003) (SURUSS study) [18]	47,053	83	5	–	–	–	–	–	–	–
Nicolaides et al. (2005) [19]	75,821	93	5	–	–	–	–	–	–	–

TABLE 12.3 Expected serum levels seen in the quadruple screen for various genetic and structural anomalies.

	Maternal serum alpha-fetoprotein (MSAFP)	Unconjugated estriol	Human chorionic gonadotropin (hCG)	Inhibin A
Trisomy 21	Low	Low	Elevated	Elevated
Trisomy 18	Low	Low	Low	N/A
Open neural tube defect	Elevated	Normal	Normal	N/A

The sequential screen can be performed in three different ways.

- *Independent sequential screen*: An FTS is performed with all three components (NT measurement, PAPP-A, and free β-hCG). The FTS is considered positive if the risk is ≥1/270. The decision to pursue diagnostic testing or not is based on the FTS result. If diagnostic testing is not done the quad screen is performed in the second trimester and the risk for aneuploidy is calculated independently of the FTS results. The detection rate is above 95% but with very high false-positive rates (>10%) as the quad screen does not take into consideration the decreased risk of trisomy 21 in the second trimester after diagnosis of aneuploid pregnancies with diagnosis in the first trimester [17,24].
- *Stepwise sequential screen*: An FTS is performed with all three components (NT measurement, PAPP-A, and free β-hCG). A high FTS risk result is used to identify those at highest risk of aneuploidy in the first trimester and they are offered diagnostic testing. The remainder go on without getting an official FTS result but knowing they were low risk and obtain a quad screen. A final risk result is then given in the second trimester using the results of both the FTS and quad screen. This method decreases the high false-positive rate of the independent sequential screen because only the highest risk patients are offered diagnostic testing after the FTS [25].
- *Contingent sequential screening*: An FTS is performed with all three components (NT measurement, PAPP-A, and free β-hCG). Those patients with a low-risk FTS result do not continue to have a quad screen. Generally, patients with a FTS risk for trisomy 21 of 1/1300 or less do not go on to second-trimester analyte analysis. Patients at high risk of aneuploidy after the FTS are offered diagnostic testing. This leaves intermediate-risk patients, approximately 15%–20%, obtaining a quad screen. The detection rate with this method is 92%–94% with a 5% false-positive rate [26,27].

Twin gestations

In general, any genetic screening is less accurate in twins, but the risk for aneuploidy is increased, unless it is a monozygotic pair. In monozygotic twins the a priori risk for aneuploidy is similar to the mother's age-related risk.

NT measurements can be obtained in any multifetal gestation; however, there may be increased technical difficulty in obtaining the measurements with multiple fetuses. Care also needs to be taken to ensure each fetus is being measured. In a dizygotic pair a separate risk can be assigned for each fetus but in a monozygotic pair with differing NT measurements it is not as clear-cut. In general, it is recommended to use the higher or average NT measurement as this has a greater detection rate compared to using the smaller NT measurement for aneuploidy risk assessment [28].

Biochemical screening in the first trimester can be combined with NT measurements in twin gestations to increase the detection rate. The maternal serum analyte levels in multiple gestations are elevated compared to singletons. The level of the analyte, either PAPP-a or free β-hCG, is translated into multiples of the median and then that number is divided by the twin median. This gives an approximate twin multiple of the median, which can be used with the NT measurement obtained in each fetus to give a separate risk assessment for each twin [29]. Some labs may adjust for chorionicity of the twins, as women with monochorionic twins have lower serum levels of PAPP-A and free β-hCG than women with dichorionic twins [29]. A metaanalysis examining sensitivity and specificity of FTS in twin gestations found sensitivity and specificity of 86.2% and 95.2%, respectively, for dichorionic twins with a similar sensitivity and specificity for monochorionic twins (87.4% and 95.4%, respectively) [30].

Second-trimester screening (triple screen and quad screen) has much lower sensitivity and specificity for twin gestations. The largest study to date in twins used a triple screen and reported a detection rate of 63% and a false-positive rate of 10.8% [31]. Performing a stepwise sequential screen may improve these results slightly but is not an option for women who present with twin gestations in the second trimester [29].

Cell-free fetal DNA screening

Background

Fetal DNA was first discovered in maternal plasma in 1997 [32]. The DNA fragments originate from apoptotic trophoblast cells and are smaller than other DNA fragments at approximately 200–450 base pairs, which allows them to be differentiated from other fragments of DNA. These DNA fragments are present in a much higher concentration than circulating fetal cells in the maternal plasma [33]. Since this discovery the technology has been evolving rapidly to utilize these fragments to test for aneuploidy and other genetic disorders in the fetus.

The fetal DNA fragments are first detectable around 7 weeks of gestation. The amount of fetal DNA in maternal circulation is calculated as the amount of fetal cell-free DNA over the total amount of cell-free DNA in any given maternal plasma sample. The result of this calculation is known as the fetal fraction. The fetal fraction increases to 3%–13% of the total maternal plasma around 10 weeks' gestation, is stable from 10 to 21 weeks' gestation, and then increases again until the third trimester when it is at its highest concentration [34]. After delivery there is rapid clearance of these fetal DNA fragments, as the half-life of the fetal DNA fragments is only 15–20 minutes.

Multiple factors can affect the fetal fraction, including maternal obesity, maternal medical conditions, gestational age, multiple gestations, and fetal aneuploidy [35]. This is important when discussing optimal timing for screening utilizing cell-free fetal DNA. For example, women with higher body mass indexes (BMIs) may benefit from screening closer to 12 weeks of gestation to ensure an adequate fetal fraction for screening and decrease the chance of the inability of the test to be performed.

The first commercially available screens for aneuploidy were available in 2011 and rapidly became the test of choice for screening for trisomy 21, with the highest reported prediction rate of any of the aneuploidy screening modalities among women at increased risk for aneuploidy.

Modalities of testing

There are various modalities used by commercial cell-free fetal DNA screening companies to screen for fetal aneuploidy. These methods can be separated into those that

TABLE 12.4 Sensitivity and false-positive rates for various methods of cell-free fetal DNA screening for trisomies 21, 13, and 18, monosomy X, and fetal triploidy.

Sensitivity (%) False-positive rate (%)	(MPSS)	Targeted MPSS	SNP
Trisomy 21	99.1	>99	>99
	0.2	0.1	0
Trisomy 18 (Edwards syndrome)	97.3– >99.9	98	>99
	0.30	0.1	<0.1
Trisomy 13 (Patau syndrome)	87.5–91.70	80	>99
	0.90	0.05	0
Monosomy X (Turner syndrome)	95	96.70	91.7
	0.50	Unreported	<0.1
Triploidy	Unable to detect	Unable to detect	>99

MPSS, Massive parallel shotgun sequencing; *SNP*, single-nucleotide polymorphism.

utilize "counting" DNA fragments and those that utilize single-nucleotide polymorphisms (SNPs). The counting methods can further be broken down into two techniques: massive parallel sequencing and targeted sequencing. These methods have their pros and cons, which are discussed below, but all three still provide the highest prediction rate for trisomy 21 in high-risk populations. Neither technique is currently proven superior in terms of detection for trisomies 13, 18, and 21. Regardless of the method used, about 5% of samples will fail to produce a result (Table 12.4) [36].

Counting

Massive parallel shotgun sequencing

This method of cell-free DNA screening utilizes universal next-generation sequencing to map the millions of free DNA pieces (massive) to their chromosome of origin. Multiple samples can be analyzed at the same time (parallel). The molecules of DNA that map to each chromosome could be maternal or fetal in origin (shotgun). The number of molecules that map to each chromosome is then determined and the fetal chromosome number is determined by comparing the absolute number of reads on chromosomes 13, 18, and 21 to the number of reads from reference chromosomes that are presumed to be disomic. The fraction of a read expected from a particular chromosome is proportional to the chromosome size; therefore, we would expect a higher fraction for chromosome 1 compared to chromosome 22. The ratio of reads belonging to a chromosome of interest, chromosome 21, for example, is compared to the total number for a sample and then compared to the mean and standard deviation in a control sample, producing a *Z*-score. The *Z*-score represents how much of chromosome 21 in the sample differs from the chromosome 21 in the control, which is known to be diploid. Manufacturers who use this method often will report positive or negative if the *Z*-score result is above or below a certain threshold. They may also have a *Z*-score range that is an indeterminant or no-call zone. The fraction of fetal DNA in the sample (fetal fraction) will affect the results of this test and samples with a low fetal fraction are more likely to give an indeterminant or no result (Fig. 12.3) [37].

The advantages of using this technology include the ability to run multiple samples at the same time, the ability to run samples without separating maternal and fetal cell-free DNA fragments, and excellent positive predictive values, especially for trisomy 21. Limitations of this method include a lower ability to predict trisomy 13 compared to trisomy 18 and trisomy 21, an adequate fetal fraction, the higher cost compared to other methods, and the need for a control sample [38,39].

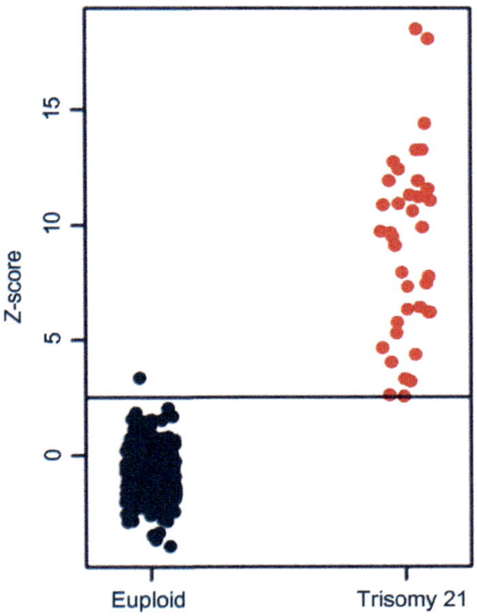

FIGURE 12.3 Mock-up of Z-score for euploid (*black*) and trisomy 21 (*red*) maternal serum samples for cell-free fetal DNA screening. A Z-score cutoff of 2.5 is shown as the *solid line*. Source: *From Ehrich M, Deciu C, Zwiefelhofer T, Tynan JA, Cagasan L, Tim R, et al. Noninvasive detection of fetal trisomy 21 by sequencing of DNA in maternal blood: a study in a clinical setting. Am J Obstet Gynecol 2011;204:205.e1–205.e11.*

Targeted massively parallel shotgun sequencing

This method of cell-free fetal DNA screening involves selective sequencing of the chromosomes of interest (13, 18, and 21) and then develops a risk calculation of sorts. This risk calculation considers fetal fraction, cell-free DNA counts, maternal age, and gestational age. The result provided is then listed as a risk rather than a negative or positive result, as with massive parallel shotgun sequencing (MPSS) [40]. The main advantage to this method is that it is cheaper than MPSS because it requires fewer counts. The primary disadvantage to this method, similar to MPSS, is that an adequate fetal fraction is needed to produce a result but, because of the fewer counts that are performed, a higher fetal fraction is needed [37].

Single-nucleotide polymorphisms targeted sequencing

The other major approach to cell-free fetal DNA screening involves the use of SNPs. SNPs occur when there is a single base-pair alteration and is a normal genetic change that occurs in every person. These genetic alterations mark where people differ from one another and account for 1.6% of the human genome [37]. This method uses SNPs with a high level of heterozygosity for comparison and thousands of SNP sequences are designed for each chromosome of interest. The initial method described required a paternal sample in addition to the maternal sample, however, a more novel approach allows for just the maternal sample, which increases the feasibility of this method. Polymerase chain reactions were performed on the maternal blood sample followed by sequencing. The product was then analyzed under different assumptions for each chromosome: one copy of the chromosome was present, two copies of the chromosome were present, or three copies were present. A maximum likelihood ratio was then calculated that the fetus was euploid, aneuploid, or triploid.

TABLE 12.5 Cell-free fetal DNA test performance characteristics in patients who receive an interpretable result at 16 weeks' gestation.

			25 years old	40 years old
	Sensitivity (%)	Specificity (%)	Positive predictive value (PPV) (%)	PPV (%)
Trisomy 21	99.3	99.8	32	85
Trisomy 18	97.4	99.8	16	59
Trisomy 13	91.6	99.9	9	57
Monosomy X	91.0	99.6	29	29

Created with noninvasive prenatal testing (NIPT) performance calculator: https://www.perinatalquality.org/Vendors/NSGC/NIPT/.

This screening method also allows for a maximum likelihood ratio calculation for uniparental disomy (all chromosomes are inherited from one parent). If no one profile fits, then no result can be produced [37].

The primary advantage for SNP analysis is less amplification variation, leading to a more accurate copy number across all chromosomes of interest. Other advantages of this method are that it allows for a very small fetal fraction, as it has been validated to a fetal fraction of 2.8%, which is smaller than MPSS or targeted MPSS and that it allows for different risk calculations for each twin in dizygotic twins, whereas MPSS and targeted MPSS do not [29]. This screening does not perform as well when there is a high degree of consanguinity between the parents. It also cannot be performed when there is a history of bone marrow transplant in the mother, or when the pregnancy is the result of egg donation, with the exception of one company [37].

Target population

The original population the cell-free fetal DNA screen was designed for was women of advanced maternal age (i.e., ≥35 years old at the time of delivery), as these women have an increased risk of aneuploidy, particularly trisomy 21, compared to younger women. The widespread availability and the attractiveness of a categorical "positive" or "negative" result, similar to a diagnostic test, have led to this screening modality being utilized outside of the originally studied population of women (Table 12.5).

The Society of Maternal-Fetal Medicine (SMFM) and American College of Obstetricians and Gynecologists (ACOG) currently recommend cell-free fetal DNA screening be used for "high-risk patients" [41]. These patients include advanced maternal age, ultrasound findings that raise concern for aneuploidy, a prior pregnancy with confirmed trisomy, positive aneuploidy screening results (i.e., quadruple screen or first-trimester screen), and a pregnancy at increased risk for trisomy 13 or trisomy 21 based on a parental balanced Robertsonian translocation [42]. Although there have been studies using cell-free fetal DNA screening in low-risk populations that have shown promising results, it is important to note their flaws, including they are underpowered, screened for trisomy 18 and trisomy 21, which have higher positive predictive values even in the high-risk population and had sample collection in the third trimester, well after most cell-free DNA screening is performed and when the fetal fraction is higher [43]. Despite this, the test is not restricted to women who are <35 years old at the time of delivery. Given these issues ACOG and SMFM recommend cell-free fetal DNA screening be reserved for those in the high-risk group they have defined.

Counseling

All women should be counseled about all their options for genetic screening in pregnancy. Those opting for cell-free DNA screening should be informed that it is still a screening test, albeit with high sensitivity and specificity, and since it is a screening test a negative screen does not guarantee an unaffected pregnancy. Low-risk women should be counseled about the potential for false-positive results. Even in women of advanced maternal age, for who the test was originally developed, this screening method will miss about 43% of anomalies because trisomies 13, 18, and 21 only make up about 50% of cytogenic abnormalities that would otherwise be detected with invasive testing [44]. A patient with a positive cell-free DNA screen should be referred for genetic counseling and offered invasive diagnostic testing, as this screening modality does not replace the accuracy and comprehensive nature of chorionic villus sampling (CVS) or amniocentesis. Women should be discouraged from pursuing pregnancy termination based on cell-free fetal DNA result alone given the risk of false-positive results. These general guidelines and recommendations have been supported by ACOG, SMFM, the American College of Medical Genetics, the International Society of Prenatal Diagnosis, and the National Society of Genetic Counselors [41,44–46].

Limitations

Despite the promise of this most recent screening test and its high detection rate, especially for trisomy 21 in high-risk populations there are important limitations to consider regarding the use of cell-free fetal DNA.

The first issue, which has been previously mentioned, is the risk of a low fetal fraction. Depending on the technology used the fetal fraction needed can be as low as 2.8% or may need to be as high as 8% before a test result can be interpreted. Certain factors affecting the fetal fraction, such as maternal BMI and fetal aneuploidy are not modifiable once there is a need for screening. Providers can help decrease the risk of a low fetal fraction by drawing the sample at the appropriate gestational age. Maternal blood draws for cell-free fetal DNA prior to 10 weeks' gestation are more likely to result in a low fetal fraction, so waiting until 10 weeks' gestation or greater will be more likely to produce an adequate sample. Additionally, in obese women (BMI $\geq 30\,\mathrm{kg/m^2}$), waiting until 11–12 weeks' gestation may produce a more reliable sample and avoid unnecessary patient anxiety and potential diagnostic testing procedures. Women who have results that are unable to be interpreted should have further genetic counseling with a detailed anatomy ultrasound and consideration of diagnostic testing given the increased risk of fetal aneuploidy in this population (Table 12.6).

A low fetal fraction may also produce a false negative and leaves a residual risk of aneuploidy [47]. This is especially true when using the targeted MPSS, which runs fewer counts. Other reasons for false negatives may include maternal genetic variation. For example, mothers with large copy number variants may have a false-negative result as the carry a higher proportion of genetic material on a particular chromosome [48]. Fetal aneuploidy can produce a false-negative result due to a low fetal fraction. In particular, trisomy 13, trisomy 18, and monosomy X have lower demonstrated fetal fractions compared to euploid fetuses and fetuses with trisomy 21. Placental mosaicism is a risk for producing false-negative and false-positive results depending on the genetic composition of the cells in the placenta compared to the fetus [49,50].

More often, placental mosaicism has been found to produce false-positive results. Other potential causes for false-positive cell-free fetal DNA results include a vanishing twin, previously unrecognized maternal aneuploidy, and maternal malignancy [51–54]. Detection of previously unrecognized maternal sex

TABLE 12.6 Test characteristics, pros and cons for common aneuploidy screening tests, and the recommended gestational ages for obtaining the tests.

Screening test	Gestational age range (weeks)	Detection rate for trisomy 21 (%)	False-positive rate (%)	Pros	Cons
Nuchal translucency	10–13 6/7	64–70	5	• No blood draws • Can be performed in multifetal gestation • Additional information gained on other fetal anomalies	• Poor detection rate when used in isolation • Requires specialized ultrasound training and good image quality
First trimester	10–13 6/7	82–87	5	• Single test/blood draw • Results in the first trimester	• Requires specialized ultrasound training and good image quality
Quad screen	15–22	69	5	• Single blood draw • No specialized ultrasound training • Provides information on other potential fetal anomalies • Option for screening for women who are late to prenatal care	• Lower detection rate than other screening tests
Integrated screen	10–13 6/7 then 15–22	96	5	• Highest detection rate for all combined tests • Provides information on other potential fetal anomalies	• Two blood draws • No results until the second trimester
Serum integrated screen	10–13 6/7 then 15–22	88	5	• No specialized ultrasound training	• Two blood draws • No results until the second trimester
Stepwise sequential screen	10–13 6/7 then 15–22	95	5	• First trimester results provided • Provides information on other potential fetal anomalies	• Two blood draws
Contingent sequential screen	10–13 6/7 then 15–22	88–94	5	• First trimester results provided as low, high, or intermediate risk • Provides information on other potential fetal anomalies	• Possibly two blood draws
Cell-free DNA	10–term	99 (if a result can be provided)	0.5	• Highest detection rate for trisomy 21 • Can be performed at any gestational age • Low chance of false positive in high-risk population	• High-risk of false positive in low-risk women • Lower sensitivity and specificity for trisomies 13 and 18

Adapted from ACOG Practice Bulletin 163 (Cuckle H, Benn P, Wright D. Down syndrome screening in the first and/or second trimester: model predicted performance using meta-analysis parameters. Semin Perinatol 2005;29:252–57 [25]; Ehrich M, Deciu C, Zwiefelhofer T, Tynan JA, Cagasan L, Tim R, et al. Noninvasive detection of fetal trisomy 21 by sequencing of DNA in maternal blood: a study in a clinical setting. Am J Obstet Gynecol 2011;204:205.e1–e11 [39]; Malone FD, Ball RH, Nyberg DA, Comstock CH, Saade GR, Berkowitz RL, et al. First-trimester septated cystic hygroma: prevalence, natural history, and pediatric outcome. FASTER Trial Research Consortium. Obstet Gynecol 2005;106:288–94 [58]; Bianchi DW, Platt LD, Goldberg JD, Abuhamad AZ, Sehnert AJ, Rava RP. Genome-wide fetal aneuploidy detection by maternal plasma DNA sequencing. MatErnal Blood IS Source to Accurately diagnose fetal aneuploidy (MELISSA) Study Group. Obstet Gynecol 2012;119:890–901[59]).

chromosome anomalies has been found with cell-free fetal DNA screening. Finally, use of this test in a low-risk population (i.e., women <35 years old at delivery) increases the risk of false-positive results, with the positive predictive value being <50% for trisomy 21 in this population [47].

Cell-free fetal DNA technology has been rapidly advancing, and some companies have branched out to include some of the more common microdeletions (e.g., 22q11.2, Prader-Willi, and Angelman). While promising, the inclusion of these microdeletion panels on cell-free fetal DNA screening tests is fraught with potential harm. The prevalence of these conditions in the general population is small, if known at all. The extremely low prevalence decreases the positive predictive value of these tests to well below where they are for screening for the common trisomies. In certain couples these tests may be warranted, for example, if there is a family history or ultrasound findings concerning for certain conditions and diagnostic testing is not desired. However, in the general, low-risk population this panel is of limited utility at the current time and may cause more patient anxiety due to the high rate of false-positive results.

The use of cell-free fetal DNA screening in twins is not recommended by ACOG and SMFM as first line, despite its availability with some companies using SNP technology. Newer data also suggest the sensitivity and specificity may continue to be as high as 99% and 100%, respectively, in a recent metaanalysis [55]. The fetal fraction in twin gestations is higher compared to gestational-age matched singletons; however, there are higher screen failure rates in twins. Additionally, when screened the fetal fractions from the twins are measured separately, when dizygotic. It is recommended that the twin with the lower fetal fraction be used to calculate the screening risk as there is an increased risk of aneuploidy with a lower fetal fraction, but this may result in a lower overall reporting rate [56,57].

Summary

Cell-free fetal DNA for screening for trisomy 21 performs better than any biochemistry test, regardless of whether NT is included; however, this test remains a screening test and is not considered diagnostic. It is also not recommended to be used in parallel with other genetic screening options (i.e., first-trimester screen, quad screen, etc.) at this time, because using multiple independent screening tests increases false-positive rates. All screen-positive cases should receive counseling and be encouraged to have confirmatory invasive diagnostic testing. It is still not recommended as first-line screening for all women in the first trimester as the prevalence of the genetic issues evaluated for cell-free fetal DNA is low in that population.

Diagnostic prenatal genetic testing

All pregnant patients have the option of diagnostic genetic testing. It is estimated that 1 in 150 live births has phenotypes associated with chromosomal abnormalities [60]. The purpose of diagnostic prenatal testing is to identify genetic abnormalities early enough in pregnancy to give the patient options regarding pregnancy continuation or coordination of pregnancy, delivery, and neonatal care. Diagnostic prenatal testing ranges from the basic karyotype for aneuploidy to whole-exome sequencing (WES). The patient's decision to pursue diagnostic genetic testing is often multilayered and dependent on the clinical situation. With varied options for the level of genetic detail examined, comprehensive genetic counseling is essential to ensure the correct testing is performed based on the patient's desires and clinical indication.

Common indications for diagnostic prenatal testing include:

- Abnormal genetic screening results;
- Abnormal ultrasound findings;

- Known parental carrier status;
- Advanced maternal age;
- Family history of genetic condition;
- Fetal demise/stillbirth;
- Parental anxiety.

Chorionic villus sampling

CVS involves sampling of the placenta at 10 0/7–13 6/7 weeks of gestation. Earlier sampling has been associated with limb reduction defects [61]. There are two routes of sampling, transabdominal or transcervical. In the transabdominal technique, using continuous ultrasound guidance, a small-gauge needle is placed through the abdomen into the placenta. Negative pressure created from an attached syringe draws the chorionic villi through the needle. Continuous motion with the needle during sampling has been thought to increase the villi yield and aid in varied sample sites. The transcervical technique utilizes a flexible plastic catheter that, under direct ultrasound guidance, is placed through the cervix and into the placenta. Villi are collected utilizing the negative suction of a syringe. An example of a transabdominal CVS needle placement is show in Fig. 12.4.

The route of CVS is determined by placental location and provider preference. In comparing both techniques, there does not appear to be any difference in pregnancy loss rates or other complications [62]. Transcervical CVS is associated with more post procedure spotting, while transabdominal CVS is felt to be more uncomfortable to the patient [63]. Subcutaneous lidocaine is administered prior to placement of the needle in the transabdominal approach, while local anesthesia is not necessary in a transcervical approach, unless a tenaculum is used to grasp the cervix, in which case a paracervical or local injection into the anterior lip of the cervix can been used. In the hands of experienced providers, CVS is relatively low risk. Reported procedure-related loss rates have ranged from 0.1% to 0.22%, and are lower at high-volume centers [62].

After the sample is obtained, the villi are placed into cell culture medium. The goal is to obtain at least 15 mg of tissue to allow for enough sample to complete all testing. Chorionic villi contain three cell lines: the outer synctiotrophoblasts, the middle cytotrophoblasts, and the inner mesenchymal cells. Cytotrophoblasts have a high mitotic index and can rapidly be examined using fluorescence in situ hybridization (FISH), which provides results in <2 days. The

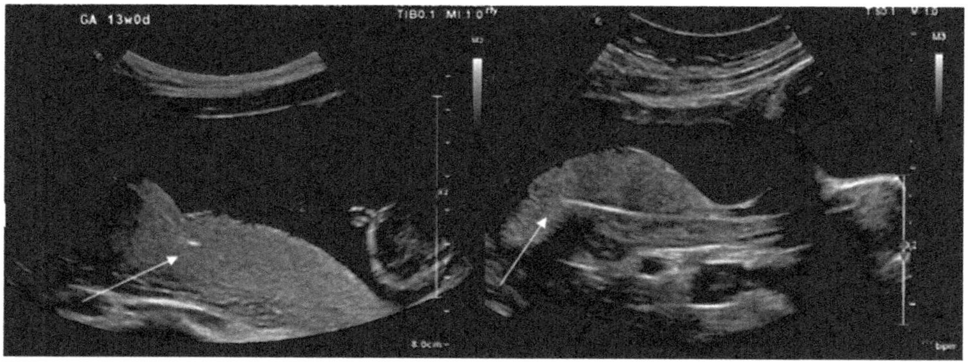

FIGURE 12.4 Sonographic examples of a transabdominal chorionic villus sampling (CVS) on the left and transcervical CVS on the right. The *arrow points* to the placement of the needle/catheter placement into the posterior placenta.

remainder of the sample is cultured to evaluate the inner mesenchymal cells. The mesenchymal cells are more closely aligned to the fetus from an embryologic standpoint, therefore awaiting karyotype from these cells is the gold standard, while the rapid karyotype from the cytotrophoblasts may exhibit a false positive. This is of importance when performing a CVS for abnormal cell-free fetal DNA, as it is the cytotrophoblasts that contribute the nucleic acids to the maternal bloodstream. It is possible to have abnormal cell-free fetal DNA from the cytotrophoblasts, and normal mesenchymal cells. Additional testing such as microarray, WES, and single-gene mutation analysis may also be performed on CVS specimens.

The primary benefit of a CVS is the early gestational age at which it is performed; giving the patient definitive genetic results at the end of the first trimester or early second trimester. Additionally, as viable cells are obtained, testing turnaround is typically faster than in amniocentesis. One of the drawbacks to a CVS is the identification of confined placental mosaicism (CPM), which occurs approximately 1% of the time [63]. Mosaicism is more often detected on direct as opposed to cultured specimens. A CPM arises when a genetic abnormality occurs after embryologic differentiation of the trophoblasts from the inner cell mass. These abnormal trophoblasts continue to replicate in the placenta, while the embryo remains genetically normal. CVS results will demonstrate some cultured cells that are normal, while some are aneuploid. Often, the normal cells are found at a much higher percentage than the abnormal, which supports the concept of trisomic rescue. Trisomic rescue occurs when a trisomic embryo loses the third copy of the affected chromosome in an attempt to return to the embryo to euploid. However, the third copy that is lost may have paternal or maternal origin, therefore it is possible to have a resulting embryo that is euploid but with two copies of a chromosome from the same parent resulting in uniparental disomy. It is important therefore, to perform testing for uniparental disomy if the results of the CVS involve chromosomes containing imprinted genes.

Patients whose results are suspicious for a CPM are advised to have an amniocentesis to more directly test the fetal compartment. Ninety percent of cases of mosaicism will demonstrate normal amniocentesis results, suggesting mosaicism confined to the placenta [64]. Isolated CPM has also been associated with abnormalities of fetal growth, therefore it is our practice to perform a follow-up fetal growth ultrasound at 32 weeks to confirm appropriate growth. The patient should also be counseled that there is still a residual risk of somatic mosaicism in a cell line not tested via amniocentesis. The clinical implication of somatic mosaicism is dependent on the cell line involved.

An additional difficulty related to CVS is in the case of multiple gestations. While pregnancy mapping is essential in assigning chorionicity and fetal nomenclature, it is possible to have genetic contamination during sampling. This is particularly true in the case of fused placentas in dichorionic diamniotic pregnancies. The risk of inadvertently sampling the same fetus twice has been estimated to be <1% [65]. In monochorionic twins only one placenta need be sampled, however, the patient should be counseled on the possibility of postsplit genetic divergence. Higher order multiples add additional challenges and CVS in this patient population should be performed by providers experienced with multifetal sampling.

Performing a CVS is contraindicated in patients with isoimmunization, as it is felt to further seed the maternal circulation with fetal antigen, thereby worsening the degree of isoimmunization. Additionally, patients with communicable diseases such as HIV or hepatitis B or C should be counseled on the possibility of vertical transmission. Transcervical CVS should not be performed in a patient with untreated gonorrhea or chlamydia.

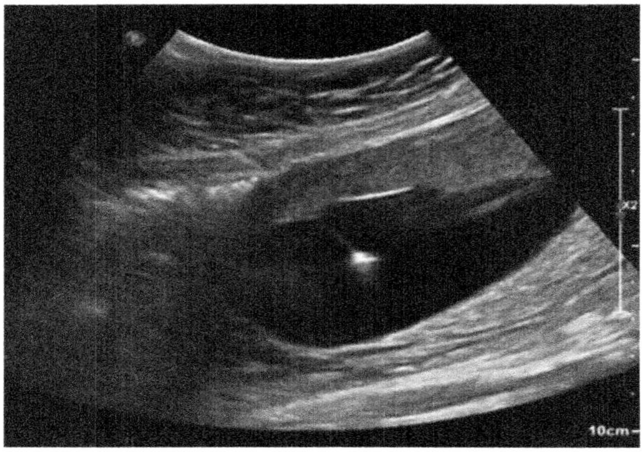

FIGURE 12.5 Example of the needle placement into the amniotic sac at time of amniocentesis.

Amniocentesis

An amniocentesis is typically performed after 15 weeks of gestation and is a direct sampling of the amniotic fluid. Within the amniotic fluid there are several fetal cell lines such as fetal skin cells, uroepithelial cells, and amniocytes. Most of these cells are nonviable as they have been sloughed off from the developing fetus. Therefore testing results take slightly longer with an amniocentesis over a CVS, as there are fewer viable cells for culture. Amniocentesis is also an ultrasound-guided procedure. A small-gauge needle, often 22 or 20 gauge, is placed into the amniotic sac, with care to avoid the fetus, umbilical cord, and when possible the placenta. An example of the needle placement during an amniocentesis is seen in Fig. 12.5. To avoid maternal contamination, the first few milliliters of fluid are discarded. Typically, 20–30 mL of amniotic fluid is collected, however, at earlier gestational ages some providers collect 1 mL of fluid per week of gestational age. An amniocentesis can be performed at any time after 15 weeks, when the amnion and chorion have fused. However, if performed in the range of periviability, test results are unlikely to be available quickly enough for the patient to exercise the option of pregnancy termination given the legal gestational age limit in most states.

Patients tolerate amniocentesis well, with minimal discomfort. The collected fluid is sent directly to the laboratory to begin the testing process. The loss rate associated with amniocentesis is low and comparable to that of CVS at high-volume centers, ranging from 0.13% to 0.27% [63]. It is difficult to truly discern procedure-related pregnancy loss from background pregnancy loss, as many patients who are pursuing diagnostic genetic testing are doing so due to fetal abnormalities that increase the risk for pregnancy complications. Amniocentesis has also been associated with procedure-related rupture of membranes. The outcome for procedure-related rupture of membranes is more favorable then nonprocedure-related rupture of membranes [66]. Amniocentesis is avoided in patients with HIV, and hepatitis B and C. However, the rates of vertical transmission in HIV patients with undetectable viral load is low.

Available testing modalities

Karyotype

Regardless of the type of procedure for obtaining the pregnancy tissue, extensive testing may be performed on the samples depending on the wishes of the family and clinical situation.

Given that aneuploidy is the most common abnormality of chromosome number, karyotype is likely sufficient to diagnose many genetically abnormal pregnancies. In fact, karyotype has a diagnostic accuracy of 99% for aneuploidy and large chromosomal abnormalities [67]. Sending the obtained sample for karyotype alone is most warranted in the setting of abnormal aneuploidy screening and/or advanced maternal age. FISH can be offered to initially evaluate for aneuploidy on uncultured cells, with initial results typically within 2 days. FISH analysis should be followed by confirmatory conventional karyotype, performed on cultured metaphase cells, as cases of false negatives and positives have been reported. FISH analysis can also be used to detect large microdeletions or duplications during karyotype analysis. This is particularly useful in the setting of known family history of a deletion or duplication, or when ultrasound findings are strongly suggestive of a known deletion/duplication syndrome.

Chromosomal microarray

Some patients desire to test beyond simple karyotype and may opt for a prenatal microarray. In the setting of a fetal anomaly, the addition of prenatal microarray has increased the yield of a pathogenic genetic variation to 6% with a normal karyotype [68]. Therefore we now routinely perform microarray for all prenatal samples in the context of increased risk of chromosomal abnormalities due to abnormal ultrasound findings. Pathogenic variants have been described as occurring in 1.7% of pregnancies with normal karyotype and ultrasound findings, therefore, microarray should be considered for all patients undergoing diagnostic genetic testing [68]. Chromosomal microarray is the preferred test for stillbirth as the test can be run on nonviable or macerated cells [69].

The prenatal microarray is performed on either uncultured tissue or on cultured cells. Microarray tests can evaluate the entire genome looking for copy number variants of >50–200 kb. These copy number variants are deletions or duplications of sections of the DNA, including variants near chromosomal breakpoints that allow for evaluation of unbalanced translocations. Microarray is also capable of detecting aneuploidy. There are two platforms available for microarray analysis: SNP arrays and comparative genomic hybridization (CGH) arrays. In prenatal microarray, a targeted panel of disease-causing regions is typically employed to reduce the risk of discovering variants of unknown significance (VOUS). It is important to know what is included on a prenatal microarray, as neonatal findings may warrant additional targeted testing. Postnatal testing via microarray is typically of higher resolution.

Most of the copy number variants detected on prenatal microarray have known associations with either pathogenic or benign variations. However, there is a risk for a VOUS to be detected. This is a DNA change that cannot be categorized as benign or pathologic due to lack of information regarding phenotypic abnormalities association with the variant, and may occur in 1.6% of pregnancies with abnormal prenatal ultrasound and normal karyotype [70]. This number has been declining as more information is available on copy number variants that were previously described as VOUS, thereby reclassifying them as benign or pathogenic. If a patient has a prior microarray that resulted in a VOUS it may be resubmitted for reclassification. In instances when a VOUS is detected, both parents should also be tested as the presence of the same VOUS in either parent indicates that the copy number variant is likely benign.

Microarray has some additional limitations, mainly an inability to detect balanced translocations or inversions. Most CGH platforms cannot detect low-level mosaicism or triploidies. The SNP-based array technique detects triploidy, uniparental disomy, and consanguinity. Given the increased yield of results, in the case of structural abnormalities, chromosomal microarray is expected to replace fetal karyotyping [71].

When counseling a patient, it is important to realize that not all resultant copy number variants have immediate clinical implications. Some results indicate an increased risk for adult-onset conditions. In fact, it may be discovered that one of the parents may also carry the same variant, thus revealing their own increased risk for disease. Chromosomal microarray can also detect consanguinity. The knowledge of these results may add undue stress during the prenatal period.

Whole-exome sequencing

As technology advances, the performance of WES has become an increasingly utilized option for prenatal genetic testing. InWES the entire genome is analyzed and the exons, or coding regions, are examined with next-generation sequencing for pathogenic variation. In the past WES was expensive and time--consuming, with meaningful results often not available for months after collection. In the setting of prenatal genetic testing, this meant its clinical value was less useful as patients would not have results in time to act. More recently results are analyzed and available much quicker, therefore the use of this test has increased. Clinically, in the prenatal period, WES is used in the case of otherwise unexplained abnormal ultrasound findings. Case series suggest a genetic abnormality may be detected in 20%–30% of fetuses with multiple anomalies when karyotype and microarray were normal [72]. A more recent prospective cohort study of pregnancies with abnormal ultrasound and normal karyotype and microarray demonstrated that targeted WES increased the diagnostic yield to 8.5% for a known pathogenic variant felt to cause the sonographic abnormality, while an additional 3.9% of fetuses had a variant of unknown significance that had potential clinical relevance [73]. This study utilized the concept of trio testing, when testing is performed on fetal, maternal, and paternal samples. This allows for determination of the origin of a mutation; either de novo or inherited. Currently it is recommended that WES be reserved for cases of multiple anomalies when all other testing has not yielded results.

Targeted gene mutation analysis

The use of targeted gene mutation analysis is reserved for cases of known familial genetic mutations. This is a targeted test of a mutation in a gene responsible for a specific disorder or category of disorders in the setting of a known familial mutation, or when both parents are discovered to be carriers of recessive conditions. Common examples include both parents being carriers for sickle cell disease or one parent being a hemophilia carrier. In the case of autosomal recessive conditions, the results of these tests may indicate that the fetus has the disease if both copies of the gene demonstrate a mutation, is a carrier of the disease if one copy has a mutation, or is neither when both copies are normal.

Additionally, targeted gene mutation analysis may be used when prenatal ultrasound findings are highly suspicious for a known condition or category of disorders. A classic example would be in the case of targeted testing for Noonan syndrome in a pregnancy with cystic hygroma. In these cases, a more targeted testing approach is used to evaluate for the most common or likely genetic condition. Some laboratories offer panels of genes with similar phenotypic findings such as skeletal dysplasia. Targeted molecular DNA testing may result as quickly as 3 days but most often takes 1–2 weeks. The testing time may be reduced if there is a known familial mutation.

References

[1] Shuttleworth G. Mongolian imbecility. Br Med J 1909;2:661.

[2] Nicolaides KH, Azar G, Byrne D, Mansur C, Marks K. Fetal nuchal translucency: ultrasound screening for chromosomal defects in first trimester of pregnancy. Br Med J 1992;304:867–9.

[3] Hyett J, Perdu M, Sharland G, Snijders RS, Nicolaides KH. Using fetal nuchal translucency to screen for major congenital heart defects at 10-14 weeks gestation: population based cohort study. BMJ 1999;31:81–5.

[4] Von Kaisenberg CS, Nicolaides KH, Brand-Saberi B. Lymphatic vessel hypoplasia in fetuses with Turner syndrome. Hum Reprod 1999;4:823–6.

[5] Brigatti KW, Malone FD. First-trimester screening for aneuploidy. Obstet Gynecol Clin North Am 2004;31:1–20.

[6] Braithwaite JM, Morris RW, Economides DL. Nuchal translucency measurements: frequency distribution and changes with gestation in a general population. Br J Obstet Gynaecol 1996;203:1201–4.

[7] NTQR: Nuchal Translucency Quality Review Program. NT measurement criteria, <https://www.ntqr.org/wfInformation.aspx> [accessed 25.02.19].

[8] Pandya PP, Altman DG, Brizot MI, Pettersen H, Nicolaides KH. Repeatability of measurement of fetal nuchal translucency thickness. Ultrasound Obstet Gynecol 1995;5:334–7.

[9] Snjders RJ, Thom EA, Zachary JM, Platt LD, Greene N, Jackson LG, et al. First-trimester trisomy screening: nuchal translucency measurement training and quality assurance to correct and unify technique. Ultrasound Obstet Gynecol 2002;19:353–9.

[10] Thornburg LL, Mulconry M, Post A, Carpenter A, Grace D, Pressman EK. Fetal nuchal translucency thickness evaluation in the overweight and obese gravida. Ultrasound Obstet Gynecol 2009;33:665–9.

[11] Rosen T, D'Alton ME. Down syndrome screening in the first and second trimesters: what do the data show? Semin Perinatol 2005;29:367–75.

[12] Cicero S, Rembouskos G, Vandecruys H, Hogg M, Nicolaides KH. Likelihood ratio for trisomy 21 in fetuses with absent nasal bone at the 11-14 week scan. Ultrasound Obstet Gynecol 2005;23:218–23.

[13] Prefumo F, Sairam S, Bhide A, Penna L, Hollis B, Thilaganathan B. Maternal ethnic origin and fetal nasal bones at 11-14 weeks of gestation. BJOG 2004;111:109–12.

[14] Tul N, Spencer K, Noble P, Chan C, Nicolaides K. Screening for Trisomy 18 by fetal nuchal translucency and maternal serum free β-hCG and PAPP-A at 10-14 weeks of gestation. Prenat Diag 1999;10:1035–42.

[15] Krantz DA, Larsen JW, Buchanan PD, Macri JN. First-trimester Down syndrome screening: free beta-human chorionic gonadotropin and pregnancy-associated plasma protein A. Am J Obstet Gynecol 1996;175:612–16.

[16] Wapner RJ, Thom E, Simpson JL, Pergament E, Silver R, Filkins K, et al. First-trimester screening for trisomies 21 and 18. N Engl J Med 2003;349:1405–13.

[17] Malone FD, Canick JA, Ball RH, Nyberg DA, Comstock CH, Bukowski R, et al. First-trimester or second-trimester screening, or both, for Down's syndrome. N Engl J Med 2005;353:2001–11.

[18] Wald NJ, Rodeck C, Hackshaw AK, Walters J, Chitty L, Mackinson AM, et al. First and second trimester antenatal screening for Down's syndrome: the results of the Serum, Urine and Ultrasound Screening Study (SURUSS). Health Technol Assess 2003;7:1–77.

[19] Nicolaides KH, Spencer K, Avgidou K, Faiola S, Falcon O. Multicenter study of first-trimester screening for trisomy 21 in 75,821 pregnancies: results and estimation of the potential impact of individual risk orientated two-stage first-trimester screening. Ultrasound Obstet Gynecol 2005;25:221–6.

[20] Merkatz IR, Nitowsky HM, Macri JN, Johnson WE. An association between low maternal serum alpha-fetoprotein and fetal chromosomal abnormalities. Am J Obstet Gynecol 1984;148:886–94.

[21] Cuckle HS, Wad NJ, Lindenbaum RH. Maternal serum alpha-fetoprotein measurement: a screening test for Down syndrome. Lancet 1984;1:926–9.

[22] Wald NJ, Watt HC, Hackshaw AK. Integrated screening for Down's syndrome based on the tests performed during the first and second trimesters. N Engl J Med 1999;341:461–7.

[23] Weisz B, Pandya P, Chitty L, Jones P, Huttly W, Rodeck C. Practical issues drawn from the implementation of the integrated test for Down syndrome screening into routine clinical practice. BJOG 2007;114:493–7.

[24] Platt LD, Greene N, Johnson A, Zachary J, Thom E, Krantz D, et al. Sequential pathways of testing after first-trimester screening for Trisomy 21. Obstet Gynecol 2004;104:661–6.

[25] Cuckle H, Benn P, Wright D. Down syndrome screening in the first and/or second trimester: model predicted performance using meta-analysis parameters. Semin Perinatol 2005;29:252–7.

[26] Reddy UM, Wapner RJ. Comparison of first and second trimester aneuploidy risk assessment. Clin Obstet Gynecol 2007;50:442–53.

[27] Benn P, Wright D, Cuckle H. Practical strategies in contingent sequential screening for Down syndrome. Prenat Diag 2005;25:645–52.

[28] Vandecruys H, Faiola S, Auer M, Sebire N, Nicolaides KH. Screening for trisomy 21 in monochorionic twins by measurement of fetal nuchal translucency thickness. Ultrasound Obstet Gynecol 2005;25:551–3.
[29] Bender W, Dugoff L. Screening for aneuploidy in multiple gestations: the challenges and options. Obstet Gynecol Clin N Am 2018;45:41–53.
[30] Prats P, Rodriguez I, Comas C, Puerto B. Systematic review of screening for trisomy 21 in twin pregnancies in first trimester combining nuchal translucency and biochemical markers: a meta-analysis. Prenat Diagn 2014;34:1077–83.
[31] Garchet-Beaudron A, Dreux S, Leporrier N, Oury JF, Muller F, ABA Study Group. Clinical Study Group. Second trimester Down syndrome maternal serum marker screening: a prospective study of 11040 twin pregnancies. Prenat Diagn 2008;28:1105–9.
[32] Lo YM, Corbetta N, Chamberlain PF, Rai V, Sargent IL, Redman CW, et al. Presence of fetal DNA in maternal plasma and serum. Lancet 1997;350:485–7.
[33] Lo YM. Fetal DNA in maternal plasma: biology and diagnostic applications. Clin Chem 2000;26:1903–6.
[34] Norton ME, Brar H, Weiss J, Karimi A, Laurent LC, Caughey AB, et al. Non-invasive chromosomal evaluation (NICE) study: results of a multicenter prospective cohort study for detection of fetal trisomy 21 and trisomy 18. Am J Obstet Gynecol 2012;207:137.e1–8.
[35] Wang E, Batey A, Struble C, Musci T, Song K, Oliphant A. Gestational age and maternal weight effects on fetal cell-free DNA in maternal plasma. Prenat Diag 2013;33:662–6.
[36] Palomaki GE, Kloza EM, Lambert-Messerlian GM, Haddow JE, Neveux LM, Erich M, et al. DNA sequencing of maternal plasma to detect Down syndrome: an international clinical validation study. Genet Med 2011;12:913–20.
[37] Dar P, Shani H, Evans MI. Cell-free DNA: comparison of technologies. Clin Lab Med 2016;36:199–211.
[38] Palomaki GE, Deciu C, Kloza EM, Lambert-Messerlian GM, Haddow JE, Neveux LM, et al. DNA sequencing of maternal plasma reliably identifies trisomy 18 and trisomy 13 as well as Down syndrome: an international collaborative study. Genet Med 2012;14:296–305.
[39] Ehrich M, Deciu C, Zwiefelhofer T, Tynan JA, Cagasan L, Tim R, et al. Noninvasive detection of fetal trisomy 21 by sequencing of DNA in maternal blood: a study in a clinical setting. Am J Obstet Gynecol 2011;204:205.e1–205.e11.
[40] Renga B. Non invasive prenatal diagnosis of fetal aneuploidy using cell free fetal DNA. Eur J Obstet Gynecol Reprod Biol 2018;225:5–8.
[41] The American College of Obstetricians and Gynecologists Practice Bulletin Number 163. Prenatal diagnostic testing for genetic disorders; May 2016, reaffirmed 2018.
[42] The Society for Maternal Fetal Medicine. SMFM statement: maternal serum cell-free DNA screening in low risk women; 2014.
[43] Bianchi DW, Parker RL, Wentworth J, Madankumar R, Saffer C, Das AF, et al. DNA sequencing versus standard prenatal aneuploidy screening. N Engl J Med 2014;370:799–808.
[44] Gregg R, Gross SJ, Best RG, Monaghan KG, Bajaj K, Skotko BG, et al. ACMG statement on noninvasive prenatal screening for fetal aneuploidy. Genet Med 2013;15:395–8.
[45] Devers PL, Cronister A, Ormond KE, Facio F, Brasington CK, Flodman P. Noninvasive prenatal testing/noninvasive prenatal diagnosis: the position of the National Society of Genetic Counselors. J Genet Couns 2013;22:291–5.
[46] Benn P, Borell A, Chiu R, Cuckle H, Dugoff L, Faas B, et al. Position statement from the aneuploidy screening committee on behalf of the board of the international society for prenatal diagnosis. Prenat Diagn 2013;33:622–9.
[47] Norton ME, Jacobsson B, Swamy GK, Laurent LC, Ranzini AC, Brar H, et al. Cell-free DNA analysis for noninvasive examination of trisomy. NEJM 2015;372:1589–97.
[48] Snyder MW, Gammill HS, Shendure J. Copy-number variation and false positive results of prenatal screening. N Engl J Med 2015;373:2585. Available from: https://doi.org/10.1056/NEJMc1507106.
[49] Grati FR, Malvestiti F, Ferreira JC, Bajaj K, Gaetani E, Agrati C, et al. Fetoplacental mosaicism: potential implications for false-positive and false-negative noninvasive prenatal screening results. Genet Med 2014;16:620–4.
[50] Mao J, Wang T, Wang BJ, Liu H, Zhang J, Cram D, et al. Confined placental origin of the circulating cell free fetal DNA revealed by a discordant non-invasive prenatal test result in a trisomy 18 pregnancy. Clin Chim Acta 2014;433:190–3.
[51] Lau TK, Jiang FM, Stevenson RJ, Lo TK, Chan LW, Chan MK, et al. Secondary findings from non-invasive prenatal testing for common fetal aneuploidies by whole genome sequencing as a clinical service. Prenat Diagn 2013;33:602–8.
[52] Wang Y, Chen Y, Tian F, Zhang J, Song Z, Wu Y, et al. Maternal mosaicism is a significant contributor to discordant sex chromosomal aneuploidies associated with noninvasive prenatal testing. Clin Chem 2014;60:251–9.

[53] Lau TK, Cheung SW, Lo PSS, Pursley AN, Chan MK, Jiang F, et al. Non-invasive prenatal testing for fetal chromosomal abnormalities by low-coverage whole-genome sequencing of maternal plasma DNA: review of 1982 consecutive cases in a single center. Ultrasound Obstet Gynecol 2014;43:254–64.

[54] Osborne CM, Hardisty E, Devers P, Kaiser-Rogers K, Hayden MA, et al. Discordant noninvasive prenatal testing results in a patient subsequently diagnosed with metastatic disease. Prenat Diagn 2013;33:609–11.

[55] Liao H, Liu S, Wang H. Performance of non-invasive prenatal screening for fetal aneuploidy in twin pregnancies: a meta-analysis. Prenat Diagn 2017;37:874–82.

[56] Bevilacqua E, Bil MM, Nicolaides KH, Ordonez E, Cirigliano V, Dierickx H, et al. Performance of screening for aneuploidies by cell free DNA analysis for maternal blood in twin pregnancies. Ultrasound Obstet Gynecol 2015;45:61–6.

[57] Samo L, Revello R, Hanson E, Akolekar R, Nicolaides KH. Prospective first-trimester screening for trisomies by cell-free DNA testing of maternal blood in twin pregnancy. Ultrasound Obstet Gynecol 2016;47:705–11.

[58] Malone FD, Ball RH, Nyberg DA, Comstock CH, Saade GR, Berkowitz RL, et al. First-trimester septated cystic hygroma: prevalence, natural history, and pediatric outcome. FASTER Trial Research Consortium. Obstet Gynecol 2005;106:288–94.

[59] Bianchi DW, Platt LD, Goldberg JD, Abuhamad AZ, Sehnert AJ, Rava RP. Genome-wide fetal aneuploidy detection by maternal plasma DNA sequencing. MatErnal Blood IS Source to Accurately diagnose fetal aneuploidy (MELISSA) Study Group. Obstet Gynecol 2012;119:890–901.

[60] Nussbaum RL, McInnes RR, Willard HF. Principles of clinical cytogenetics and genome analysis. Thompson & Thompson genetics in medicine. Philadelphia, PA: Elsevier; 2016. p. 57–74.

[61] Botto LD, Olney RS, Mastroiacovo P, Khoury MJ, Moore CA, Alo CJ, et al. Chorionic villus sampling and transverse digital deficiencies: evidence for anatomic and gestational-age specificity of the digital deficiencies in two studies. Am J Med Genet 1996;62:173–8.

[62] Akolear R, Beta J, Picciarelli G, Ogilvie C, D'Antonio F. Procedure-related risk of miscarriage following amniocentesis and chorionic villus sampling: a systematic review and meta-analysis. Ultrasound Obstet Gynecol 2015;45:16–26.

[63] The American College of Obstetricians and Gynecologists Practice Bulletin Number 162. Prenatal diagnostic testing for genetic disorders; May 2016, reaffirmed 2018.

[64] Goldberg JD, Wohlferd MM. Incidence and outcome of chromosomal mosaicism found at the time of chorionic villus sampling. Am J Obstet Gynecol 1997;176:1349–52.

[65] van den Berg C, Braat AP, Van Opstal D, Halley DJ, Kleijer WJ, den Hollander NS, et al. Amniocentesis or chorionic villus sampling in multiple gestations? Experience with 500 cases. Prenat Diagn 1999;19:234–44.

[66] Borgida AF, Mills AA, Feldman DM, Rodis JF, Egan JF. Outcome of pregnancies complicated by ruptured membranes after genetic amniocentesis. Am J Obstet Gynecol 2000;193:937–9.

[67] Jackson LG, Zachary JM, Fowler SE, Desnick RJ, Golbus MS, Ledbetter DH, et al. A randomized comparison of transcervical and transabdominal chorionic villus sampling. The U.S. National Institute of Child Health and Human Development Chorionic-Villus Sampling and Amniocentesis Study Group. N Engl J Med 1992;327:594–8.

[68] Wapner RJ, Martin CL, Levy B, Ballif BC, Eng CM, Zachary JM, et al. Chromosomal microarray versus karyotyping for prenatal diagnosis. N Engl J Med 2012;367:2175–84.

[69] Dugoff L, Norton M, Kuller J. Society for Maternal-Fetal Medicine. The use of chromosomal microarray for prenatal diagnosis. SMFM Consult Series #41.

[70] Brady PD, Delle Chiaie B, Christenhusz G, Dierickx K, Van Den Bogaert K, Menten B, et al. A prospective study of the clinical utility of prenatal chromosomal microarray analysis in fetuses with ultrasound abnormalities and an exploration of a framework for reporting unclassified variants and risk factors. Genet Med 2014;16:469–76.

[71] The American College of Obstetricians and Gynecologists Committee Opinion Number 682. Microarrays and Next Generation Sequencing Technology: the use of Advanced Genetic Diagnostic Tools in Obstetrics and Gynecology; December 2016.

[72] Drury S, Williams H, Trump N, Boustred C, GOS Gene, Lench N, et al. Exome sequencing for prenatal diagnosis of fetuses with sonographic abnormalities. Prenat Diagn 2015;35:1010–17.

[73] Lord J, McMullan D, Eberhardt R, Rinck G, et al. Prenatal exome sequencing analysis in fetal structural abnormalities detected by ultrasonography (PAGE): a cohort study. Lancet 2019;393(10173):747–57 [Epub ahead of print].

CHAPTER

13

Expanded carrier screening in reproductive medicine

Jeffrey S. Dungan

Division of Clinical Genetics, Department of Obstetrics & Gynecology, Northwestern University Feinberg School of Medicine, Chicago, IL, United States

Expanded carrier screening (ECS) is the successor to traditional genetic carrier screening for couples seeking, or with, a pregnancy. The goal is to identify those couples who are at risk for transmitting genetic disorders to their offspring, specifically single-gene, or Mendelian, disorders. Such screening is elective, and patients should always have the option to forego such analysis. For the most part, disorders included in carrier screening protocols are inherited in an autosomal recessive (AR) pattern, meaning both parents must be carriers in order to produce affected offspring. A couple identified as being at-risk (both carriers) have a 1 in 4 (25%) chance of this occurring. Women may also be asymptomatic carriers of X-linked recessive disorders and an increasing number of these disorders are appearing on ECS panels. Transmission of such alleles may result in an affected son (50% chance for male offspring to be affected). Most X-linked recessive disorders are manifested in male offspring only because of their hemizygous state, having only a single X chromosome, although exceptions exist. For example, females who are heterozygous for a full fragile X mutation may display some features of that neurologic disorder.

The preconception phase of reproduction is the ideal time to pursue such screening [1], as the pregnancy options are wider. If carrier screening is performed prenatally, there may be time constraints to performing a full evaluation of carrier status of both partners, as well as subsequent prenatal diagnosis if elected.

Carrier screening fills a gap in reproductive medicine, because most individuals found to be carriers have no family history of that disorder. This is in part due to the fact that asymptomatic carriers of AR disorders will transmit the disease-causing allele through several generations with no family awareness, given the low probability of a mating with another unrelated carrier. Historically, carrier testing was only provided to couples after the birth of a child affected with some AR disorder, essentially confirming what was already self-evident. Preconception carrier screening is thus an important tool to help couples better plan reproduction with the goal of avoiding the birth of an affected offspring.

Human Reproductive Genetics
DOI: https://doi.org/10.1016/B978-0-12-816561-4.00013-2

Traditional carrier screening has been based on limiting analysis to those populations with a given disorder prevalence higher than in the general population. In this way, limited resources (money) would be used for populations with the greatest chance of identifying a carrier. The disorders included on lists of genes for which carrier screening was performed relate to the higher carrier prevalence amongst certain ethnic and cultural backgrounds.

Principles of carrier screening

Table 13.1 lists examples of those disorders for which preconception/prenatal carrier screening (hereafter referred to generically as carrier screening) are typically offered. Common features of these disorders have been defined based on long-standing principles of carrier screening originally spelled out by Wilson and Jungner for the WHO in 1968 [2], although their original statement was designed for screening individuals for disease, not carrier status. Nonetheless, such considerations help guide decision-making about the design of carrier screening programs with the goal of helping couples avoid transmitting severe, life-threatening, or debilitating disorders for which treatment has no or minimal impact.

TABLE 13.1 Common Mendelian disorders for which carrier screening is available.

Disorder	Target population
Tay-Sachs disease	Ashkenazi Jewish and French Canadian
Cystic fibrosis	All individuals
Hemoglobinopathies	
Sickle cell disease	African and African-American
Beta-thalassemia	Mediterranean, Asian, Middle Eastern, Hispanic, and West Indian
Alpha-thalassemia	Southeast Asian, African, West Indian, and Mediterranean
Fragile X syndrome	Positive family history of ID, ASD, or POI
Spinal muscular atrophy	All individuals

ASD, Autism spectrum disorder; *ID*, intellectual disability; *POI*, premature ovarian insufficiency.
Adapted from Committee Opinion #691, ACOG.

Several tenets have been put forth addressing various elements of carrier screening that warrant consideration [3–5]. While interpretation of these guidelines may vary from a laboratory or patient perspective, these principles exist to help guide laboratories and clinicians in using sound clinical reasoning when offering screening for different disorders. Traditionally, application of carrier screening was straightforward, because the disorders being screened have been serious, common (in specific populations), and for the most part are untreatable or have ineffective treatments. As will be discussed later, the introduction of ECS has put some of these long-held practices in question, and introduced new debate as to what categories of genetic disease should be included in these protocols.

While a later section of this chapter will address some elements of carrier screening related to specific disorders, some general principles include such aspects as the voluntary nature of carrier screening, clinical and analytic validity, confidentiality, ability to take action based on results, cost-effectiveness, and clinical utility. Other important points address the diseases to be included. In general, diseases should be serious, of notable prevalence in a population, have reasonable genotype–phenotype correlation, and well-defined natural history [6].

Historic perspectives

The prototype for widespread reproductive carrier screening was the program to identify carriers of Tay-Sachs disease (TSD) (OMIM

#272800), a deficiency of hexosaminidase A, found more commonly in individuals of Ashkenazi Jewish (AJ) descent. Given the severe and nontreatable nature of TSD, identifying couples at risk provides an opportunity to apply a disease-reducing strategy on a population known to be at high risk, but with individual members frequently of unknown carrier status. Initial screening was performed by measurement of enzyme levels. Despite the caveats of using an enzyme assay (such as indeterminate enzyme levels, pseudodeficiency, and others), the program was immensely successful in lowering the birth incidence of children with TSD in this population [7].

Carrier screening for hemoglobinopathies in the United States slowly gained widespread use in the 1980s, after reliable diagnosis could be established prenatally through amniotic fluid cells or chorionic villi. However, uptake for prenatal testing for certain hemoglobinopathies has not been high. Early studies indicate fewer than half of couples at risk for sickle cell disease in their offspring chose to undergo prenatal testing [8]. Higher rates for uptake of prenatal testing however have been reported for beta-thalassemia, with a corresponding reduction in birth incidence in high-risk populations, such as in Sardinia [9].

In the early 2000s, after considerable debate, universal screening for cystic fibrosis (CF) carriers was introduced into clinical practice in the United States. While over 2500 known mutations in the cystic fibrosis transmembrane regulator gene (*CFTR*) have been associated with some form of CF, a small handful are responsible for the majority of serious "classic" CF. A panel of 23 mutations within this gene has been endorsed by the American College of Obstetricians and Gynecologists (ACOG) and the American College of Medical Genetics and Genomics (ACMG) [5], and now constitutes the recommended approach to identifying carriers. However, detection rates vary among different ethnicities, and are usually lower in populations that are not of northern European descent. Such a distribution of mutations within certain populations affects the "residual risk" that exists for someone to carry an undetected disease-causing variant within this gene, which will be described later. In some populations the residual risk remains relatively high. It is for this reason that some entities, such as commercial laboratories, prefer to include a larger number of mutations in their *CFTR* testing assays.

For years, ACOG and ACMG recommended offering screening to populations with higher carrier rates (northern Europeans and AJ) while making it "available" for other ethnicities. However, over time it was clear that such an approach was cumbersome and often misapplied by clinicians. Therefore in 2011 their guidelines were changed to recommending universal screening for all individuals regardless of ethnicity, either prenatally or preconceptionally.

Other aspects of traditional ethnicity-based screening

Certain populations are known to have higher carrier frequencies for some single-gene disorders than the general population. This fact has served as the basis for developing ethnicity-based carrier screening (see Table 13.1). The objective is to limit screening to those populations where the prevalence is considered sufficiently high to warrant performance of lab testing, thereby maintaining a favorable cost-effectiveness balance. This approach has been the mainstay of reproductive carrier screening for decades. In addition to those disorders mentioned above, other examples include additional heritable conditions found more commonly in the AJ population. For example, ACOG endorses screening this population not only for TSD, but also for CF, Canavan disease, and familial dysautonomia [5]. One key feature of an ethnicity-based approach using DNA analysis is that only a limited number of mutations needs to be assessed, given the predominance of "founder" mutations in this population, which tends to be endogamous.

Such a philosophy also applies to screening for a variety of hemoglobinopathies, including beta- and alpha-thalassemias. Screening for these disorders traditionally involves inspection of red blood cell indices and/or hemoglobin electrophoresis. These assays are relatively inexpensive but can be prone to erroneous interpretation from conditions such as iron deficiency. When results from these screens identify individuals with concerning parameters, then DNA analysis can be used to confirm (or rule out) carrier status at the molecular level.

While these approaches have worked reasonably well for years, new technologies warrant a reconsideration of this traditional approach. As will be discussed later, one feature of ECS using DNA sequencing techniques is that hemoglobin analysis can essentially be bypassed, and detection of carriers is accomplished by finding sequence variants.

There is not universal agreement among professional societies as to which disorders should be included on ethnicity-based panels. For example, ACOG and ACMG recommendations contain different lists of conditions to screen the AJ population; ACOG's recommended set was described above. The list of AJ disorders that ACMG recommends screening [10] also includes Fanconi anemia (group C), Niemann-Pick type A, Bloom syndrome, mucolipidosis IV, and Gaucher disease type I. Commercial laboratories frequently create their own versions of a "Jewish heritage" panel, and thus the clinician is left to choose from a variety of options, with no clear basis for deciding which panel is optimal.

Universal screening

The term "universal carrier screening" has been defined as offering assessment of a given set of genes to all individuals, regardless of ethnicity [11]. The basis for such an approach lies in two principal realms: reproductive justice, and perhaps more pragmatically, the fact that many individuals are now of mixed ethnicity, or uncertain ethnicity. The principle of justice in this context implies that all individuals should have access to the same content and level of care. Such an approach likely simplifies the offering of carrier screening for the clinician (one test that applies for everyone) as well as taking into account the possibility of mixed ethnicity in the patients. An example of this is the recommendation by ACOG and ACMG that all patients should be offered mutation analysis of *CFTR*, and more recently, of *SMN1*, the gene responsible for spinal muscular atrophy [5].

Role of expanded carrier screening

As previously stated, ECS is defined as assessment of genetic carrier status beyond traditional, ethnicity-based approaches. The number of genes that is now offered commercially by some laboratories has exceeded 250. While this "more is better" approach has some appeal, there are also important caveats that the clinician must understand when deciding whether to incorporate it into routine clinical practice.

In order to correctly assess the benefits and limitations of ECS, numerous organizations have weighed in on the properties of such an approach. A statement from the European Society of Human Genetics is summarized in Box 13.1 and was described by Hennemann et al. [12]. As stated in this box, carrier screening is primarily designed to "facilitate reproductive decision making" for couples. This mandates that well-informed clinicians need to be able to provide appropriate pre and posttest counseling to patients and couples. It is widely recognized that a knowledge gap exists related

BOX 13.1

Principles and objectives of expanded carrier screening

Primary goal of carrier screening is to facilitate informed reproductive decision-making

Education

All options for reproductive management should be considered

Increased equity and reduced stigmatization by offering same testing to all

Ideally performed preconceptionally

Source: *Adapted from Henneman L, Borry P, Chokoshvili D, Cornel MC, van El CG, Forzano F, et al. Responsible implementation of expanded carrier screening. Eur J Hum Genet 2016;24:e1–12.*

BOX 13.2

Summary of joint statement on expanded carrier screening in reproductive medicine

Carrier screening is voluntary

Conditions vary in severity

A negative screen does not eliminate risk to offspring

Pretest education and counseling should be provided

The condition should encompass one or more of the following:

- Cognitive disability
- Need for surgical or medical intervention
- Detrimental effect on quality of life
- Prenatal diagnosis of the disorder would impact further pregnancy management

The genes and variants should have a well-understood genotype–phenotype association

Residual risk estimates should be provided to individuals with negative screening results

Source: *Adapted from: Edwards JG, Feldman G, Goldberg J, Gregg AR, Norton ME, Rose NC, et al. Expanded carrier screening in reproductive medicine—points to consider. A joint statement of the American College of Medical Genetics and Genomics, American College of Obstetricians and Gynecologists, National Society of Genetic Counselors, Perinatal Quality Foundation, and Society for Maternal-Fetal Medicine. Obstet Gynecol 2015;1225:653–62.*

to genetic carrier screening that is being addressed by several professional organizations, such as ACOG, ACMG, and others.

One source of providing that needed education is a consensus statement that was issued by several American professional societies in 2015 [4]. In this "Points to Consider" statement, several aspects of counseling for carrier screening were delineated (see Box 13.2). These included such points as the elective nature of screening, the variable severity of conditions, the inability to eliminate all risk, the potential for multiple conditions to be identified, and the potential to be identified as having personal health risks. Another major aspect of this statement had to do with selection of disorders that are included on ECS panels.

BOX 13.3

Criteria for disease inclusion on expanded carrier screening (ECS) panel: ACOG

1. Carrier frequency of 1 in 100 or greater
2. Well-defined phenotype
3. Has detrimental effect on quality of life
4. Causes cognitive or physical impairment
5. Requires surgical or medical intervention
6. Onset early in life

Source: *Adapted from American College of Obstetricians and Gynecologists. Committee Opinion 690. Carrier screening in the age of genomic medicine. Obstet Gynecol 2017;129:595–6.*

These guidelines are meant in part to add some rationale and logic into approaches to carrier screening, particularly in the decisions about what disorders/types of disorders are appropriate to include on the panels. The technology now clearly outstrips the understanding of how best to approach these questions. This consensus statement spells out many aspects of reproductive carrier screening that are essential for providing informed and balanced counseling for patients prior to undergoing such testing.

ACOG has also delineated characteristics of disorders that would be appropriate in deciding which to include on ECS panels (see Box 13.3). One may argue there are some disease characteristics that are poorly defined by this list and are somewhat subjective. One couple's definition of "detrimental effect on quality of life" may differ considerably from another couple. Nonetheless, the basic premise behind these criteria is that the disorder should be serious, and have neonatal/childhood onset. Adult-onset disorders are not typically considered appropriate for inclusion on ECS panels for reproductive purposes. (This is in contradistinction to the offering of preconception assessment of autosomal dominant cancer predisposition syndromes in individuals from high-risk families.)

Diseases included should have serious and early ramifications for the affected individual. The disorders may be such that delivery should occur in tertiary center, with availability of specialists to manage the anticipated newborn issues. Alternatively, the condition may be such that couples choose to end the pregnancy. Another consideration is to be prepared to render only palliative care to the newborn, an option that should be planned in conjunction with neonatologists.

Undertaking ECS should be elective and presented to couples as an option, not a mandatory medical test. Not all couples wish to face the choices that knowledge of carrier status would entail. Others believe they would not change pregnancy management regardless of results. An important point to recognize is that different patients will make different decisions regarding such testing. The critical piece for the clinician offering the test is to ensure those decisions are made with accurate comprehension of the benefits and limitations of carrier screening.

The disorders on the panel should have reasonably predictable phenotype. This aspect becomes muddled for many disorders in which expressivity may be highly variable, even within a family. For many Mendelian disorders, there is poor or poorly understood genotype–phenotype correlation. Discussing possible variability in prognosis for a fetus found to have inherited such a disorder can be extremely complex and vexing for the family to understand. This is a key feature to include in counseling, because uncertainty in medical testing is likely a foreign concept for most patients. The inability to accurately provide predictions about phenotype may also be a compelling reason to exclude a disorder from the panel.

Another consideration about which disorders to include is whether couples would actually alter their reproductive planning or management if found to be a carrier. Experience indicates that partners of recently identified carriers may not follow through on determining their own carrier status, for a variety of reasons. This is an aspect of carrier screening that should be explored prior to initiating such testing.

Some ECS panels include disorders that are also found on some newborn screening (NBS) panels, depending on where the infant is born. This may appear to be paradoxical, as the objectives of the two screening protocols differ. A major difference between NBS and prenatal/preconception screening is the inclusion of disorders on NBS panels are potentially manageable with dietary or environmental adjustments postnatally. For example, biotinidase deficiency is on most states' NBS panel, given the management of affected children is biotin supplementation, which essentially corrects the metabolic issues, and leads to normal phenotypic outcomes. Yet, some ECS panels contain evaluation of *BTD* mutations, the genetic abnormality behind biotinidase deficiency.

There is no compelling reason to include disorders that are mild, readily treatable, or that appear only with late onset. For example, hereditary hemochromatosis is an adult-onset disorder of variable penetrance, and inclusion on prenatal carrier screening is of dubious value. This disorder was explicitly mentioned in the Consensus Statement described earlier as one that should not be included on ECS panels [4].

As studies and experience have shown, identification of carrier couples will provide information that can lead to avoiding the birth of an offspring afflicted with a serious disorder. In couples choosing to undergo this type of screening, such an option has implications for not only their immediate family, but other family members will also be identified as potentially being a carrier, and thus can choose to undergo confirmatory or exclusionary testing [13]. This is referred to as cascade testing, and clinicians should be aware that counseling patients about this opportunity is an important part of holistic care.

Mutation screening versus gene sequencing

Laboratories differ as to the molecular genetic analyses performed in their ECS panels. There are two general approaches: mutation screening (genotyping) and sequencing. Mutation screening is designed to detect a known and limited number of pathogenic variants within the gene, which can range from only one to dozens. Sequencing is more comprehensive in that essentially any sequence variant (with some exceptions) will be detected.

The advantage of mutation screening is that only known disease-causing variants are identified and reported. The primary disadvantage is *not* detecting a sequence variant that may be pathogenic. Thus the residual risk of being a carrier will be higher with mutation screening than with a sequencing approach. However, there will be no identification of variants of uncertain significance (VUS), which therefore simplifies counseling about results.

A major advantage of sequencing is full analysis of the gene and variants in coding regions, splice-site disruptions, and other potential disruptors of gene function. Depending on the protocol used, some of those insertion-deletions (indels, short sequences) or deletion-duplications (del-dups, long sequences) may not be detected [14]. While full analysis will result in the lowest possible residual risk of being a carrier, there is a higher likelihood of identifying a VUS. From a clinical standpoint, a high VUS rate is undesirable as it leads to a greater proportion of patients left with less reassurance about their own status, which makes counseling a challenge.

No professional society guidelines exist that state a clear recommendation for one form of analysis over the other. Many factors go into selection of the laboratory to provide mutation analysis, and in general the clinicians are responsible for making those determinations. On occasion, there may be a preferred laboratory provider based on third-party payor arrangements, and thus the decision may not lie solely with the clinician.

Genotype–phenotype correlations

There are two aspects of characterizing genomic disorders that, for clinical purposes, will lead to counseling dilemmas as it relates to reproductive medicine. One has to do with the phenomena of reduced penetrance and variable expressivity. Reduced penetrance means that not all individuals harboring the same gene variant will manifest any features of the disorder. If a gene variant is, for example, 50% penetrant, then 50% of the carriers of that variant will demonstrate some feature(s) of the associated disorder. Variable expressivity means that the same gene variant can lead to different phenotypic features, even within a family. These characteristics may be due in part to age of patient, unrecognized modifiers within a genome, or environmental influences that lead to differing phenotypes among individuals who carry the same pathogenic variant.

The other feature that is important to recognize is the less-than-perfect interpretation of pathogenicity of a novel or uncommon variant when it is detected in a laboratory. One criticism of sequencing analysis for ECS is the lack of well-established phenotype predictions of novel variants that are thought to be pathogenic, or likely pathogenic. According to ACMG guidelines [15], laboratories classify variants as "pathogenic" if there is a >99% probability of disruption of gene function [16]. If there is 90%–99% likelihood of disruption of gene functions, the finding is designated as "likely pathogenic." If the variant is <10% likely to be disease causing, it is considered benign. As will be described later, the remaining variant interpretations fall into a category known as "variants of uncertain significance."

Laboratories use a multitude of tools to help establish the pathogenicity of novel variants. While detailed discussion of these methods is beyond the scope of this chapter, the interested reader is directed to the most recent Standards and Guidelines for the interpretation of sequence variants, a joint consensus statement from ACMG, Association for Molecular Pathology, and the College of American Pathologists [15].

However, establishing pathogenicity is not synonymous with phenotype correlation. Thousands of variants may be classified as pathogenic, but the expressivity and penetrance may be unclear. In addition, the phenotype may be highly dependent on the second mutation on the other chromosome, and individuals homozygous for a given variant may have a noticeably different presentation than individuals who are compound heterozygous. Even within families with the same inherited mutations, expressivity can be highly variable for a number of disorders.

Determination of residual risk

Some ECS panels use mutation screening/genotyping as the analytic method. Depending on the number of mutations analyzed, there may remain a significant proportion of potential disease-causing variants that are undetected, however, this varies based on the ethnic distribution of mutations. For example, by use of the 23-mutation CFTR panel endorsed by ACOG and ACMG, an individual of African descent is predicted to have 64% of disease alleles detected [5]. Contrast that detection rate with the 94% detection rate using the same panel in an AJ patient. The CF carrier incidence in individuals of African descent is about 1 in 60, and in AJ individuals it is 1 in 24. The residual risk for still carrying a pathogenic variant in the AJ patient after negative screening with that panel is 1 in 380, but for the African-American patient, the residual risk is 1 in 170. Residual risk is determined by the equation: carrier frequency × (1−detection rate). The ability to determine residual risk requires knowledge of the disease (or carrier) prevalence of the disorder in the population being tested, and the proportion of disease alleles in that population that are analyzed by mutation screening. Providing residual risk estimates is an important feature of both pretest and posttest counseling.

If a sequencing assay is used, the residual risk will be inherently lower, given the high detection rate (large majority of sequence variants are detected, typically 98%−99 + %). One caveat is if the sequencing assay used by a lab has low or no detection of other genomic alterations, such as nondetection of del-dups, genomic rearrangements that require different technologies to detect. For many disorders, the proportion of disease alleles caused by del-dups may not be known:

Clinical utility of expanded carrier screening

Introducing a new clinical paradigm into practice is only of benefit if the target patient population accepts it and makes use of it. This is the definition of clinical utility. There are few studies which have examined the clinical utility of ECS. These reports focus primarily on whether couples choose to undergo such screening, and what they do with the information they receive.

To put the utility of ECS into perspective, it should be compared to the high clinical utility demonstrated with TSD carrier screening described earlier. Carrier frequency in the AJ population is around 1 in 30 (so birth incidence had been about 1 in 3600). With the use of routine carrier screening, the birth incidence has dropped by 90% in the US Ashkenazi population. Of note, detection of TSD carriers in the AJ population has traditionally been with enzyme analysis, and/or limited genotyping, but a small residual risk for carrier status remains. The residual risk is higher in non-Jewish populations. With sequencing, >99% of disease alleles are detected regardless of ethnic background, although labs differ as to reported detection rates.

Similar reductions in birth incidence have been reported with other "high"-prevalence diseases in other populations. Such an example is the impact of CF carrier screening, with couples identified as having an affected fetus generally choosing to terminate those pregnancies [17]. Use of preimplantation genetic diagnosis (PGD), donor gametes, or choosing not to have offspring are outcomes that also would reduce the birth incidence of a given disorder, and have been used by couples at risk for CF.

Haque et al. demonstrated a notable increase in identification of at-risk couples using a universal ECS platform compared to guideline-based approaches [18]. These investigators, from a large commercial lab performing ECS, demonstrated increased identification using modeling based on carrier frequencies among different ethnicities determined from their testing of over 346,000 individuals submitting samples. Of note, most of the testing from this lab at the time of this analysis was done by mutation screening, although a sequencing approach was introduced for the later specimens. Across all populations reported, there was an increase in identifying fetuses at risk that would not have been identified with guideline-based testing alone. These figures are depicted in Table 13.2. These data assume all carriers will ultimately have their partner tested, one aspect of carrier screening in general that has been underanalyzed.

Initial reports have emerged examining the utility of ECS by couples seeking assisted reproductive technologies. A study by Franasiak et al. [19] examined change in reproductive choices among couples pursuing in vitro fertilization (IVF). In a cohort of 6643 individuals (3738 couples), there were eight couples identified as being at risk. While the percentage of couples from the cohort is low, those at-risk couples did choose alternate reproductive interventions. The ECS assays used in this study were primarily genotyping, and thus may have not have identified carrier status in some people.

Another study from a large ECS lab in the United States examined reproductive behaviors in couples identified as being at risk because both parents were carriers of pathogenic variants in the same gene [20]. Using a survey of these couples, this group identified 391 respondents that were either already pregnant when ECS results were available, or were planning

TABLE 13.2 Predicted number of affected fetuses and risk of recessive disease by screening panel utilized.

Racial/ethnic category of both parents	Mean no. of fetuses/100,000 pregnancies expected to be affected			
	ACOG + ACMG panel only	Adding severe + profound conditions	Cumulative risk for couple of disease on ACOG + ACMG panel only	Cumulative risk for couple of all severe + profound
African/African-American	316.5	363.6	1/316	1/275
Ashkenazi Jewish	174.8	392.2	1/571	1/255
East Asian	7.6	129.9	1/13158	1/770
Hispanic	19.9	94.5	1/5025	1/1058
Middle Eastern	17.7	193.8	1/5650	1/516
Mixed/other Caucasian	48.8	153.8	1/2049	1/649
Northern European	55.2	159.2	1/1812	1/628
South Asian	20.3	111.5	1/4926	1/896
Southeast Asian	165.3	207.9	1/605	1/481
Southern European	54.9	171.2	1/1821	1/583
Unknown	38.5	150.4	1/2597	1/655

ACOG, American College of Obstetricians and Gynecologists. Carrier screening recommendations in Ref. [5].
ACMG, American College of Medical Genetics and Genomics.
"Severe + profound" refer to disease classification provided by Counsyl, Inc. on their promotional material.
Adapted from Haque IS, Lazarin GA, Kang P, Evans EA, Goldberg JD Wapner RJ. Modeled fetal risk of genetic diseases identified by expanded carrier screening. JAMA 2016;316:734–42.

pregnancy. Of those who were pregnant, 37% reported undergoing prenatal diagnosis (either chorionic villus samplingor amniocentesis) for the condition. In the 36% found to have an affected fetus, 40% of the pregnancies were terminated. In couples identified during the preconception, 77% reported that interventions would be taken to avoid an affected pregnancy, including preimplantation genetic testing for monogenic (PGT-M) (59%), prenatal diagnosis (20%), or other measures, such as donor gamete use, adoption, or avoidance of pregnancy altogether. There was also a direct correlation between frequency of planned interventions and the severity of the disorder, with the highest proportions taken if the couple was at risk for "profound" conditions. These data indicate that couples receiving appropriate counseling pretest and posttest make sound clinical decisions, and do indeed use the information provided by ECS in reproductive planning.

Options for carrier couples

The preconception state is ideal for carrier screening. If a couple is identified as being at risk, then plans can be made to circumvent the 25% chance of producing affected children. Such options include preimplantation genetic diagnosis (now termed preimplantation genetic testing—monogenic, PGT-M), use of donor gametes, adoption, or becoming pregnant and undergoing prenatal diagnosis to determine whether the fetus is affected.

The ability to undertake PGT-M requires that the lab have the knowledge of the relevant mutations, and the capability to perform the molecular analysis on pretransfer embryos [21]. This is nearly always the case, but some exceptions will arise due to the complexity and structure of some gene variants.

There is also the question about PGT-M for patients/partners identified with a VUS. In general, that is not medically warranted. However, there may be instances where one of the reproductive pair carries a pathogenic variant, and the other carries a VUS. In order to minimize the chance of transferring an embryo that may actually end up affected with the disease, some parents will opt to not transfer those embryos that inherited the two nonnormal alleles.

If a pregnancy is already established, the only method of determining whether the fetus is affected is through diagnostic testing, such as amniocentesis or chorionic villus sampling. In order for this to be achieved, knowledge of the DNA variants is essential. Such couples will need genetic analysis prior to undertaking the test. New assays involving noninvasive approaches to analyzing cell-free DNA fragments in the detection of Mendelian disorders may ultimately be a method for fetal analysis that may result in the ability to forego invasive testing procedures.

Carrier screening for X-linked disorders

Many laboratories include X-linked disorders on their panels. The most widespread of these is for fragile X screening. The *FMR1* gene contains a trinucleotide repeat (–CGG–) at its 5′ end, which can expand during female meiosis (but only rarely during male meiosis). The size of the trinucleotide repeat dictates the impact on gene function. A normal-size allele is up to 44 repeats, and is associated with normal gene function. A fully expanded mutation contains over 200 repeats, and leads to inhibition of gene function. Such an expansion results in fragile X syndrome in males who carry a full mutation (and about half of females that carry a full mutation). Phenotypic features of fragile X syndrome are described in several excellent reviews [22,23]. Carrier screening is designed to detect "premutation" allele sizes, which are comprised of 55–200 repeats. These are considered an unstable allele size, and are prone to expansion to full mutation size during female meiosis. There is a direct correlation between premutation triplet repeat number and likelihood of expansion to full mutation, with larger premutation alleles being more prone to expand. Finally, there is also an "intermediate" or "gray zone" repeat size (45–54) that is more stable than the premutation, but has potential for adding a small number of repeats during meiosis, possibly into the premutation range.

Health implications for female carriers of premutation *FMR1* alleles are well characterized, and should be discussed with patients prior to initiating carrier screening. There is approximately a 15% risk for premature ovarian insufficiency before age 40 [24], but primary ovarian insufficiency may occur as early as the 20 seconds in some carriers. In addition, other manifestations of *FMR1* premutations are related to risk for fragile X tremor-ataxia syndrome (FXTAS), which is more likely to affect men with a premutation allele than women. By age 70, about half of men with a fragile X premutation may manifest with FXTAS.

Counseling about the likelihood of *FMR1* expansion can be confusing to patients and clinicians alike. One source of this confusion is the variability of likelihood of expansion based on additional molecular alterations within the repeat region. Within the –CGG– repeat region, there may be interruptions with –AGG– repeats. These interruptions reduce the likelihood of expansion into the next higher category of *FMR1* disease alleles, at least at the lower end of –CGG– repeat numbers [25]. Testing for these –AGG– repeats may provide women with additional information as they decide whether to pursue PGD or prenatal diagnosis for fragile X-related conditions.

Another important feature of X-linked recessive disorders is the fact that many heterozygous female carriers may manifest some features of the disorder, although typically not to the same extent as in hemizygous affected males. One such example is Duchenne muscular dystrophy, due to mutation within the *DMD* gene. Female carriers have up to a 20% risk of developing a cardiomyopathy [26], and should undergo echocardiographic surveillance over the course of their lifespan [27]. It is also important to note that approximately one-third of males diagnosed with Duchenne muscular dystrophy are the result of de novo mutations within *DMD*, and thus absence of *DMD* mutation in the female parent does not eliminate the possibility of having an affected son.

Finally, it is relevant to note that for X-linked disorders, males are not typically screened, nor is it indicated to perform partner testing if the female patient is found to carry such a mutation. Her daughters will have a 50% chance of being a carrier (like the mother), and overall there is a 25% chance of having an affected son (50% chance of producing a male, and 50% chance of transmitting the X-linked disease allele).

Counseling for consanguineous couples

Couples who are comprised of third-degree relatives (the most common form of consanguinity reported) share approximately 12.5% of their genomes [28]. This in turn translates into a higher likelihood that both would carry the same recessive alleles (if present in the family's genome) and thus such pairings are associated with higher rates of AR disorders in their offspring. ECS offers such couples far more information than would ethnicity-based approaches, so consideration should be given to use the more comprehensive screening.

Once again, the preconception period is the ideal time to perform such screening, and some studies have suggested that performance of ECS prior to accepting a marital partner would be accepted by some [29].

Counseling regarding variants of uncertain significance

This term applies to a DNA sequence variant that has not been convincingly demonstrated to be disease causing, nor has it been proven to be a benign polymorphism. Most carrier screening laboratories do not report the finding of VUS given the obvious conundrum of how to use such information clinically. (A VUS will be reported in other clinical genomic applications, such as in attempting to make a diagnosis in an individual with some form of abnormal phenotype.) Such sequence alterations should generally not be utilized in clinical decision-making when identified during carrier screening, as association with disease status is unclear.

Software programs exist to predict what effect a given variant might have on protein structure or function. While nonsynonymous changes, that is, the resulting amino acid is different from the wild type, may be of concern, a synonymous change (no amino acid change) is less likely to result in disruption of protein structure or function. Those variants which are "nonsense," that is, result in a truncated protein, are more likely to be of clinical significance. Occasionally family studies can be helpful in assigning pathogenicity to a given variant, but this is not usually available in a timely fashion. Therefore the majority of laboratories and clinicians will not seek out, nor take action on, a VUS.

One possible exception is the setting where one of the reproductive partners carries a known pathogenic variant in the gene in question. If a couple is seeking out preimplantation genetic diagnosis, disclosure of a VUS may be relevant in identifying those embryos which should not be transferred that have inherited both the VUS and the pathogenic variant. Given the uncertainty of disease state in those offspring, some couples would choose not to transfer those embryos.

A VUS is typically only encountered from a lab that performs full gene sequencing as opposed to one that uses a mutation screening platform. Additionally, if a couple is determined to potentially be at risk because of the presence of a pathogenic variant and a VUS, one should consult with the lab that will be performing PGD, to ensure it is willing to test for the presence of the VUS, because that is not universally available.

Gamete donors

There is considerable debate over the role of the ECS for gamete donors. Current American Society for Reproductive Medicine guidelines [30] endorse utilization of the same guidelines for carrier screening that have been delineated by ACOG for biologic parents. The issue has to do with rejecting potential donors solely on the basis of carrying a pathogenic variant for a given disorder. Since most people harbor two to three variants in AR genes, the pool of "eligible" donors so deemed because of the absence of any pathogenic variants will inherently dwindle to very few. Some ECS panels identify pathogenic variants in >75% of individuals screened.

One approach that has been considered is to not use donor gametes from carriers only for a recipient that has also undergone screening and has a variant in the same gene. This is an instance when preconception testing of the recipient would thus allow carriers of nonmatching disorders to serve as suitable gamete donors. While this may seem straightforward, logistically this approach entails several challenges.

Another option is for the IVF clinical service to retain the ability to check donor genetic status in the event a recipient is found to carry a pathogenic mutation. Again, this would require significant infrastructure to manage such potentialities.

Ethical arguments in favor of expanded carrier screening

The ethical principle of patient autonomy should lead to a mandate that ECS be made available if patients desire such [31]. As ECS has now been available for several years, clinicians should have an awareness of its potential benefits, and be prepared to offer it to patients. ACOG [1] states that ECS is an option to which patients should have access, if requested.

The principle of justice supports any person having access to the same testing options as others. In settings where payor-mandated rules dictate clinical practice, this becomes problematic. On the other hand, costs for ECS continue to drop, and experience at our center indicates that some labs are willing to offer payment plans to make ECS accessible to more individuals. Of more pragmatic importance, individuals may be of mixed ethnicity, or unknown ethnicity, and using rigid guidelines to determine which patient should be offered which screening becomes not only impractical but unjust.

Practical arguments opposing expanded carrier screening

As with many new technologies being introduced into clinical practice, several arguments revolve around cost-effectiveness, cost–benefit, potential for harm, and clinical utility [32].

Payors want some indication of the value of a lab test or new approach to screening prior to agreeing to cover such tests. Unlike screening for high-prevalence disorders in select populations (typically ethnic based), using ECS across all populations represents a significant change in screening protocols. Countries with state-sponsored health care seek out the same reassurance of value before deciding about using limited resources for a new program [33]. There are limited data on the cost-effectiveness of ECS.

Most of the disorders on ECS panels are individually rare. Carrier frequencies will vary considerably based on an individual's ethnic background. Even with relatively common disorders, such as CF, reported carrier prevalence ranges from 1 in 30 for northern European Caucasian, to 1 in 94 for Asians, which is close to the minimum "acceptable" carrier frequency of 1 in 100 delineated by the ACOG/ACMG consensus statement.

Counterarguments to the rarity of single conditions, though, include the fact that, as a group, there is indeed a high likelihood of finding carrier status for some condition. As a reminder, single-gene disorders account for 20% of infant mortality, and a high proportion of pediatric hospitalizations occur as a direct result of genetic disease, so endeavors aimed at lowering those rates seem appropriate.

Perhaps a more compelling argument, however, is that new technologies (such as next-generation sequencing) allow for analysis of a large number of genes for essentially the same cost as doing analysis of a single gene. The costs have dropped so dramatically, that from an economic standpoint, it makes little sense to only perform analysis for one or two disorders. More importantly, identification of fetuses at risk is more frequently accomplished by using ECS versus guideline-based screening as shown earlier.

Genes on expanded carrier screening panels with additional implications

There are a number of genes which appear on ECS panels that convey health risks to the patient beyond those relevant to producing affected offspring. These are genes that, even when in a heterozygous state for a pathogenic variant, have been associated with direct health implications to the carrier. Identifying variants in these genes raises additional counseling dilemmas.

TABLE 13.3 Genes appearing on some expanded carrier screening (ECS) panels that are associated with health risk to the heterozygous carrier.

Gene	Health risks to carriers
Autosomal recessive (AR)	
ATM	Increased cancer risk, especially breast
NBN	Increased cancer risk, especially breast
GBA	Parkinson's disease
X-linked recessive	
FMR1	Premature ovarian insufficiency and FXTAS
DMD	Cardiomyopathy
GLA	Cardiac disease and hypertension
OTC	Hyperammonemia and neurocognitive deficits

FXTAS, Fragile X-related tremor-ataxia syndrome.

Some of the genes that are included in currently available panels that bear such concerns are listed in Table 13.3. Testing such genes could be considered a form of presymptomatic testing given that it is likely the individual seeking ECS may not have symptoms of a genetic disorder. Including these disorders warrants special attention, as usually patients seeking out ECS are already pregnant, and introducing the possibility of previously unrecognized health risks at such a vulnerable state is likely to produce anxiety. Identification of carriers of X-linked genes on this list poses particular counseling challenges, as many biologic phenomena, such as skewed X-inactivation, may play a role in the likelihood of manifesting any symptoms. Most commercial labs offering such testing include descriptions of carrier health risks on their websites or informational material.

Identifying individuals with two pathogenic variants

Some disorders on commercially available ECS panels are so variable in phenotype that identification of an affected (but presumably asymptomatic) individual is a possibility. On occasion, someone may be found to carry two pathogenic variants, and this may indicate that both copies of the gene are mutated, that is, the variants are in "*trans*." Alternatively, both pathogenic variants may reside on the same chromosome ("*cis*") and the other gene allele is normal, and the patient thus is indeed just a carrier. In either circumstance, partner testing should be offered.

These patients may be able to get clarification of their status by performing family studies (e.g., parental testing) to determine whether the variants are in *cis* or *trans*. If both parents are heterozygous for a single variant, then the proband is molecularly affected, if not clinically. All offspring will be at least carriers of the disorder. However, if one parent is identified with the same genotype (i.e., harbors both mutations) or carries neither, then there is either nonpaternity, or the proband's two mutations are in *cis*.

If family testing is not an option, the patient should consider undergoing evaluation to assess the disease state. Many such disorders are inborn errors of metabolism, and further characterization of status may be possible by additional laboratory analysis. Such individuals would likely benefit by consulting with a metabolic specialist.

Conclusion

As ECS becomes increasingly utilized in reproductive settings, additional evidence of its benefits and utility, as well as limitations and unanticipated consequences, will accumulate. Current barriers to widespread implementation now include cost and utility concerns. There is no reason why ECS cannot achieve the same success as have other single-gene oriented screening programs in providing personal and public health benefits. It is incumbent, however, on clinicians to become well-versed in the tenets and application of ECS, in order to provide optimal care for their reproductive patients. As there are many aspects of carrier screening that may be less than self-evident, keeping abreast of changes to the preconception and prenatal testing landscape is critical.

References

[1] American College of Obstetricians and Gynecologists. Committee Opinion 690. Carrier screening in the age of genomic medicine. Obstet Gynecol 2017;129:595–6.

[2] Wilson JMG, Jungner G. Principles and practice of screening for disease. Geneva: WHO; 1968. Available from: <http://www.who.int/bulletin/volumes/86/4/07-050112BP.pdf> Accessed 17.01.19.

[3] Grody WW, Thompson BH, Gregg AR, Bean LH, Monaghan KG, Schneider A, et al. ACMG position statement on prenatal/preconception expanded carrier screening. Genet Med 2013;15:482–3.

[4] Edwards JG, Feldman G, Goldberg J, Gregg AR, Norton ME, Rose NC, et al. Expanded carrier screening in reproductive medicine—points to consider. A joint statement of the American College of Medical Genetics and Genomics, American College of Obstetricians and Gynecologists, National Society of Genetic Counselors, Perinatal Quality Foundation, and Society for Maternal-Fetal Medicine. Obstet Gynecol 2015;1225:653–62.

[5] American College of Obstetricians and Gynecologists. Carrier screening for genetic conditions. Committee Opinion No.691. Obstet Gynecol 2017;129:e41–55.

[6] Ram KT, Klugman SD. Best practices: antenatal screening for common genetic disorders other than aneuploidy. Curr Opin Obstet Gynecol 2010;22:139–45.

[7] McGinniss MJ, Kaback MM. Heterozygote testing and carrier screening. In: Rimoin DL, Pyeritz RC, Korf BR, editors. Emery and Rimoin's principles and practice of medical genetics. 6th ed. Philadelphia: Elsevier; 2013 [chapter 24].

[8] Rowley PT, Loader S, Sutera CJ, Walden M, Kozyra A. Prenatal screening for hemoglobinopathies. I. A prospective regional trial. Am J Hum Genet 1991;48:439–46.

[9] Cao A, Kan YW. The prevention of thalassemia. Cold Spring Harb Perspect Med 2013;3:a011775.

[10] Gross SJ, Pletcher BA, Monaghan KG, for the Professional Practice Guidelines Committee. Carrier screening in individuals of Ashkenazi Jewish descent. Genet Med 2008;10:54–6.

[11] van der Hout S, Holtkamp KCA, Henneman L, de Wet G, Dondorp WJ. Advantages of expanded universal carrier screening: what is at stake? Eur J Hum Genet 2017;25:17–21.

[12] Henneman L, Borry P, Chokoshvili D, Cornel MC, van El CG, Forzano F, et al. Responsible implementation of expanded carrier screening. Eur J Hum Genet 2016;24:e1–e12.

[13] American College of Obstetricians and Gynecologists. Committee Opinion No. 693. Counseling about genetic testing and communication of genetic test results. Obstet Gynecol 2017;129:e96–e101.

[14] Muzzey D, Evans EA, Lieber C. Understanding the basics of NGS: from mechanism to variant calling. Curr Genet Med Rep 2015;3:158–65.

[15] Richard S, Aziz N, Bale S, Bick D, Das S, Gastier-Foster J, et al. Standards and guidelines for the interpretation of sequence variants: a joint consensus recommendation of the American College of Medical Genetics and Genomics and the Association for Molecular Pathology. Genet Med 2015;17:405–24.

[16] Biesecker LG, Nussbaum RL, Rehm H. Distinguishing variant pathogenicity from genetic diagnosis: how to know whether a variant causes a condition. JAMA 2018;320:1929–30.

[17] Ioannou L, McClaren BJ, Massie J, Lewis S, Metcalfe SA, Forrest L, et al. Population-based carrier screening for cystic fibrosis: a systematic review of 23 years of research. Genet Med 2014;16:207–16.

[18] Haque IS, Lazarin GA, Kang P, Evans EA, Goldberg JD, Wapner RJ. Modeled fetal risk of genetic diseases identified by expanded carrier screening. JAMA 2016;316:734–42.

[19] Franasiak JM, Olcha M, Bergh PA, Hong KH, Werner MD, Forman EJ, et al. Expanded carrier screening in an infertile population: how often is clinical decision making affected? Genet Med 2016;18:1097–101.

[20] Johansen Taber KA, Beauchamp KA, Lazarin GA, Muzzey D, Arjunan A, Goldberg JD. Clinical utility of expanded carrier screening: results-guided actionability and outcomes. Genet Med 2018;21(5):1041–8. Available from: https://doi.org/10.1038/s41436-018-0321-0 [Epub ahead of print].

[21] Vaz-de-Macedo C, Harper J. A closer look at expanded carrier screening from a PGD perspective. Hum Reprod 2017;32:1951–6.

[22] Saul RA, Tarleton JC. FMR1-related disorders. In: Adam MP, Ardinger HH, Pagon RA, et al., editors. GeneReviews® [Internet]. Seattle, WA: University of Washington; 1998 [Updated 2012 Apr 26]. Seattle; 1993–2019. Available from: <https://www.ncbi.nlm.nih.gov/books/NBK1384/>.

[23] Jacquemont S, Hagerman RJ, Hagerman PJ, Leehey MA. Fragile-X syndrome and fragile X-associated tremor/ataxia syndrome: two faces of FMR1. Lancet Neurol 2007;6:45–55.

[24] Allen EG, Sullivan AK, Marcus M, Small C, Dominguez C, Epstein MP, et al. Examination of reproductive aging milestones among women who carry the FMR1 premutation. Hum Reprod 2007;22:2142–52.

[25] Nolin SL, Glicksman A, Ersalesi N, Dobkin C, Brown WT, Cao R, et al. Fragile X full mutation expansions are inhibited by one or more AGG interruptions in premutation carriers. Genet Med 2015;17:358–64.

[26] Ishizaki M, Kobayashi M, Adachi K, Matsumura T, Kimura E. Female dystrophinopathy: review of current literature. Neuromuscul Disord 2018;28:572–81.

[27] Buddhe S, Cripe L, Friedland-Little J, Kertesz N, Eghtesady P, Finder J, et al. Cardiac management of the patient with Duchenne muscular dystrophy. Pediatrics 2018;142(s2):s72–81.

[28] Hamtamy H. Consanguineous marriages. J Community Genet 2012;3:185–92.

[29] Verdonk P, Metselaar S, Storms O, Bartels E. Reproductive choices: a qualitative study of Dutch Moroccan and Turkish consanguineously married women's perspectives on preconception carrier screening. BMC Women's Health 2018;18:79. Available from: https://doi.org/10.1186/s12905-018-0574-4.

[30] Practice Committee of the American Society for Reproductive Medicine and the Practice Committee of the Society for Assisted Reproductive Technology. Recommendations for gamete and embryo donation. A Committee Opinion. Fertil Steril 2013;99:47–63.

[31] Capalbo A, Chokoshvili D, Dugoff L, Franasiak J, Gleicher N, Pennings G, et al. Should the reproductive risk of a couple aiming to conceive be tested in the contemporary clinical context? Fertil Steril 2019;111:229–38.

[32] Burke W. Genetic tests: clinical validity and clinical utility. Curr Protoc Hum Genet 2015;81:9.15.1–9.15.8. Available from: https://doi.org/10.1002/0471142905.hg0915s81.

[33] Molster CM, Lister K, Metternick-Jones S, Baynam G, Clarke AJ, Straub V, et al. Outcomes of an international workshop on preconception expanded carrier screening: some considerations for governments. Front Public Health 2017;5:25. Available from: https://doi.org/10.3389/fpubh.2017.00025.

PART C

How to Analyze an Embryo

CHAPTER

14

Preimplantation genetic testing for monogenic diseases

Ana Cervero and Julio Martín

Igenomix, Valencia, Spain

Introduction

Preimplantation genetic testing for monogenic diseases (PGT-M) is an alternative to prenatal diagnosis for those patients with a known risk of transmitting a Mendelian or single-gene disorder to their offspring. Oocytes and/or preimplantation embryos obtained by in vitro fertilization (IVF) are analyzed and only those embryos free of the condition under study are transferred to the uterus to achieve pregnancy. Therefore the main advantage of PGT-M is to increase the likelihood of having an unaffected pregnancy, avoiding the difficult decision of pregnancy termination after an invasive prenatal diagnosis if results are unfavorable.

Edwards and Gardner carried out the early research in PGT-M [1], determining, in 1968, the gender in some biopsies coming from rabbit blastocysts. The first fruitful application of PGT-M in humans was performed by Handyside and colleagues in 1990 [2], who carried out sexing of embryos by polymerase chain reaction (PCR) using primers for amplifying Y-chromosome-specific DNA sequences to avoid males affected with an X-linked disorder. Those embryos identified as female were selectively transferred to the uterus [2]. Later, successful PGT-M was reported for cystic fibrosis [3], based on the amplification of a DNA fragment containing the causative mutation and its detection by fragment analysis [3].

PGT-M is performed in laboratories worldwide and its indications have been progressively expanded. The exact number of PGT-M cycles that have been performed to date is unknown and can only be estimated. The European Society for Human Reproduction and Embryology (ESHRE) PGT-M consortium has collected data about PGT-M cycles since 1999, showing thousands of PGT-M cycles performed, allowing the births of hundreds of healthy children. The last compilation between January and December 2010, reported a total of 5732 IVF cycles with PGT-M or preimplantation genetic screening (PGS), including PGS-sex selection. Of these, 2753 (48%) were carried out for PGT-M purposes, in which 1574 cycles were performed for single-gene disorders, including human leukocyte antigen (HLA) typing [4]. These ESHRE

Human Reproductive Genetics
DOI: https://doi.org/10.1016/B978-0-12-816561-4.00015-6

data represent only a partial record of the PGT-M cases performed worldwide, and are indicative of the general trend in the field.

A multidisciplinary team and a deep collaboration between the assisted reproduction unit and the genetic laboratory are required for PGT-M. Both units can either be colocated within the same institute or geographically separate. This latter situation requires an effective transportation and logistics process; IVF treatment (controlled ovarian stimulation, oocyte retrieval and IVF, embryo culture, and embryo transfer) is carried out in an assisted reproduction unit and only the biopsied embryonic samples are transported to the genetic unit where the PGT-M analysis is performed.

Regarding clinical results of PGT-M, the last data collection carried out for the ESHRE consortium showed that embryo transfer was achieved in 81% of PGT-M cycles. The clinical pregnancy rate obtained for the cycles was 28% per oocyte retrieval and 36% per embryo transfer, giving an overall implantation rate of 27%. Finally, the delivery rate was 24% per oocyte retrieval and 31% per embryo transfer, and the miscarriage rate was 10% [4]. Nevertheless, it is very important to note that there may be significant differences in the clinical outcomes between different IVF centers.

Finally, it is important to know that PGT-M is regulated or even prohibited in many countries based on national or local laws. In many countries, PGT-M can be applied only for serious conditions and, sometimes, especially for adult-onset conditions, HLA compatibility or even for a previously untested disorder, it is necessary to apply to a specific national committee to obtain approval for performing the PGT-M [5].

Indications for preimplantation genetic testing for monogenic diseases

PGT-M is recommended when couples are at risk of transmitting a known genetic abnormality to their children. Therefore its indication is equivalent to conventional prenatal diagnosis. PGT-M has been mainly used to analyze well-known autosomal dominant, autosomal recessive, or X-linked single-gene disorders. Nevertheless, almost all single-gene disorders that can be diagnosed in adults can be also identified in the embryo. Indeed, the conditions for which PGT-M has been applied increase annually. Finally, other uses for PGT-M include gender selection, HLA typing, and late-onset genetic diseases including the identification of embryos at risk for hereditary cancers. It is worth mentioning here that some of these are forbidden or regulated by law in certain countries, and sometimes considered controversial for some actors.

Mendelian conditions or single-gene disorders

According to the latest ESHRE PGT-M consortium data, the most common indications for autosomal dominant diseases are myotonic dystrophy type 1, neurofibromatosis 1, and Huntington's disease (HD) [4]. In this disorders, one mutated copy of the gene is enough for a person to be affected. In some cases, the affected member of the couple has inherited the condition from an affected parent. In others, there is no history of the disorder in the patient's family and the condition results from a new mutation in the gene. When the patient requesting PGT-M has a de novo mutation it is mandatory to identify the pathogenic variant causing the disease. Once the mutation has been characterized, this variant can be analyzed in the embryo.

For autosomal recessive conditions, the presence of two mutated copies from each healthy carrier parent are required for a person to be affected. Cystic fibrosis, spinal muscular atrophy, and hemoglobinopathies are the three most frequently requested indications for this mode of inheritance [4].

X-linked disorders are produced by mutations in genes located on the X chromosome. Recessive X-linked conditions are passed through the maternal line with the condition appearing in males and being carried in females, but not usually expressed. Affected males will not have risk of affected offspring; none of their sons will be affected since they inherit the Y-chromosome and all their daughters will be obligate carriers. Duchenne's muscular dystrophy, hemophilia A, and fragile X syndrome [4] are some of the most common conditions for which PGT-M has been carried out. Sexing with fluorescent in situ hybridyzation (FISH) was initially widely applied for X-linked disorders in order to select female embryos for transfer [6]. However, specific testing of the molecular defect has replaced FISH due to several advantages. First, it allows the identification and subsequent transfer of those healthy male embryos that by FISH diagnosis would be discarded. Second, female carriers may be identified that can be excluded from transfer or not, according to law or center policy and patient wishes. Indeed, this is significant for X-linked dominant disorders (e.g., fragile X syndrome), where it is possible that carrier females may manifest some symptoms of the disease.

Late-onset diseases and cancer predisposition

PGT-M has been also applied for single-gene diseases that do not develop until adulthood and for cancer predisposition genes [7]. For cancer predisposition syndromes that are not fully penetrant and for which some form of therapeutic measures may be available, prenatal diagnosis and termination of pregnancy remain controversial and PGT-M appears as an attractive option, preventing the difficult decision of termination of an established pregnancy. In this sense, the Ethics Committee of the American Society for Reproductive Medicine published that PGT-M for adult-onset conditions of lesser severity and penetrance is ethical for reasons of reproductive liberty [8]. Nevertheless, PGT-M for adult-onset diseases of less serious or of variable penetrance should be considered only after patients are carefully and thoroughly counseled to weigh the risks of PGT-M and IVF for the patient. The counseling should also address the patient-specific prognosis for achieving pregnancy and birth, if known, through IVF with PGT-M [8]. Despite these ethical and legal issues [9], the number of PGT-M cycles reported for this type of conditions is increasing [4], and the procedure has already been carried out for several diseases, including the common syndromes of genetic predisposition to colon and breast cancer [7,10].

For some adult-onset conditions [e.g., Huntington's disease—(HD)], it may happen that patients at risk do not want to perform the genetic study to avoid knowing their real genetic status in advance (presymptomatic), but still they would like to make sure that their children do not inherit the mutation in case they are true carriers. Unlike prenatal diagnosis, PGT-M for HD allows maintaining the status of the carrier of the mutation blinded [11] either by nondisclosure or the less ethically and troublesome exclusion tests. In the former, the mutation is analyzed but the results are not revealed to the patient. This approach has several practical and ethical issues including the need of not giving any details of the IVF cycle in order to avoid a potential clue about the patient's carrier status. Moreover, a mock transfer could be necessary if there are not any embryos for transfer so that the patients do not guess they are carriers. In the exclusion test, those embryos inheriting the haplotype coming from the affected grandparent are ruled out for the transfer. The drawback in this case is that unaffected embryos could be rejected if the patient is not a real carrier, which statistically happens in 50% of cases.

Recently, an even more controversial step forward has been taken by Treff et al. [12], who have employed the PGT to screen embryos for a couple of polygenic disorder risks, hypothyroidism and type I diabetes. According to the authors, this additional testing may be used to prioritize available embryos for transfer and to provide actionable information for long-term monitoring [12]. This new approach, regardless of other legal or controversial considerations, will require comprehensive genetic counseling to support its understanding by patients and final clinical implementation.

Human leukocyte antigen typing or testing for family matching

Another controversial but well-established indication is *HLA matching* in which PGT-M is employed to conceive a child (with or without a specific genetic risk) having a specific HLA combination for future sample donation; that is, compatible cord blood or hematopoietic stem cells for transplantation to save an affected sibling [13]. Hematopoietic stem cell transplantation (HSCT) from an HLA-identical donor is the best therapeutic option for genetic diseases affecting the hematopoietic and/or immune system in children (e.g., β-thalassemia, Fanconi anemia, and others), and can also be an effective therapeutic option for acquired diseases (e.g., leukemia, acquired medullary aplasia) [14,15]. Due to the difficulty of finding HLA-identical donors for affected children within the corresponding families or in hematopoietic stem cell banks, PGT-M for HLA typing is a realistic therapeutic approach for some patients.

It is important to highlight that the law regulating the PGT-M for HLA matching depends on the country and, in some, HLA-PGT-M cases have to be approved case by case by a national committee after evaluating the clinical and therapeutic characteristics and weighing carefully the potential risks and benefits to all those involved [5].

PGT-M for HLA typing alone is performed for acquired diseases or can be performed in conjunction with a single-gene disorder, in order to select an embryo free of the inherited condition and HLA-matched to an existing affected child [13–16]. This approach was applied for the first time in 2001 for Fanconi anemia [13] and since then has been carried out for several different diseases affecting the hematopoietic system. HLA testing on preimplantation embryos is usually performed by indirect analysis, using short tandem repeat markers (STRs) or single-nucleotide polymorphisms (SNPs) as there are many of them throughout the HLA region, allowing 100% accuracy HLA typing and detecting possible recombination events [17,18].

It should be noted that the clinical results for this indication are expected to be worse than those obtained for the classic ones, mainly due to the low number of embryos available for transfer. In a standard case, where PGT-M will be used to select embryos that are both free of a specific disease and a HLA match, the chance of finding an embryo, that is, both healthy and a suitable match is only 18.75% in the case of autosomal recessive conditions, such as beta-thalassemia. Moreover, most of the patients requesting preimplantation HLA typing are of advanced reproductive age and, therefore, the outcome of the procedure has limited success. Indeed, many patients could require several attempts before they become pregnant and deliver an HLA-identical offspring. Thus patients should be counseled deeply to have realistic expectations about the procedure and should be also well informed about the possible risks and complications. Since the development of HLA testing, establishing pregnancy, and pregnancy itself are time consuming, sadly the death of the affected baby may happen before the HSCT becomes available [18]. Moreover, as reported by Kahraman et al. [18], the stem-cell dose obtained from umbilical cord blood is frequently insufficient, and extra time is needed for the child to gain enough weight to be able to donate his or her bone marrow cells. All these limitations might increase the time it will take for the sick sibling to undergo the transplant, aside from the fact that 9 months are required for delivery of a successfully implanted embryo.

Regardless of ethical objections, including the instrumentalization of the future child (the new child is considered by certain people as an instrument to cure another child), the results show that this clinical procedure is an option, with recognized positive outcomes [13–16].

Technologies and testing methods

Polymerase chain reaction and capillary electrophoresis

Multiplex PCR using fluorescently labeled primers designed specifically for the mutation of interest combined with primers for closely linked STR markers has been traditionally the gold standard to perform the PGT-M [19]. The method for allele discrimination depends on the mutation nature. Thus fragment analysis by capillary electrophoresis on an automated sequencer is usually performed for those insertion/deletion mutations and for the analysis of the STR markers. The genotyping of point mutations requires a postamplification step, with minisequencing being the most frequently used method for the detection of this kind of variant [20]. In the minisequencing technique, a primer extension reaction is performed, allowing rapid and accurate detection of point mutations. The minisequencing primer is designed to anneal one base before the target site, and it can only be elongated with one specific dideoxynucleotide. The four different dideoxynucleotides are labeled with different fluorochromes, and the products can be analyzed on an automated DNA sequencing system. Other strategies, such as amplification refractory mutation system [21], restriction enzyme digestion [22], and real-time PCR [23], have been also applied in PGT-M.

The use of multiplex PCR for linkage markers alone (so-called preimplantation genetic haplotyping) has become widespread in PGT-M for monogenic disorders [19] and HLA typing [17]. The main advantage is that such protocols can be used for several couples, independent of the mutation they carry, thus saving time and resources in pre-PGT-M workups. However, the ability to use such indirect testing depends on the availability of appropriate family samples to determine the "at-risk haplotype." Thus in cases where no such samples are available or in de novo mutation cases, this approach cannot be applied alone, and it is necessary to identify the disease-causing mutation directly in the embryos.

It is highly recommended to perform a pre-PGT-M work up with the samples from the requesting couple and from other family members to assess the feasibility of the testing strategy and to identify the informative STR markers that will be used during the PGT-M. The analysis of polymorphic markers in DNA samples from patients and other relatives identifies which alleles are expected in the embryos, and the specific marker alleles which cosegregate with the mutation. This combined approach improves accuracy, minimizing potential errors caused by undetected allele drop out (ADO) or contamination [24]. ADO refers to the amplification failure (or extreme preferential nonamplification) of one of the two alleles, making a heterozygous locus appear homozygous, and potentially leading to misdiagnosis.

Whole-genome amplification for single or few embryo cells

As indicated, PCR methods for DNA variation detection, that is, to discriminate the risk allele(s) from the normal allele(s), are still widely used for PGT-M despite the extensive work-up required for each new disorder tested. For day 3 cleavage-stage biopsy, direct mutation analysis in combination with microsatellite markers (STRs) flanking the gene or indirect analysis with only multiple STRs can be used without initial genomic amplification. The advent of trophectoderm (TE) biopsy widens the implementation of alternative high-throughput genotyping methods in parallel with the use of methods for genome-wide DNA amplification.

Following cell lysis and without prior DNA purification, whole-genome amplification (WGA) was implemented [25] to provide sufficient DNA template to carry out subsequent DNA amplifications or downstream techniques including multiple PCR testing, avoiding the necessity of extensive optimization of multiplex PCR protocols [26], and genome-wide PGT-M methods. These included array-based comparative genomic hybridization, SNP array, and more recently the use of next-generation sequencing (NGS) for low-coverage whole-genome sequencing (WGS). Moreover, with the use of WGA, combining PGT-M with genome-wide embryo testing for aneuploidy (PGT-A) was possible using the same sample; the aim of the combined approach was to improve the clinical results [27]. Finally, WGA facilitates repeat testing of the same samples, for example, after prenatal confirmation, use in proficiency testing, validation, or in the case of run failure during a clinical case.

Several methods for WGA have been developed over time and are now available as commercial kits. Remarkably, any WGA technique still should be evaluated and selected in functioning of the downstream application, and this is especially true when a single blastomere is biopsied as, despite the large quantities of amplified DNA produced, it is well established that certain WGA methods yield relatively high ADO rates for many *loci* [28]. This potential limitation can be circumvented with the application of enough linked markers to avoid misdiagnosis; alternatively, it can be reduced with the use of TE biopsies [27]. Regarding clinical indications, multiple displacement amplification (MDA) is recommended for haplotyping, whereas displacement degenerate oligonucleotide-primed PCR is the method of choice for detection of chromosomal copy number variation. Nevertheless, proper evaluation regarding genomic coverage and potential technical errors like ADO will indicate which method performs better in each laboratory, also depending on the available infrastructure, equipment, and staff expertise.

Single-nucleotide polymorphisms arrays

SNP arrays are high-density oligo arrays containing probes for SNPs located throughout the entire genome. These arrays are scanned, and SNP genotypes are called based on the fluorescence and the ratio of hybridization intensities for the two SNP alleles. The best known SNP array is a commercial array known as *karyomapping*. This is commercialized as a comprehensive, robust, off-the-shelf method for linkage-based testing of almost any single-gene disorder [29]. A set of informative SNP markers are identified for each of the four parental chromosomes by means of the analysis of several hundred thousand SNPs throughout the genome in the parents [29]. The phase of the alleles for each informative SNP locus along each chromosome and linkage of the risk alleles with the parental chromosomes can then be established by reference to the genotype of a relative of known disease status [29]. The main advantage of this platform is that it is applicable to any familial single-gene disorder, or any combination of loci, within the chromosome regions covered by informative SNP loci, eliminating the need for developing patient- or disease-specific tests [29].

Currently, it is possible to determine both monogenic diagnosis and aneuploidy detection (plus HLA haplotyping) by PGT-M using the same sample. For this reason, a single assay using the same platform to detect simultaneously both chromosomal and monogenic disorders is desirable. Since *karyomapping* defines unique sets of SNP markers for each of the four parental chromosomes, it is such a method by allowing accurate identification of the region of interest containing the mutation and simultaneous high-resolution molecular cytogenetic analysis [30,31]. Meiotic trisomies can be identified by the presence of both haplotypes from one parent in segments of the chromosome, resulting from the inheritance of two chromosomes with different patterns of recombination, in combination with a single haplotype from the other parent. Moreover, monosomies or deletions can be identified by the absence of one of the parental haplotypes [29,32]. However, at present *karyomapping* is not commercially validated for aneuploidy screening and does not readily detect mitotic trisomies nor simple copy number variation.

The main disadvantages of the *karyomapping* approach are that diagnosis is challenging or even not possible when insufficient informative SNP markers are available (e.g., in some telomeric genes), or when pseudogenes are involved. Moreover, it cannot be used for de novo mutation cases or when other tested family members are not available to provide samples as a reference or are not informative owing to recombination [29]. In such cases, direct mutation testing from at least one embryo is necessary to establish the phase [32]. This limitation will be even more relevant as more carrier screening tests are performed which identify cocarriage of mutations in the same gene among couples with no family history or affected children—the historic source of referrals for PGT-M.

Next-generation sequencing -based haplotyping

In general, NGS is currently used and gradually being optimized for the detection of rare and common genetic variants due to its broader coverage and decreasing cost per genomic data. As before, the implementation of the TE biopsy and DNA amplification methods (WGA) allowed testing the use of NGS for PGT-M. NGS, also known as massive parallel sequencing, implies the analysis of multiple genetic loci (sequencing data or reads) for multiple (embryo) samples simultaneously. As with previous high-throughput strategies, NGS also allows the combined testing of aneuploidy and single-gene disorders from the same TE biopsy using a single platform. Several approaches have been developed, including targeted locus-specific and genome-wide haplotyping-based methods

Regarding PGT-M, early published studies showed the possibility of NGS to test embryo cells. In 2013, Treff et al. evaluated a targeted NGS protocol to test DNA from TE biopsy [33]. Results were consistent with two conventional methodologies of PGT-M [33]. However, a major concern at that time was errors due to an intrinsic sequencing process and insufficient sequencing depth, potentially causing a false positive or a failure to identify a mutation (false negative), that is, false results due to the presence of sequencing artifacts and ADO, respectively. Another proof-of-concept study for the use of NGS used WGS to detect de novo single-nucleotide and short indel mutations, by sampling 5 to 10 cells from blastocyst-stage embryos [34]. As indicated by the authors, >95% of each embryo genome was called, thus allowing detection and phasing for up to 82% of de novo single-base variants with a false-positive rate of about one error per gigabyte (of sequencing) data, that is, about 10 sequencing errors per embryo or about a 100-fold lower error rate than previously published. As suggested by the authors, phased WGS could be used as part of the PGT process to comprehensively detect disease-causing mutations in order to reduce the incidence of genetic diseases. Almost simultaneously,

Yan et al. published a combined PGT strategy using an NGS procedure that was able to simultaneously detect a single-gene disorder and aneuploidy [35]. The MARSALA strategy "Mutated Allele Revealed by Sequencing with Aneuploidy and Linkage Analyses" combined NGS and single-cell WGA methodologies. The main limitation of this approach was the requirement for private adaptation of the protocol to each family mutation.

An interesting genome-wide approach was presented by Del Rey et al. [36]. Using TE biopsies and testing different WGA methods, the authors applied a commercially available in solution capture kit to recover and sequence DNA fragments specific for more than 4800 disease-associated genes. Aiming to develop a new diagnostic tool to increase the implantation rate in the PGT cycles, they used this strategy for a single workflow for direct detection of family mutations, an indirect approach through linkage analysis of heterozygous SNPs, together with the evaluation of the cytogenetic status of the embryo. The authors indicated that by using this new method, no set up for the direct and indirect mutation detection is needed and it simultaneous allows detection of any cytogenetic imbalance independently from their origin.

Although several NGS solutions are available commercially, their clinical use remains limited when compared to alternative methods. Also, technical constraints of the main NGS strategy (so called short-read NGS) limit the use of this technology for direct testing of certain types of mutations such as dynamic mutations (trinucleotide repeats), certain frameshift and gene rearrangements, and/or copy number variations. In addition, bias introduced during the DNA amplification process may lead to misinterpretations; indeed, WGA methods perform differentially for efficient aneuploidy testing when compared to single-gene or mutation testing. Finally, biological scenarios like embryo mosaicism need better knowledge to understand the potential impact for clinical diagnosis accuracy. Therefore further studies and new developments are needed to achieve a universal NGS protocol to be used routinely in most clinical cases of PGT-M to be combined with PGT-A.

Simultaneous embryo testing for preimplantation genetic testing for monogenic diseases and preimplantation genetic testing for aneuploidies

The high incidence of chromosomal abnormalities in human embryos obtained by assisted reproduction techniques leading to miscarriages and implantation failures has been well described [37,38]. Couples requesting PGT-M to avoid transmission of single-gene disorders are not without these same problems even though they are often considered as "fertile." For this reason, the simultaneous analysis of the disease and the presence of aneuploidies, selecting for transfer those PGT-M "unaffected" and simultaneously euploid embryos can be a benefit from them also.

Several studies have shown significant improvement in rates of pregnancy and live births following testing for aneuploidy in patients undergoing IVF for infertility [38,39]. The use of WGA product provides a straightforward solution for performing the simultaneous analysis of PGT-M and aneuploidy screening using the same sample. In this sense, the clinical use of simultaneous detection of monogenic and chromosomal disorders using different technologies has been reported several times [30,35,40,41]. Rechitsky et al. published one of the first articles where the simultaneous detection of cytogenetic disorders and cystic fibrosis was described [40]. In 2015, the first systematic study of PGD combined with aneuploidy screening was published by the same group, demonstrating an increase in the pregnancy rate from 45.4% in the conventional PGD to 68.5%

with combined aneuploidy screening and a threefold reduction in spontaneous abortion (5.5% vs 15%) [41].

Our retrospective data indicate that 43.6% of the embryos diagnosed at blastocyst stage as normal for the genetic disease have some chromosome abnormalities [42]. Specifically, 16.3% of those PGT-M normal embryos showed trisomies or monosomy X that could lead to miscarriage if transferred. A further 20.2% of PGT-M normal embryos were carrying some monosomies that could result in implantation failure. Therefore these results, in line with other studies [41,43], indicate that the combination of accurate PGT-M and detection of chromosome aneuploidy may improve implantation and rates of healthy live births.

Limitations

As with any genetic test, PGT-M presents certain limitations. First, it is mandatory that the disorder which is intended to be diagnosed has a comprehensive and accurate genetic characterization to at least identify the gene responsible for the condition. Thus some conditions, including autism and some immunological disorders, where the causes remain unidentified are not suitable for PGT-M.

Moreover, as PGT-M involves both an IVF procedure and a selection procedure based on genetic testing, it is important to predict the number of unaffected embryos expected for transfer prior to starting the procedure. There are several factors that may affect that number. Thus it will depend on the embryo quality and the theoretical risk according to the genetic disorder (e.g., dominant, recessive, and X-linked). On the other hand, it is well known that chromosome aneuploidy is the major cause of IVF failure and miscarriage. In this sense, the woman's age and the presence of other additional factors, including male factors, are aspects to consider during the treatment, as they increase the production of incompetent gametes. In conclusion, a sufficient number of embryos should be analyzed to obtain nonaffected embryos for transfer and to benefit patients. Advances in vitrification procedures have made it feasible to batch oocytes or embryos to reach a minimum number of embryos for analysis if needed.

One final significant point regarding PGT-M concerns patient and clinician expectations. PGT-M minimizes the risk for the disease for which the couple has a high risk of transmitting to their offspring but does not provide a guarantee of a completely healthy baby. There is always a small risk of misdiagnosis due to the existence of biological and technical limitations (mosaicism, ADO, recombination, and contamination), and therefore couples should always be advised about the possibility of prenatal diagnosis to confirm results. Moreover, sometimes couples assume that they will have a normal healthy child following successful PGT-M for a specific disorder, forgetting that a more cryptic disorder may be present which was not what was causing the disease identified previously in the family. Furthermore, no other genes or even mutations within the same gene are analyzed and, if chromosomes are not analyzed, an aneuploid but genetically unaffected embryo may be transferred. The entire procedure should always be explained in detail before the treatment to ensure that couples are informed about the potential risks and limitations.

Conclusion

PGT-M can be used to screen embryos for almost any kind of genetic disorder in which the genetic cause is characterized, increasing, year by year, the number of indications and the total number of PGT-M cases. The implementation of preconception carrier screening tests for couples with no family history of a specific genetic disease will increase the number of PGT-M cases further. With the improvements in the technologies, best practice guidelines, and the implementation of external quality assessment and laboratory accreditation programs [44–46] PGT-M analysis has reached a high level of accuracy and has enabled the possibility of performing multiple diagnoses from the same sample. The diagnosis of a monogenic disease can be combined with HLA typing and/or with the detection of chromosomal abnormalities allowing reproductive outcomes to be improved.

References

[1] Gardner RL, Edwards RG. Control of the sex ratio at full term in the rabbit by transferring sexed blastocysts. Nature. 1968;218(5139):346–9.

[2] Handyside AH, Kontogianni EH, Hardy K, Winston RM. Pregnancies from biopsied human preimplantation embryos sexed by Y-specific DNA amplification. Nature 1990;344(6268):768–70.

[3] Handyside AH, Lesko JG, Tarín JJ, Winston RM, Hughes MR. Birth of a normal girl after in vitro fertilization and preimplantation diagnostic testing for cystic fibrosis. N Engl J Med 1992;327(13):905–9.

[4] De Rycke M, Belva F, Goossens V, Moutou C, SenGupta SB, Traeger-Synodinos J, et al. ESHRE PGD Consortium data collection XIII: cycles from January to December 2010 with pregnancy follow-up to October 2011. Hum Reprod 2015;30(8):1763–89.

[5] Soini S. Preimplantation genetic diagnosis (PGD) in Europe: diversity of legislation a challenge to the community and its citizens. Med Law 2007;26(2):309–23.

[6] Harper JC, Coonen E, Ramaekers FC, Delhanty JD, Handyside AH, Winston RM, et al. Identification of the sex of human preimplantation embryos in two hours using an improved spreading method and fluorescent in-situ hybridization (FISH) using directly labelled probes. Hum Reprod 1994;9(4):721–4.

[7] Rechitsky S, Verlinsky O, Chistokhina A, Sharapova T, Ozen S, Masciangelo C, et al. Preimplantation genetic diagnosis for cancer predisposition. Reprod Biomed Online 2002;5(2):148–55.

[8] Ethics Committee of the American Society for Reproductive Medicine. Use of preimplantation genetic testing for monogenic defects (PGT-M) for adult-onset conditions: an Ethics Committee opinion. Fertil Steril 2018;109(6):989–92.

[9] Clancy T. A clinical perspective on ethical arguments around prenatal diagnosis and preimplantation genetic diagnosis for later onset inherited cancer predispositions. Fam Cancer 2010;9(1):9–14.

[10] Spits C, De Rycke M, Van Ranst N, Verpoest W, Lissens W, Van Steirteghem A, et al. Preimplantation genetic diagnosis for cancer predisposition syndromes. Prenat Diagn 2007;27(5):447–56.

[11] Sermon K, De Rijcke M, Lissens W, De Vos A, Platteau P, Bonduelle M, et al. Preimplantation genetic diagnosis for Huntington's disease with exclusion testing. Eur J Hum Genet 2002;10(10):591–8.

[12] Treff NR, Zimmerman R, Bechor E, Hsu J, Rana B, Jensen J, et al. Validation of concurrent preimplantation genetic testing for polygenic and monogenic disorders, structural rearrangements, and whole and segmental chromosome aneuploidy with a single universal platform. Eur J Med Genet 2019;62 (8):103647.

[13] Verlinsky Y, Rechitsky S, Schoolcraft W, Strom C, Kuliev A. Preimplantation diagnosis for Fanconi anemia combined with HLA matching. JAMA. 2001;285 (24):3130–3.

[14] Kuliev A, Rechitsky S, Verlinsky O, Tur-Kaspa I, Kalakoutis G, Angastiniotis M, et al. Preimplantation diagnosis and HLA typing for haemoglobin disorders. Reprod Biomed Online 2005;11(3):362–70.

[15] Verlinsky Y, Rechitsky S, Sharapova T, Laziuk K, Barsky I, Verlinsky O, et al. Preimplantation diagnosis for immunodeficiencies. Reprod Biomed Online 2007;14(2):214–23.

[16] Kakourou G, Kahraman S, Ekmekci GC, Tac HA, Kourlaba G, Kourkouni E, et al. The clinical utility of PGD with HLA matching: a collaborative multi-centre ESHRE study. Hum Reprod 2018;33(3):520–30.

[17] Fiorentino F, Kahraman S, Karadayi H, Biricik A, Sertyel S, Karlikaya G, et al. Short tandem repeats haplotyping of the HLA region in preimplantation HLA matching. Eur J Hum Genet 2005;13(8):953–8.

[18] Kahraman S, Beyazyurek C, Yesilipek MA, Ozturk G, Ertem M, Anak S, et al. Successful haematopoietic stem cell transplantation in 44 children from healthy siblings conceived after preimplantation HLA matching. Reprod Biomed Online 2014;29(3):340–51.

[19] Fiorentino F, Biricik A, Nuccitelli A, et al. Strategies and clinical outcome of 250 cycles of preimplantation genetic diagnosis for single gene disorders. Hum Reprod 2006;21(3):670–84.

[20] Fiorentino F, Magli MC, Podini D, Ferraretti AP, Nuccitelli A, Vitale N, et al. The minisequencing method: an alternative strategy for preimplantation genetic diagnosis of single gene disorders. Mol Hum Reprod 2003;9(7):399–410.

[21] Moutou C, Gardes N, Nicod JC, Viville S. Strategies and outcomes of PGD of familial adenomatous polyposis. Mol Hum Reprod 2007;13(2):95–101.

[22] Spits C, De Rycke M, Verpoest W, Lissens W, Van Steirteghem A, Liebaers I, et al. Preimplantation genetic diagnosis for Marfan syndrome. Fertil Steril 2006;86(2):310–20.

[23] Vrettou C, Traeger-Synodinos J, Tzetis M, Palmer G, Sofocleous C, Kanavakis E. Real-time PCR for single-cell genotyping in sickle cell and thalassemia syndromes as a rapid, accurate, reliable, and widely applicable protocol for preimplantation genetic diagnosis. Hum Mutat 2004;23(5):513–21.

[24] Harton GL, De Rycke M, Fiorentino F, Moutou C, SenGupta S, Traeger-Synodinos J, et al. ESHRE PGD consortium best practice guidelines for amplification-based PGD. Hum Reprod 2011;26(1):33–40.

[25] Handyside AH, Robinson MD, Simpson RJ, Omar MB, Shaw MA, Grudzinskas JG, et al. Isothermal whole genome amplification from single and small numbers of cells: a new era for preimplantation genetic diagnosis of inherited disease. Mol Hum Reprod 2004;10 (10):767–72.

[26] Renwick P, Trussler J, Lashwood A, Braude P, Ogilvie CM. Preimplantation genetic haplotyping: 127 diagnostic cycles demonstrating a robust, efficient alternative to direct mutation testing on single cells. Reprod Biomed Online 2010;20(4):470–6.

[27] Rechitsky S, Pakhalchuk T, San Ramos G, Goodman A, Zlatopolsky Z, Kuliev A. First systematic experience of preimplantation genetic diagnosis for single-gene disorders, and/or preimplantation human leukocyte antigen typing, combined with 24-chromosome aneuploidytesting. Fertil Steril 2015;103(2):503–12.

[28] Spits C, Le Caignec C, De Rycke M, Van Haute L, Van Steirteghem A, Liebaers I, et al. Optimization and evaluation of single-cell whole-genome multiple displacement amplification. Hum Mutat 2006;27(5):496–503.

[29] Handyside AH, Harton GL, Mariani B, Thornhill AR, Affara N, Shaw MA, et al. Karyomapping: a universal method for genome wide analysis of genetic disease based on mapping crossovers between parental haplotypes. J Med Genet 2010;47(10):651–8.

[30] Natesan SA, Handyside AH, Thornhill AR, Ottolini CS, Sage K, Summers MC, et al. Live birth after PGD with confirmation by a comprehensive approach (karyomapping) for simultaneous detection of monogenic and chromosomal disorders. Reprod Biomed Online 2014;29(5):600–5.

[31] Thornhill AR, Handyside AH, Ottolini C, Natesan SA, Taylor J, Sage K, et al. Karyomapping-a comprehensive means of simultaneous monogenic and cytogenetic PGD: comparison with standard approaches in real time for Marfan syndrome. J Assist Reprod Genet 2015;32(3):347–56.

[32] Konstantinidis M, Prates R, Goodall NN, Fischer J, Tecson V, Lemma T, et al. Live births following Karyomapping of human blastocysts: experience from clinical application of the method. Reprod Biomed Online 2015;31(3):394–403.

[33] Treff NR, Fedick A, Tao X, Devkota B, Taylor D, Scott Jr. RT. Evaluation of targeted next-generation sequencing-based preimplantation genetic diagnosis of monogenic disease. Fertil Steril 2013;99 (5):1377–84.

[34] Peters BA, Kermani BG, Alferov O, Agarwal MR, McElwain MA, Gulbahce N, et al. Detection and phasing of single base de novo mutations in biopsies from human in vitro fertilized embryos by advanced whole-genome sequencing. Genome Res 2015;25 (3):426–34.

[35] Yan L, Huang L, Xu L, Huang J, Ma F, Zhu X, et al. Live births after simultaneous avoidance of monogenic diseases and chromosome abnormality by next-generation sequencing with linkage analyses. Proc Natl Acad Sci USA 2015;112:15964–9.

[36] Del Rey J, Vidal F, Ramírez L, Borràs N, Corrales I, Garcia I, et al. Novel Double Factor PGT strategy analyzing blastocyst stage embryos in a single NGS procedure. PLoS One 2018;13(10):e0205692.

[37] Rodrigo L, Mateu E, Mercader A, Cobo AC, Peinado V, Milán M, et al. New tools for embryo selection: comprehensive chromosome screening by array comparative genomic hybridization. Biomed Res Int 2014;2014:517125.

[38] Rubio C, Bellver J, Rodrigo L, Bosch E, Mercader A, Vidal C, et al. Preimplantation genetic screening using fluorescence in situ hybridization in patients with repetitive implantation failure and advanced maternal age: two randomized trials. Fertil Steril 2013;99 (5):1400–7.

[39] Scott Jr RT, Upham KM, Forman EJ, Hong KH, Scott KL, Taylor D, et al. Blastocyst biopsy with comprehensive chromosome screening and fresh embryo transfer significantly increases in vitro fertilization implantation and delivery rates: a randomized controlled trial. Fertil Steril 2013;100(3):697–703.

[40] Rechitsky S, Verlinsky O, Kuliev A. PGD for cystic fibrosis patients and couples at risk of an additional genetic disorder combined with 24-chromosome aneuploidy testing. Reprod Biomed Online 2013;26 (5):420–3040.

[41] Rechitsky S, Pakhalchuk T, San Ramos G, Goodman A, Zlatopolsky Z, Kuliev A. First systematic experience of preimplantation genetic diagnosis for single-gene disorders, and/or preimplantation human

leukocyte antigen typing, combined with 24-chromosome aneuploidy testing. Fertil Steril 2015;103 (2):503–12.

[42] Cervero A, Martínez-Conejero JA, Mir P, Rodrigo L, Rubio C, Al Asmar N, et al. Clinical outcome of preimplantation genetic diagnosis for single-gene disorders could be improved with simultaneous comprehensive chromosome screening. In: Paper Presented at the 14th international conference on PGDIS, Chicago; May 2015.

[43] Minasi MG, Fiorentino F, Ruberti A, Biricik A, Cursio E, Cotroneo E, et al. Genetic diseases and aneuploidies can be detected with a single blastocyst biopsy: a successful clinical approach. Hum Reprod 2017;32(8):1770–7.

[44] Harper JC, Sengupta S, Vesela K, Thornhill A, Dequeker E, Coonen E, et al. Accreditation of the PGD laboratory. Hum Reprod 2010;25(4):1051–65.

[45] Harton G, Braude P, Lashwood A, Schmutzler A, Traeger-Synodinos J, Wilton L, et al. ESHRE PGD consortium best practice guidelines for organization of a PGD centre for PGD/preimplantation genetic screening. European Society for Human Reproduction and Embryology (ESHRE) PGD Consortium. Hum Reprod 2011;26(1):14–24.

[46] SenGupta SB, Dhanjal S, Harper JC. Quality control standards in PGD and PGS. Reprod Biomed Online 2016;32(3):263–70.

CHAPTER

15

Future technologies for preimplantation genetic applications

Nada Kubikova[1] *and Dagan Wells*[1,2]

[1]Nuffield Department of Women's and Reproductive Health, John Radcliffe Hospital, University of Oxford, Oxford, United Kingdom [2]Juno Genetics, Oxford, United Kingdom

Preimplantation genetic testing

Preimplantation genetic testing (PGT) encompasses a wide variety of methods for the analysis of genetic material sampled from early human embryos, prior to the establishment of a pregnancy. Thus far, PGT has been used almost exclusively in combination with in vitro fertilization (IVF) treatment, and is deployed either to avoid the transmission of inherited disorders or in an attempt to improve IVF treatment outcomes. In the former case, embryos from couples known to be at high risk of passing on a familial condition are tested and only those found to be free of the disorder are considered for transfer to the mother's uterus. Since genetically abnormal embryos are never transferred, any pregnancies established are expected to be free of the condition and pregnancy terminations and affected births are thus avoided. When applied to the detection and avoidance of conditions caused by mutation of a single gene, this strategy is referred to as preimplantation genetic testing for monogenic disease (PGT-M). The use of PGT to enhance IVF outcomes has focused on the detection of chromosome abnormalities, which are common in human preimplantation embryos and are the principal cause of failed embryo implantation and miscarriage. The transfer of embryos found to be chromosomally normal, in preference to those that are aneuploid, has been reported to lead to a higher probability of a live birth per embryo transferred and lower rates of miscarriage [1–3]. This approach is known as preimplantation genetic testing for aneuploidy (PGT-A).

Essentially, PGT can be divided into two components: (1) embryological, which involves many aspects of routine IVF, but also a method of collecting DNA from the embryos; (2) genetic, which involves the processing and analysis of the genetic material in order to yield a clinically useful result. Both of these aspects of PGT have seen considerable evolution in the 30 years since the first cases. For many years the dominant method for obtaining genetic material involved the biopsy of cells (blastomeres) from cleavage-stage embryos. In most cases, only one cell was removed for

Human Reproductive Genetics
DOI: https://doi.org/10.1016/B978-0-12-816561-4.00016-8

testing. However, the last decade has seen a dramatic shift in practice, with blastomere biopsy increasingly abandoned in favor of sampling several trophectoderm cells at the blastocyst stage. The reason for the change in practice is related in part to the fact that genetic tests are more accurate and robust when several cells are available for analysis, rather than just one. Nonetheless, a more important explanation is the growing evidence that removal of a single blastomere at the relatively fragile cleavage stage has the potential to impair subsequent development, leading to lower pregnancy rates for biopsied embryos [4].

Noninvasive preimplantation genetic testing

While existing data suggest that trophectoderm biopsy has little impact on blastocyst viability, methods vary widely and there is no consensus concerning the optimal technique for cell removal. It would be naïve to think that blastocyst biopsy is entirely without risk to the embryo, although any danger might be minimal when carried out by an experienced embryologist working in a well-optimized laboratory. The desire to test preimplantation embryos without negatively impacting their viability has led to interest in noninvasive methods of obtaining genetic material from cultured IVF embryos. Additionally, embryo biopsy typically necessitates investment in specialist equipment (e.g., a laser), as well as requiring the skills of an experienced embryologist. The training of staff, purchase and maintenance of equipment, as well as ongoing salary expenses, add greatly to the costs of PGT. The possibility of an approach to PGT that avoids the need to biopsy embryos is therefore also desirable from an economic perspective.

Some research has focused on obtaining an indirect evaluation of the genetic competence of oocytes or embryos, such as by attempting to establish correlations between chromosomal status and patterns of gene expression in cumulus cells [5], or associating proteomic signatures with aneuploidy [6]. However, most studies undertaken with the aim of delivering a noninvasive genetic assessment of embryos have focused their attention on embryonic DNA found in the culture medium or in the blastocoel cavity.

The first indication that the blastocoel cavity might contain DNA suitable for genetic analysis was published by Palini et al. [7]. The sampling procedure, sometimes termed "blastocentesis," involves piercing the trophectoderm using an ICSI pipette and careful aspiration of the fluid within [6,8]. The collapse of the blastocoel cavity is a standard part of some blastocyst cryopreservation techniques and is not thought to be damaging to the embryo [9,10]. Thus, blastocentesis can be considered a minimally invasive method, which requires less skill than embryo biopsy and can be undertaken without a laser.

Efforts to perform PGT using genetic material from blastocoel fluid (BF) have encountered some technical challenges, likely related to the low quantity and degraded condition of the DNA [7,11,12]. To date, most studies have employed whole-genome amplification (WGA) in order to increase the total amount of DNA available prior to analysis of individual genetic loci or chromosomal copy number. This approach has met with variable success, with published amplification rates ranging from 34.8% to 87.5% for the blastocoel samples studied [7,8,11–16]. In general, results suggest that DNA amplification from BF is achieved less often than from biopsied cells, but that when WGA is successful the proportion of the genome accessible is similar to that obtained from cell specimens, and that the DNA is suitable for downstream analysis of specific genetic loci. However, most studies have only assessed small numbers of samples and at least one report indicated lower concordance when blastocoel fluid-DNA (BF-DNA) and trophectoderm biopsies were compared in the context of PGT-M [15].

While there are currently insufficient data showing the suitability of BF-DNA for PGT-M for this to be considered clinically, results for chromosomal analysis have been somewhat more encouraging. An analysis of BF from 116 blastocysts [8] achieved successful WGA in 82% of samples, which although lower than rates typically observed for trophectoderm biopsy specimens nonetheless represents one of the best series of results reported thus far for BF. The cytogenetic concordance (considering a simple euploid or aneuploid classification) of BF with respect to polar bodies, blastomeres, and trophectoderm biopsies, was 97.9%, 97.7%, and 98.4%. Recently, the same group compared paired BF samples and trophectoderm biopsies from 256 blastocysts and reported 96% concordance for euploid versus aneuploid diagnosis. However, some groups have found it more difficult to obtain meaningful results from BF samples, with concordance rates varying from ~30% to 60% [13,15]. It is unclear whether variations in the results of BF analysis are related to differences in procedure (some of which may damage cells and enhance the likelihood of DNA release), differences in patient populations, or simply related to the small sample sizes in many published studies.

Perhaps a more promising noninvasive preimplantation genetic testing (niPGT) approach could be examination of the embryonic DNA present in the media in which embryos are cultured. Several studies have investigated molecules secreted into the medium by embryos (the secretome) and considered their potential to provide information concerning viability. Factors analyzed have included metabolites, proteins, interleukins, and micro-RNAs [17–20]. In the case of genetic analysis, the detection of embryonic DNA in spent culture medium (SCM) has been reported as early as days 2 and 3 of development [21–26]. Most analyses of DNA in SCM have been carried out after culture from day 3 to days 5 or 6. The amplification rates achieved from such samples have typically been superior to those reported after blastocentesis, but still inferior to those obtained following cellular biopsy, suggesting that while DNA in the SCM is of low abundance and/or degraded it is a less challenging substrate to work with than genetic material from the blastocoel [24,27]. Attempts to perform WGA using SCM have yielded encouraging results, with 81.8%–100% of samples amplifying [28–33]. Individual loci can be amplified from WGA products with high efficiency, although appreciable rates of allele dropout (ADO), and a high incidence of maternal DNA contamination in some studies, indicate that there still remain substantial obstacles to the use of cell-free DNA for PGT-M [15,24,30]. In one study of 72 SCM samples, 89.7% of loci were successfully amplified, less than accomplished using trophectoderm biopsy (100%), but superior to results from BF samples (27.4%). Unfortunately, the accuracy of the genotyping results obtained was impacted by DNA contamination, only 20.8% of SCM samples displaying full concordance with paired trophectoderm biopsy specimens.

Initial investigations into the use of SCM for PGT-A demonstrated that DNA was present in the majority of cases [31]. However, while amplification rates for SCM samples often exceeded 90%, the cytogenetic concordance with the corresponding embryos was often low. Subsequent studies using different amplification methods have improved amplification and accuracy rates. In a recent study by Xu and coworkers [33], a chromosome copy number evaluation was successfully obtained in 100% of samples and the concordance with respect to associated embryos was 85.7% (when defined as euploid or chromosomally abnormal). It is clear that methods for PGT-A using SCM still require optimization. For example, the ideal volume of culture medium, the optimal DNA amplification method, and the correct time for SCM sampling, all remain unknown. Thus far, results suggest that PGT-A data from SCM samples are better when culture volumes are smaller than typically used in IVF clinics, and when the embryos are more advanced in their development. In a study by Lane et al. [29], 178 embryos and associated SCM samples were examined. Amplification was successful in 94% of SCM samples and, while rates of ploidy concordance with corresponding trophectoderm biopsies were low (65.4%) for day 3 to day 5 cultures, they exceeded 95% when culture commenced on day 4.

Technical optimizations will also have to take into consideration how best to avoid DNA contamination. The scale of this problem was highlighted by Vera-Rodriguez et al. [32], in a study involving analysis of days 3–5 SCM from 60 embryos. Chromosome copy number information was obtained from 91.6% of SCM samples, while 100% of trophectoderm biopsies from the corresponding embryos yielded a result. Only 33.3% of informative paired samples were concordant in their aneuploidy diagnosis (the lowest concordance rate reported among SCM studies), while the remaining samples displayed chromosomal patterns consistent with maternal contamination. This suggests that contamination may be the predominant cause of discordant results between SCM and embryo biopsy specimens, at least in some published studies.

In summary, the recent identification of embryonic DNA in the BF and SCM has led to substantial interest in the potential for minimally invasive PGT. By avoiding embryo biopsy, it is anticipated that the costs of PGT could be reduced and any risks to the embryo of genetic testing almost entirely removed. However, questions remain concerning the accuracy of current niPGT strategies. The quantity of DNA in BF and SCM samples is low and the integrity is likely to be relatively poor, presenting challenges for genetic analysis. Optimal methods for the collection, amplification, and analysis of extraembryonic DNA all remain to be defined. Furthermore, it is not yet certain whether routine embryo culture techniques will have to be altered in an effort to concentrate the DNA in media samples and reduce the risks of contamination. It will also be important to confirm the origin of extraembryonic DNA: whether it derives from the inner cell mass, the trophectoderm, or both; whether aneuploid cells in mosaic embryos undergo apoptosis more often than euploid cells, thus contributing disproportionately to the DNA in the medium/blastocoel. While there is no guarantee that niPGT will ever be able to replace embryo biopsy for clinical diagnosis, the potential benefits of such a technique, if proven accurate, are substantial and consequently it is inevitable that this will remain an active and interesting area of research over the next few years.

Future perspectives in preimplantation genetic testing for monogenic disease

The amount of DNA obtained from a preimplantation embryo biopsy is too low to permit a direct analysis and consequently some form of DNA amplification is necessary. Conventional approaches for PGT-M utilize multiplex PCR, simultaneously amplifying several distinct loci that together provide the information necessary for an accurate diagnosis. Typically, the DNA fragments amplified include the mutation site and several linked informative polymorphisms. The inclusion of polymorphisms, situated in close proximity to the affected gene, provides an indirect means of detecting inheritance of the chromosome carrying the mutation. Since individual polymerase chain reaction (PCR) fragments can suffer allele dropout (ADO—the failure of amplification from one of the two chromosomes in a cell), the utilization of redundant tests, which analyze several amplified fragments and provide additional opportunities to detect the presence of the mutant gene, are of great importance. Furthermore, if multiple polymorphisms are used, they have the potential to provide a DNA fingerprint for the embryo, which can help to reveal the presence of contamination when it occurs.

Multiplex-PCR strategies used for PGT-M frequently require an extensive investigation, prior to clinical application, in order to identify polymorphic markers that are informative in the family seeking PGT. Additionally, simultaneous amplification of several separate polymorphic sites, as well as parental mutations, all from an extremely small number of cells, presents technical challenges and requires optimization of reaction conditions. The need to develop optimized, family-specific tests often leads to a delay in the initiation of patients' cycles and increases the cost of PGT-M, with consequent reductions in patient access. The introduction of genome-wide single-nucleotide polymorphism (SNP) arrays for PGT-M has succeeded in streamlining the delivery of tests, providing a universal linkage-based system for diagnosis of most monogenic disorders. By reducing the need for patient-specific PGT-M protocols, the time required for the preparation of new tests has been greatly reduced. The best known SNP-array approach for PGT-M is known as "karyomapping," a technique in which parents and a close relative of known disease status are genotyped for ~300,000 SNPs scattered across the genome [34–36]. Sets of informative SNPs in the vicinity of the gene of interest are genotyped for each of the four parental chromosomes and their phase (i.e., which alleles are inherited together and are therefore located on the same parental chromosome) is determined by examining the genotypes of the same SNPs in different members of the same family. These phased combinations of linked polymorphisms, known as haplotypes, are sufficient to deduce the status of any embryos produced by the couple, without having to directly detect the causative mutation(s). A similar technique called haplarithmisis, utilizes a next-generation sequencing approach in order to reveal the genotypes of polymorphisms and to reveal haplotypes across the entire genome, thus providing the linkage data needed to diagnose embryos [37].

Although genome-wide SNP arrays and NGS-based haplotyping save considerable labor in the PGT laboratory, they remain relatively expensive, and the requirement of a DNA sample from an additional close relative can sometimes prove problematic. With the continuous reduction in the cost of sequencing, there is hope that tests such as haplarithmisis could be carried out at significantly lower cost in the future. However, for the time being the lowest costs for PGT-M may rely on harnessing NGS technology in other ways. Approaches for PGT-M utilizing NGS are now emerging and a few have already been validated and implemented clinically [38–41]. Some tests utilize multiplex PCR amplification followed by sequencing of a large number of linked polymorphic markers as well as mutation sites. The *HBB* gene, in which the mutations for β-thalassemia and sickle cell anemia (SSA) are found, is an example where such an approach has been applied clinically. Sequencing of the entirety of the *HBB* gene (both exonic and intronic regions), along with numerous intragenic and extragenic linked SNPs provides a single protocol, which is universally applicable despite the vast diversity of mutations found within the *HBB* gene [41]. Such a generic protocol eliminates the need for all but the simplest preclinical work-up, reducing costs and accelerating the pathway to treatment. The cost savings provided are especially relevant in less affluent parts of the world, which often coincide with areas where β-thalassemia and SSA are of high prevalence. There is also some evidence to suggest that the extreme sensitivity of NGS-based methods may result in lower ADO rates, allowing detection of alleles that are difficult to detect due to extremely poor amplification [41].

Preimplantation genetic testing for polygenic disease

The easy access to genomic technologies and the continuous decrease in their cost is accelerating the development of more comprehensive testing platforms. Recently, a single universal platform was developed and validated to test for aneuploidies, structural rearrangements, specified monogenic diseases, and certain traits controlled by polygenic inheritance [42]. The aim of this methodology is to rank embryos, prioritizing those at lower risk of polygenic diseases such as hypothyroidism and type I diabetes. It can be argued that polygenic disease risk prediction in preimplantation embryos is desirable and should be considered a valuable addition to the important health-related data revealed during the course of PGT. However, expansion of embryo testing to cover multiple genetic variants that together confer a degree of risk, sometimes interacting with each other and with the environment in ways that are not fully understood, represents a significant deviation from the traditional application of PGT.

For the most part, the last 30 years have seen PGT utilized for the same range of inherited conditions for which prenatal testing has generally been considered appropriate—monogenic disorders that have a clear association between mutation and phenotype. Where PGT has diverged from prenatal diagnosis has been in its wider application to late-onset disorders (e.g., Huntington disease) and conditions associated with incomplete penetrance (e.g., *BRCA* mutations that predispose to breast cancer) and, most strikingly, the use of preimplantation testing to identify embryos that are HLA compatible with an affected sibling, who is in need of stem cell transplantation [43]. The introduction of PGT for polygenic disease raises technical, logistic, and ethical questions. It will inevitably require an expansion of genetic counseling efforts to support its clinical utilization, and some might argue that it is ethically questionable to test for such conditions. As new predictors become available, it likely that all of the embryos tested will have an increased risk of something, be it cardiovascular disease, diabetes, cancer, or other medically important problems. How will an embryo with an increased risk for one condition be weighed against a sibling embryo with an elevated risk for a different disease. There are fears that prioritizing embryos that are "genetically superior" based on their disease risk scores might create a hostile environment, potentially stigmatizing those who develop disease or those who suffer from disabilities. On the other hand, if predictions related to the development of serious health issues are demonstrated to be accurate, some might argue in favor of protecting the right for reproductive autonomy and parental choice. Most controversial of all, at least one company promoting the use of PGT to manage polygenic disease risk has proposed testing to predict intellectual capacity, with a view to avoiding transfer of embryos at risk of producing individuals with a low IQ. As technologies continue to evolve, this area will clearly remain an active area of ethical debate.

Whole-genome sequencing of the preimplantation embryo

Considering the decreasing cost of sequencing-based methodologies, one might envisage a day when the most economical and straightforward strategy for PGT is simply to sequence the entire genome of each embryo. This would eliminate the need to develop patient-specific or disease-specific tests [44].

Any chromosomal abnormalities would be revealed as well as any gene mutations (essentially delivering PGT-M and PGT-A in a single test) and, if desired, polygenic risk scores and information about long-term health could be acquired from the same data. It is likely that mutations that impair embryonic development would also be detected in some embryos, assisting in the prioritization of viable embryos for transfer to the uterus during IVF cycles. The frequency of such mutations is currently unknown, but their presence may provide a partial explanation for the fact that at least one-fourth of chromosomally normal and morphologically perfect embryos fail to produce a viable pregnancy after transfer to the uterus. In terms of the cost of the technology, there are already commercially available sequencers that do not require a large capital investment and it is only a matter of time before the cost of sequencing an individual genome falls to a level where it is conceivable that all embryos suitable for biopsy could be examined.

In the past, deficiencies in methods of genome amplification and DNA sequencing precluded the application of whole-genome sequencing to human preimplantation embryos. However, these technological hurdles have been largely overcome. One of the few challenges still remaining is the requirement for data storage. This may well become the single most important factor on the clinical scale, especially when considering that some regulatory bodies currently require the data obtained from genetic testing to be stored for decades or even indefinitely. The human genome consists of over 3 gigabases (> 3,000,000,000 base pairs), which means that genetic laboratories will face significant and ongoing capital investments into IT infrastructure and data storage. Given the highly sensitive nature of genetic information, back-up systems and robust data privacy protection mechanisms will all need to be in place.

Higher resolution and increased genomic coverage would, without doubt, lead to an even more comprehensive analysis of the embryo's genetic status. However, considering that in any given embryo, only a fraction of loci will be directly relevant to disease and that many (perhaps the majority) of the variants discovered would have an uncertain impact on health, the balance between the additional value provided by WGS and the great increase in the bioinformatic and patient counseling burden might not be favorable at the current time [44]. Nonetheless, as understanding of the genome and how it functions improves, the depth of information provided by whole-genome sequencing will have growing clinical utility and it seems certain that it will eventually improve embryo diagnosis and IVF success rates. For the most part, the argument that remains to be debated, as with polygenic disease, is an ethical one.

Germline genome editing

Undoubtedly, PGT for monogenic disease continues to be a valuable reproductive option for couples who are at high risk of transmitting heritable genetic disorders to their children. Yet despite its growing clinical implementation over the last two decades, PGT-M has a number of limitations. First, there is a finite number of embryos created in an IVF cycle and the majority of these embryos will usually be discarded, either as a result of inadequate development or because they are diagnosed as being affected by the inherited condition for which they were being tested [45]. Indeed, published data indicate that 16%–20% of PGT cycles do not reach the point of uterine transfer and that fewer than 25% of cycles result in a healthy ongoing pregnancy [46,47]. This means that the physically, psychologically, and often financially, demanding process of PGT-M frequently fails to produce the much wanted pregnancy. Currently, alternatives to PGT-M include the use of donor oocytes, sperm, or embryos and adoption, all of which sacrifice the possibility of having a genetically related child. The other option is to try to conceive naturally (assuming the couple is fertile) and undergo prenatal testing. Of course, if the prenatal test reveals the presence of genetic disease in the fetus, a choice will have to be made between pregnancy termination and the birth of an affected child.

The reproductive options discussed above have, for the past 30 years, been the only available strategies that couples have at their disposal when trying to avoid transmission of an inherited disorder. More recently, dramatic advances in genome analysis and engineering technologies have opened up another possibility: germline genome editing (GE). While heritable GE is not currently recommended as a reproductive strategy, it has potential to become one in the future. The application of GE for the avoidance of inherited disease would involve the modification of a mutant gene in order to restore a wild-type sequence. Such an approach would shift the paradigm of the current reproductive strategies away from diagnosis and exclusion and toward cure.

From a technical perspective, conducting genome-editing interventions at the time of fertilization or during early preimplantation embryonic stages, can be viewed as ideal, since it is easier to ensure that the active components used for GE will be delivered to all cells. This is important because many inherited conditions affect multiple tissues or organs and a return to normal function will often require the mutant gene to be corrected in most, if not all, cells. It may be extremely difficult to access the genomes of cells later in life, when the target cells are potentially numbered in the millions and populate hard-to-reach internal organs. A fertilized oocyte or embryo that underwent GE would ultimately give rise to an individual carrying the edited gene in all cells of their body. This would not only include all of the somatic cells, but the germ cells also, a fact which has been the basis of some ethical concerns (as discussed below). Genome-editing interventions, performed on human embryos, are without a doubt ethically controversial; however, some might argue that the current practice of discarding affected but otherwise viable embryos is wasteful and perhaps no better from ethical, moral, as well as certain religious perspectives [45]. With GE, embryos previously diagnosed as affected could become eligible for transfer, thus rescuing them from being destroyed and increasing the number of IVF embryos available to the couple, which would likely lead to improved chances of a pregnancy during that treatment cycle. In one scenario, if GE could be combined with natural cycle IVF, in which only a single oocyte is collected and fertilized with the partner's sperm, perhaps no viable embryo would need to be discarded.

How far are we from (safe) clinical application of genome editing?

CRISPR-Cas9 (clustered regularly interspaced short palindromic repeat-Cas9) is currently the leading approach for GE of cells, tissues, and whole organisms. It has been successfully applied in microorganisms, plants, animals, and most recently in human embryos donated for research [48–53]. Cas9 is an endonuclease of bacterial origin, which can be guided to specific "target" DNA sequences by a single-stranded RNA containing a specified sequence ($\sim$12 bases in length) complimentary to the target DNA. Upon successful recognition of a protospacer-adjacent motive sequence, Cas9 flanks the targeted region and cleaves each DNA strand, generating a double-stranded break (DSB) [48]. Most cells resolve the induced DSB predominantly by two mechanisms: error-prone nonhomologous end joining (NHEJ) and, less frequently, homology-directed repair (HDR). During the process of reconnecting the two ends of the broken DNA strand, NHEJ introduces insertions and deletions (indels), which typically results in disruption of the targeted gene and a consequent loss of function. In contrast, HDR rebuilds the site of breakage using a homologous DNA molecule as a template. In diploid cells, the second, undamaged copy of the gene is usually employed as the template for HDR, leading to replacement and correction of the copy in which Cas9 has induced a DSB. However, it is also possible to supply an exogenous DNA sequence, with homology to the targeted site, which the cell can utilize as a template for repair [48].

Genome-editing technology has already been applied to correct pathogenic mutations such as those causing Duchenne muscular dystrophy and β-thalassemia in cellular and animal models [54,55]. In 2017, a proof-of-concept study demonstrated the possibility of targeted correction of germline mutations in human preimplantation embryos for the first time, using a CRISPR-Cas9-based technology to remove a dominant heterozygous *MYBPC3* mutation, responsible for an inherited form of cardiomyopathy [49]. In the same year, researchers in the United Kingdom edited a group of human zygotes donated for research in order to study the role of an important developmental regulator OCT4 using a similar CRISPR-Cas9-based approach, but in this case deployed to knockout gene function rather than correct a mutation [48]. Together, these studies mark the beginning of a new era, in which germline GE is used with the intention of answering basic biological questions related to embryonic development. The results also shed light on significant drawbacks and substantial difficulties associated with potential clinical application of GE tools in their current formats. Despite achieving relatively high targeting efficiency, it appears that only a proportion of embryos are able to resolve the DSBs by HDR, and therefore succeed in correcting the mutant gene. A significant proportion of the edited embryos might harbor additional indels, further disrupting the targeted gene. Even more deleterious could be the induction of large deletions and/or complex structural rearrangements, extending over many kilobases of DNA from the cut site, which could possibly lead to genomic instability and mitotic arrest.

The mechanisms of DNA repair after the introduction of DSBs specific to human preimplantation embryos remain largely unknown. There are questions whether such mechanisms are fully active and concerning the extent to which embryo cells can cope with the DNA strand breaks induced by GE techniques. Studies in cell lines have demonstrated that the efficiency of CRISPR-Cas9 is greatly enhanced by tumor suppressor p53 inhibition [56,57]. Whether the same applies to human preimplantation embryos is not known, but if there was a need to inhibit p53 in embryos in order to achieve efficient GE, this would likely be problematic for clinical application. The *p53* gene is a master regulator of the cell cycle, DNA repair, and apoptosis and its disruption, even if only temporary, might well have serious consequences for embryonic development.

Large deletions and chromosomal aberrations, as well as any form of mosaicism (i.e., where some cells are successfully edited and others are not, or where a proportion of the cells harbor additional deleterious indels produced by NHEJ) might be difficult to detect in preimplantation embryos subjected to GE, and would also present a serious safety concern for clinical application. It remains to be determined whether mosaicism in gene editing can be reduced by modulating the cell cycle stage at which DSBs are induced and whether this approach can yield 100% uniformity in the desired genotype. A new generation of GE tools using catalytically impaired CRISPR-Cas9, known base editors, has recently been developed [58,59]. Base editors could potentially achieve more specific and better refined editing, avoiding the problematic introduction of DSBs altogether, instead inducing alterations through the direct irreversible conversion of one base to another (e.g., a single mutant base could be substituted for the wild-type equivalent). In addition to developing a precise GE tool, it is essential to examine the potential off-target consequences of GE technologies, particularly their capacity to induce mutations in unintended regions of the genome, which have close homology to the targeted locus. The approaches that investigate the off-target effects of GE have thus far relied on the use of in silico modeling as they are rapid, easy to use, and inexpensive. However, they have only a predictive value and their estimates are far from definitive. With the prospect of clinical implementation, one might foresee that whole-genome sequencing of the edited embryo might become an inevitable and essential accessory to identify and exclude any embryos affected by off-target mutagenesis and to ensure the delivery of safe and efficacious treatment.

Ethical considerations for germline genome editing

Technological advances, particularly in the area of molecular biology and genomics, have outpaced the regulatory frameworks set-up to govern them and present a serious ethical concern for many people. Until recently, human GE was in the realm of science fiction. However, the advent of CRISPR-Cas9 technologies together with reports of the birth of the first genome-edited children in China in 2018 have prompted a wide societal debate. Even prior to the application of CRISPR-Cas9 to human embryos, multiple bodies charged with providing guidelines and advice on medical issues had already launched inquiries into the ethics of germline GE in the context of human reproduction.

As discussed above, the application of GE technologies to gametes or preimplantation embryos, in order to correct an inherited disorder, maximizes the likelihood that the mutation will be successfully eliminated from all of the cells. Yet it is this apparent benefit that also makes the use of GE during the preimplantation stage contentious, since any alterations would be present in the germline and could, in theory, be propagated through future generations. For some this would mean crossing a perceived line. Nevertheless, from a purely clinical perspective, the successful editing of all cells, including the germ cells, would make it possible to permanently eliminate a deleterious mutation from a family, and therefore free future generations from the burden of disease transmission and from the need for further medical interventions. It could be argued that this protects the interest and welfare of the future individual.

As treatments improve, more individuals suffering from genetic disease will survive into reproductive age and may want to have genetically related children [60]. The desire to avoid the transmission of a mutation, without discarding potentially viable embryos following PGT-M, can surely be appreciated in these cases, and has indeed been recognized by the UK Nuffield Council on Bioethics and the US National Institute of Sciences' in their recent reports on the subject. After careful deliberation, the Nuffield Council came to the view that "there are circumstances in which gene editing of human embryos should be permissible." It is likely that, to begin with, PGT and GE would have to be carried out in tandem, in order to confirm successful correction and an absence of unintended edits, but it is possible to imagine that if GE evolves into a precise and safe tool, PGT might eventually become superfluous.

Although GE technologies might not be ready for clinical trials in human embryos at this time, it would be irresponsible for science not to explore the possibility that they could, in the future, deliver a major advancement in precision medicine, with the capacity to eliminate the majority of inherited diseases. The recently published results obtained from studies using the new-generation base editors suggest that these might be significantly safer because of the avoidance of DSBs [58,59]. Furthermore, it should be remembered that there are few medical interventions that are entirely without risk and that these must be weighed against the potential benefits of treatment. It is also worth recalling that some procedures that are almost universally embraced today, such as organ transplantation, were once considered controversial.

While conversations about the legitimacy of germline GE continue, there is already at least one assisted reproductive treatment that has been successfully implemented in order to permanently correct an inherited genetic defect. Mitochondrial disorders, where a proportion of the mitochondria in each cell harbors a deleterious mutation leading to a dysfunction in ATP production and clinical consequences that are frequently severe, have been addressed by removing the meiotic spindle from an affected oocyte (or pronuclei from a fertilized egg) and transferring into the "healthy" cytoplasm of a donor oocyte. This procedure has already been licensed for use in the United Kingdom (by the Human Fertilisation and Embryology Authority) and, internationally, has led to the birth of at least one child who appears to be free of mitochondrial disease [61]. The spindle transfer procedure has also been proposed as a method to assist in the treatment of infertile patients with a history of unsuccessful IVF treatment due to poor in vitro embryo development. Data from a mouse model, characterized by high rates of embryo developmental arrest, have shown encouraging results, with rescue of the phenotype after transfer of meiotic spindles to donor oocytes from a different mouse strain [62].

With new and powerful technologies always comes the fear of abuse. These concerns should not be lightly dismissed and need to be the subject of an inclusive public debate. In terms of GE being used as a therapeutic intervention, some argue that there is potential for the technique to be applied for nonmedical reasons: introducing genetic variants that do not exist in either parent, for the purpose of enhancement rather than cure. Such modifications could be aimed at conferring resistance to pathogens, increasing tolerance to environmental conditions or enhancement of physical or mental attributes. To address these concerns, it is necessary to build a consensus and decide which traits would be ethically justifiable and acceptable for alteration. It is possible that in well-regulated areas of the world the use of GE would always be confined to treatment of serious medical illness. In line with this notion, it is the view of the Nuffield Council that the use of heritable GE interventions should be "consistent with social justice and solidarity so that it should not be expected to increase disadvantage, discrimination, or division in society." From a technical perspective, it is worth noting that most traits are controlled by polygenic inheritance and as such the enhancement would be technically challenging using the existing approaches, which focus on the correction of a single mutation. Public attitudes and prevailing social norms will likely shape how germline GE will be used, positions that might conceivably change over time [60]. If GE is to be used at all, adequate guidelines and a regulatory framework need to be developed, setting out minimal conditions that would have to be met in respect to clinical and technical issues surrounding the gene to be edited, the need and justification for such modification, and the criteria for the efficacy, precision, and safety of the tool.

Since the introduction of PGT, the methods available for genetic analysis have undergone rapid and sustained evolution. Today, these advances promise to provide universal protocols for the simultaneous detection of all inherited defects caused by gene mutations or chromosome abnormalities. Such methods could provide PGT at lower costs, with shorter patient waiting times, and deliver enhanced accuracy. If combined with noninvasive methods of testing, costs would fall further still and risks to the embryos (already low) would be essentially eliminated. However, with powerful new genetic technologies also come new clinical and ethical questions. As we enter an era of whole-genome sequencing, we must ask how much information we really want to obtain from each embryo. If we learn all aspects of an embryo's genetics, how will patients be counseled and what elements should be considered appropriate for embryo selection. Finally, there has been great excitement over the development of effective genome-editing methods. Such techniques offer the hope that mutations causing inherited conditions could one day be corrected during the preimplantation stage, although considerable public consultation, ethical debate, and assessment of safety still need to take place before such methods enter clinical practice.

References

[1] Yang Z, Liu J, Collins GS, Salem SA, Liu X, Lyle SS, et al. Selection of single blastocysts for fresh transfer via standard morphology assessment alone and with array CGH for good prognosis IVF patients: results from a randomized pilot study. Mol Cytogenet 2012;5(1):24.

[2] Scott RT, Upham KM, Forman EJ, Hong KH, Scott KL, Taylor D, et al. Blastocyst biopsy with comprehensive chromosome screening and fresh embryo transfer significantly increases in vitro fertilization implantation and delivery rates: a randomized controlled trial. Fertil Steril [Internet] 2013;100(3):697–703. Available from: http://dx.doi.org/10.1016/j.fertnstert.2013.04.035.

[3] Forman EJ, Hong KH, Ferry KM, Tao X, Taylor D, Levy B, et al. In vitro fertilization with single euploid blastocyst transfer: a randomized controlled trial. Fertil Steril [Internet] 2013;100(1):100–107.e1. Available from: http://dx.doi.org/10.1016/j.fertnstert.2013.02.056.

[4] Scott RT, Upham KM, Forman EJ, Zhao T, Treff NR. Cleavage-stage biopsy significantly impairs human embryonic implantation potential while blastocyst biopsy does not: a randomized and paired clinical trial. Fertil Steril 2013;100(3):624–30.

[5] Fragouli E, Wells D, Iager AE, Kayisli UA, Patrizio P. Alteration of gene expression in human cumulus cells as a potential indicator of oocyte aneuploidy. Hum Reprod [Internet] 2012;27(8):2559–68. Available from: <http://www.ncbi.nlm.nih.gov/pubmed/22617123>.

[6] Poli M, Ori A, Child T, Jaroudi S, Spath K, Beck M, et al. Characterization and quantification of proteins secreted by single human embryos prior to implantation. EMBO Mol Med 2015;7(11):1465–79.

[7] Palini S, Galluzzi L, De Stefani S, Bianchi M, Wells D, Magnani M, et al. Genomic DNA in human blastocoele fluid. Reprod Biomed Online 2013;26(6):603–10.

[8] Magli MC, Pomante A, Cafueri G, Valerio M, Crippa A, Ferraretti AP, et al. Preimplantation genetic testing: polar bodies, blastomeres, trophectoderm cells, or blastocoelic fluid? Fertil Steril 2016;105(3):676–683e5.

[9] Mukaida T, Oka C, Goto T, Takahashi K. Artificial shrinkage of blastocoeles using either a micro-needle or a laser pulse prior to the cooling steps of vitrification improves survival rate and pregnancy outcome of vitrified human blastocysts. Hum Reprod 2006;21(12):3246–52.

[10] Vanderzwalmen P, Bertin G, Debauche C, Standaert V, van Roosendaal E, Vandervorst M, et al. Births after vitrification at morula and blastocyst stages: effect of artificial reduction of the blastocoelic cavity before vitrification. Hum Reprod 2002;17(3):744–51.

[11] Gianaroli L, Magli MC, Pomante A, Crivello AM, Cafueri G, Valerio M, et al. blastocentesis: a source of DNA for preimplantation genetic testing. Results from a pilot study. Fertil Steril 2014;102(6):1692–9.

[12] Zhang Y, Li N, Wang L, Sun H, Ma M, Wang H, et al. Molecular analysis of DNA in blastocoele fluid using next-generation sequencing. J Assist Reprod Genet 2016;33(5):637–45.

[13] Tobler KJ, Zhao Y, Ross R, Benner AT, Xu X, Du L, et al. Blastocoel fluid from differentiated blastocysts harbors embryonic genomic material capable of a whole-genome deoxyribonucleic acid amplification and comprehensive chromosome microarray analysis. Fertil Steril 2015;104(2):418–25.

[14] Tšuiko O, Zhigalina DI, Jatsenko T, Skryabin NA, Kanbekova OR, Artyukhova VG, et al. Karyotype of the blastocoel fluid demonstrates low concordance with both trophectoderm and inner cell mass. Fertil Steril 2018;109(6):1127–1134.e1.

[15] Capalbo A, Romanelli V, Patassini C, Poli M, Girardi L, Giancani A, et al. Diagnostic efficacy of blastocoel fluid and spent media as sources of DNA for preimplantation genetic testing in standard clinical conditions. Fertil Steril 2018;110(5):870–879.e5.

[16] Magli MC, Albanese C, Crippa A, Tabanelli C, Ferraretti AP, Gianaroli L. Deoxyribonucleic acid detection in blastocoelic fluid: a new predictor of embryo ploidy and viable pregnancy. Fertil Steril 2018;111(1):77–85.

[17] Capalbo A, Ubaldi FM, Cimadomo D, Noli L, Khalaf Y, Farcomeni A, et al. MicroRNAs in spent blastocyst culture medium are derived from trophectoderm cells and can be explored for human embryo reproductive competence assessment. Fertil Steril 2016;105 (1):225–235.e1-3.

[18] Huang G, Zhou C, Wei C, Zhao S, Sun F, Zhou H, et al. Evaluation of in vitro fertilization outcomes using interleukin-8 in culture medium of human preimplantation embryos. Fertil Steril 2017;107(3):649–56.

[19] Katz-Jaffe MG, McReynolds S, Gardner DK, Schoolcraft WB. The role of proteomics in defining the human embryonic secretome. Mol Hum Reprod 2009;271–7.

[20] Sánchez-Ribas I, Diaz-Gimeno P, Quiñonero A, Ojeda M, Larreategui Z, Ballesteros A, et al. NGS analysis of human embryo culture media reveals miRNAs of extra embryonic origin. Reprod Sci 2018;26(3) 193371911876625.

[21] Stigliani S, Persico L, Lagazio C, Anserini P, Venturini PL, Scaruffi P. Mitochondrial DNA in Day 3 embryo culture medium is a novel, non-invasive biomarker of blastocyst potential and implantation outcome. Mol Hum Reprod 2014;20(12):1238–46.

[22] Stigliani S, Anserini P, Venturini PL, Scaruffi P. Mitochondrial DNA content in embryo culture medium is significantly associated with human embryo fragmentation. Hum Reprod 2013;28(10):2652–60.

[23] Assou S, Aït-Ahmed O, El Messaoudi S, Thierry AR, Hamamah S. Non-invasive pre-implantation genetic diagnosis of X-linked disorders. Med Hypotheses 2014;83(4):506–8.

[24] Galluzzi L, Palini S, Stefani De S, Andreoni F, Primiterra M, Diotallevi A, et al. Extracellular embryo genomic DNA and its potential for genotyping applications. Future Sci OA 2015;1(4):FSO62.

[25] Hammond ER, McGillivray BC, Wicker SM, Peek JC, Shelling AN, Stone P, et al. Characterizing nuclear and mitochondrial DNA in spent embryo culture media: genetic contamination identified. Fertil Steril 2017;107 (1):220–228.e5.

[26] Yang L, Lv Q, Chen W, Sun J, Wu Y, Wang Y, et al. Presence of embryonic DNA in culture medium. Oncotarget. 2017;8(40):67805–9.

[27] Capalbo A, Bono S, Spizzichino L, Biricik A, Baldi M, Colamaria S, et al. Sequential comprehensive chromosome analysis on polar bodies, blastomeres and trophoblast: insights into female meiotic errors and chromosomal segregation in the preimplantation window of embryo development. Hum Reprod 2013;28 (2):509–18.

[28] Feichtinger M, Vaccari E, Carli L, Wallner E, Mädel U, Figl K, et al. Non-invasive preimplantation genetic screening using array comparative genomic hybridization on spent culture media: a proof-of-concept pilot study. Reprod Biomed Online 2017;34(6):583–9.

[29] Lane M, Zander-Fox DL, Hamilton H, Jasper MJ, Hodgson BL, Fraser M, et al. Ability to detect aneuploidy from cell free DNA collected from media is dependent on the stage of development of the embryo. Fertil Steril 2017;108(3):e61.

[30] Liu WQ, Liu JQ, Du HZ, Ling JW, Sun XF, Chen DJ. Non-invasive pre-implantation aneuploidy screening and diagnosis of beta thalassemia IVSII654 mutation using spent embryo culture medium. Ann Med 2017;49(4):319–28.

[31] Shamonki MI, Jin H, Haimowitz Z, Liu L. Proof of concept: preimplantation genetic screening without embryo biopsy through analysis of cell-free DNA in spent embryo culture media. Fertil Steril 2016;106 (6):1312–18.

[32] Vera-Rodriguez M, Diez-Juan A, Jimenez-Almazan J, Martinez S, Navarro R, Peinado V, et al. Origin and composition of cell-free DNA in spent medium from human embryo culture during preimplantation development. Obstet Gynecol Surv 2018;33(4):745–56.

[33] Xu J, Fang R, Chen L, Chen D, Xiao J-P, Yang W, et al. Noninvasive chromosome screening of human embryos by genome sequencing of embryo culture medium for in vitro fertilization. Proc Natl Acad Sci USA 2016;113(42):11907–12.

[34] Natesan S a, Bladon AJ, Coskun S, Qubbaj W, Prates R, Munne S, et al. Genome-wide karyomapping accurately identifies the inheritance of single-gene defects in human preimplantation embryos in vitro. Genet Med [Internet] 2014;16(January):1–8. Available from: <http://www.ncbi.nlm.nih.gov/pubmed/24810687>.

[35] Handyside AH, Harton GL, Mariani B, Thornhill AR, Affara N, Shaw M-A, et al. Karyomapping: a universal method for genome wide analysis of genetic disease based on mapping crossovers between parental haplotypes. J Med Genet 2010;47(10):651–8.

[36] Konstantinidis M, Prates R, Goodall N-N, Fischer J, Tecson V, Lemma T, et al. Live births following Karyomapping of human blastocysts: experience from clinical application of the method. Reprod Biomed

Online [Internet] 2015;31(3):394–403 [cited 2017 Sep 6]; Available from: <http://www.ncbi.nlm.nih.gov/pubmed/26206283>.

[37] Zamani Esteki M, Dimitriadou E, Mateiu L, Melotte C, Van der Aa N, Kumar P, et al. Concurrent whole-genome haplotyping and copy-number profiling of single cells. Am J Hum Genet 2015;96(6):894–912.

[38] Yan L, Huang L, Xu L, Huang J, Ma F, Zhu X, et al. Live births after simultaneous avoidance of monogenic diseases and chromosome abnormality by next-generation sequencing with linkage analyses. Proc Natl Acad Sci USA [Internet] 2015;112(52):15964–9. Available from: <http://www.pnas.org/lookup/doi/10.1073/pnas.1523297113>.

[39] Chen S-C, Xu X-L, Zhang J-Y, Ding G-L, Jin L, Liu B, et al. Identification of PKD2 mutations in human preimplantation embryos in vitro using a combination of targeted next-generation sequencing and targeted haplotyping. Sci Rep [Internet] 2016;6(1):25488 [cited 2017 Sep 6]; Available from: <http://www.ncbi.nlm.nih.gov/pubmed/27150309>.

[40] Ren Y, Zhi X, Zhu X, Huang J, Lian Y, Li R, et al. Clinical applications of MARSALA for preimplantation genetic diagnosis of spinal muscular atrophy. J Genet Genomics [Internet] 2016;43(9):541–7. Available from: http://dx.doi.org/10.1016/j.jgg.2016.03.011.

[41] Kubikova N, Babariya D, Sarasa J, Spath K, Alfarawati S, Wells D. Clinical application of a protocol based on universal next-generation sequencing for the diagnosis of beta- thalassaemia and sickle cell anaemia in preimplantation embryos. Reprod Biomed Online [Internet] 2018;37(2):136–44. Available from: https://doi.org/10.1016/j.rbmo.2018.05.005.

[42] Treff NR, Zimmerman R, Bechor E, Hsu J, Rana B, Jensen J, et al. Validation of concurrent preimplantation genetic testing for polygenic and monogenic disorders, structural rearrangements, and whole and segmental chromosome aneuploidy with a single universal platform. Eur J Med Genet 2019;62(8):103647.

[43] Verlinsky Y, Rechitsky S, Schoolcraft W, Strom C, Kuliev A. Preimplantation diagnosis for fanconi anemia combined with hla matching. J Am Med Assoc 2001;285(24):3130–3.

[44] Spath K, Wells D. Deep impact: sequencing embryo biopsy specimens at increasing depth. Reprod Biomed Online 2015;31(1):1–3.

[45] Wells D, Vermeesch JR, Simpson JL. Current controversies in prenatal diagnosis 3: gene editing should replace embryo selection following PGD. Prenat Diagn 2019;39(5):344–50.

[46] Gutiérrez-Mateo C, Sánchez-García JF, Fischer J, Tormasi S, Cohen J, Munné S, et al. Preimplantation genetic diagnosis of single-gene disorders: experience with more than 200 cycles conducted by a reference laboratory in the United States. Fertil Steril 2009;92(5):1544–56.

[47] De Rycke M, Goossens V, Kokkali G, Meijer-Hoogeveen M, Coonen E, Moutou C, et al. Consortium data collection XIV-XV: cycles from January 2011 to December 2012 with pregnancy follow-up to October 2013. Hum Reprod 2017;32(10):1974–94.

[48] Fogarty NME, McCarthy A, Snijders KE, Powell BE, Kubikova N, Blakeley P, et al. Genome editing reveals a role for OCT4 in human embryogenesis. Nature [Internet] 2017;550(7674):67–73. Available from: <http://www.nature.com/doifinder/10.1038/nature24033>.

[49] Ma H, Marti-Gutierrez N, Park S-W, Wu J, Lee Y, Suzuki K, et al. Correction of a pathogenic gene mutation in human embryos. Nature [Internet] 2017;548(7668):413–19 [cited 2017 Nov 15]; Available from: <http://www.ncbi.nlm.nih.gov/pubmed/28783728>.

[50] Maddalo D, Manchado E, Concepcion CP, Bonetti C, Vidigal JA, Han Y-C, et al. In vivo engineering of oncogenic chromosomal rearrangements with the CRISPR/Cas9 system. Nature [Internet] 2014;516(7531):423–7 [cited 2017 Nov 15]; Available from: <http://www.ncbi.nlm.nih.gov/pubmed/25337876>.

[51] Wang Y, Cheng X, Shan Q, Zhang Y, Liu J, Gao C, et al. Simultaneous editing of three homoeoalleles in hexaploid bread wheat confers heritable resistance to powdery mildew. Nat Biotechnol [Internet] 2014;32(9):947–51 [cited 2017 Nov 15]; Available from: <http://www.ncbi.nlm.nih.gov/pubmed/25038773>.

[52] Yin H, Xue W, Chen S, Bogorad RL, Benedetti E, Grompe M, et al. Genome editing with Cas9 in adult mice corrects a disease mutation and phenotype. Nat Biotechnol [Internet] 2014;32(6):551–3 [cited 2017 Nov 15]; Available from: <http://www.ncbi.nlm.nih.gov/pubmed/24681508>.

[53] Dever DP, Bak RO, Reinisch A, Camarena J, Washington G, Nicolas CE, et al. CRISPR/Cas9 β-globin gene targeting in human haematopoietic stem cells. Nature [Internet] 2016;539(7629):384–9 [cited 2017 Nov 15]; Available from: <http://www.nature.com/doifinder/10.1038/nature20134>.

[54] Long C, McAnally JR, Shelton JM, Mireault AA, Bassel-Duby R, Olson EN. Prevention of muscular dystrophy in mice by CRISPR/Cas9-mediated editing of germline DNA. Sci (80–) [Internet] 2014;345(6201):1184–8. Available from: <http://www.sciencemag.org/cgi/doi/10.1126/science.1254445>.

[55] Song B, Fan Y, He W, Zhu D, Niu X, Wang D, et al. Improved hematopoietic differentiation efficiency of gene-corrected beta-thalassemia induced pluripotent

stem cells by CRISPR/Cas9 system. Stem Cell Dev [Internet] 2015;24(9):1053–65. Available from: <http://online.liebertpub.com/doi/10.1089/scd.2014.0347>.

[56] Haapaniemi E, Botla S, Persson J, Schmierer B, Taipale J. CRISPR-Cas9 genome editing induces a p53-mediated DNA damage response. Nat Med 2018;24 (7):927–30.

[57] Ihry RJ, Worringer KA, Salick MR, Frias E, Ho D, Theriault K, et al. P53 inhibits CRISPR-Cas9 engineering in human pluripotent stem cells. Nat Med 2018;24 (7):939–46.

[58] Gaudelli NM, Komor AC, Rees HA, Packer MS, Badran AH, Bryson DI, et al. Programmable base editing of A•T to G•C in genomic DNA without DNA cleavage. Nat [Internet] 2017;24(9):1053–65 [cited 2017 Nov 15];. Available from: <http://www.nature.com/doifinder/10.1038/nature24644>.

[59] Komor AC, Kim YB, Packer MS, Zuris JA, Liu DR. Programmable editing of a target base in genomic DNA without double-stranded DNA cleavage. Nature [Internet] 2016;533(7603):420–4 [cited 2017 Nov 15]; Available from: <http://www.ncbi.nlm.nih.gov/pubmed/27096365>.

[60] Lovell-Badge R. CRISPR babies: a view from the centre of the storm. Development. 2019;146(3). Available from: http://dx.doi.org/10.1242/dev.175778.

[61] Zhang J, Liu H, Luo S, Lu Z, Chávez-Badiola A, Liu Z, et al. Live birth derived from oocyte spindle transfer to prevent mitochondrial disease. Reprod Biomed Online 2017;34(4):361–8.

[62] Costa-Borges NL, Mestres E, Miguel-Escalada I, Basalmeda R, Garcia M, Vanrell I, et al. Meiotic spindle transfer overcomes embryo developmental arrest in compromised oocytes: proof of concept in the mouse model. Fertil Steril 2017;108(3):e41.

PART D

Reproductive genetic counseling

CHAPTER

16

Psychological aspects of reproductive genetic screening and diagnoses

Dorothy A. Greenfeld

Yale University School of Medicine, New Haven, CT, United States

Genetic screening has become an increasingly important tool for diagnosis and treatment in reproductive medicine [1]. Advances in genetic testing with improved diagnostic accuracy have reformed clinical practice and led to innovations in treatment. The integration of genetic screening technology and assisted reproductive technology (ART) has expanded at an accelerating rate and as a result fertility treatment centers now routinely incorporate genetic testing as a complement to diagnosis and treatment of their patients. However, the acceleration of genetic testing is not without its controversy. Historically, innovations in ART such as in vitro fertilization (IVF) with attendant offshoots such as oocyte donation and gestational surrogacy have led to successes that raised patients' hopes and introduced new family constellations. At the same time, they provoked public and patient concern about moral and ethical implications of the technology. These concerns are now echoed by the advent of reproductive genetic testing in fertility care where the spectrum of possible effects extends from the reassurance of preconception knowledge of a healthy pregnancy to the creation of embryos for the purpose of sex selection [2].

Whether the world of ART is already well known to couples entering into fertility treatment or represents a new and fearsome experience, the bond they all share is the hope for a healthy pregnancy and a healthy baby. The psychological experience of IVF has been well described and is generally acknowledged to be a rigorously emotional journey for participants but, while the medical aspects of reproductive genetic screening have been well described in the literature, a greater examination of the psychological impact and emotional demands of screening for ART patients is needed. This chapter describes selected reproductive genetic tests and their psychological concomitants, with illustrative cases provided. Where needed, the differentiation between genetic counseling and psychological counseling is identified as their roles may overlap but are mutually beneficial.

Human Reproductive Genetics
DOI: https://doi.org/10.1016/B978-0-12-816561-4.00017-X

Reproductive genetic screening

Patients treated for infertility typically absorb a new treatment language replete with acronyms such as (IVF and intracytoplasmic sperm injection (ICSI). Similarly, reproductive genetics has introduced an array of rapidly evolving screening options with changes in accompanying acronyms. These include preconception carrier screening (PCS), extended preconception carrier screening (ECS), preimplantation genetic testing for aneuploidy (PGT-A) (formerly known as PGS), and preimplantation genetic testing for monogenic defects (PGT-M) (formerly known as PGD). As a result of this panoply of screening options ART programs increasingly encounter a broader variety of patients. Some learn through routine PCS that they are carriers of a gene that may or definitely will affect the health of their child and are referred for preimplantation PGT-M of their embryos created through IVF. Other patients referred for PGT-M have a family history of genetic disorder(s), have given birth to a genetically affected child, or have otherwise experienced reproductive trauma. Additionally, patients of mature age, patients with a history of recurrent pregnancy loss (RPL), and patients with previous IVF implantation failure are currently screened for embryo chromosome number through preimplantation PGT-A.

Preconception carrier screening

The purpose of PCS has been described as "increasing reproductive autonomy of individuals and couples by providing preconception knowledge that could inform them of available treatment options" [3]. A growing number of physicians support the practice of PCS for their patients, and expanding public awareness of genetic screening has led to greater patient acceptance of the process. Originally PCS was emphasized for certain ethnic groups more likely to carry a gene for diseases such as Tay-Sachs in Ashkenazi Jews and thalassemia in Italians. Currently, because we now live in what has been described as a "pan-ethnic society" with increasing intermingling of ethnic groups, PCS is recommended for all patients and partners considering pregnancy. Fertility treatment programs routinely utilize PCS for recessive disorders such as cystic fibrosis and fragile X, and increasingly make use of ECS for hundreds of other diseases with different levels of diagnostic capacity [4]. However, when testing results suggest that the couple has a good chance of having a baby with a genetic disorder, the knowledge can be devastating and the treatment options may not be practical or affordable, or may be otherwise emotionally charged. Couples may decide to accept the risk of having a child with an inherited illness, remain childless, pursue adoption, choose gamete donation, or utilize PGT-M of embryos created through IVF. Undertaking any of these choices is typically emotionally challenging.

Because PCS will lead to more instances where one or both partners test positive for being a carrier, their understanding of the implications of the results underscores the need for both education and psychosocial support. Mental health professionals (here referred to as infertility counselors) working in ART have long understood and emphasized the importance of pretreatment education and patients' comprehension of the process as critical in the alleviation of apprehension. The psychological impact of screening is lessened when there is counseling pre and posttesting since "improved genetic knowledge is inversely correlated with the testee's anxiety" [5]. The importance of the tester's knowledge and ability to impart that knowledge in a way that is understandable should be assumed, but a study of PCS administered to obstetric practices cited a lack of knowledge among physicians and the lay public as a major problem. The authors also cited a lack of guidance for patients both pre and post screening, and costs of testing that may not be covered by insurance as part of the problem [6].

What the introduction to PCS means to patients involved in the testing can be quite variable. For example, some may be aware of a genetic deficiency among family members and expect a result which confirms this history. A patient with a diagnosis of unexplained infertility, typically someone haunted by the need to find a reason, upon learning that the cause is likely to be genetic may feel some relief [7]. For many patients, however, such results can be wholly unanticipated, causing anxiety and distress.

Lewis et al. reviewed 20 studies published between 1990 and 2007 that addressed the psychosocial impact of carrier testing for autosomal and x-linked genetic disorders. The review identified a number of factors that appear to influence the emotional impact of carrier testing such as anxiety, guilt and stigmatization, effect on family relationships, effect on self-image, active coping mechanisms, and reproductive issues. Anxiety was a factor in all studies whether a subject was a carrier or a noncarrier. While women experienced greater anxiety than men, the anxiety dissipated over time, generally within 6 months. Several of the studies reviewed credit clear written instructions and explanations and high-quality genetic counseling as important factors in alleviating anxiety. Guilt was also an issue that emerged, especially if the carrier already had an affected child, and guilt was stronger in women than in men. Additionally, women who did not have an affected child but had the condition in the family experienced what was identified as "survivor guilt" [8]. Typically, patients with no known history of genetic defect when being screened expect negative results and those who are known to be at high risk or who perceive themselves at high risk, expect positive results. This may explain why those at risk tend to experience less distress after a positive result than those unaware of the risk [5].

Case Example

Ann and Bill, a couple in their early 30s, were referred for IVF after months of failing to conceive. The pretreatment work-up included routine PCS for both partners and the couple, with no known family history of genetic disorders, assumed that their results would be negative. When results revealed that both were carriers of cystic fibrosis, they were dumbfounded and confused. The genetics counselor met with them and explained the disorder and what the results meant, and when the couple learned that their chances for having an affected child were 1 in 4 (25%) and what the disease would mean for that child, Ann became distraught and inconsolable. Bill took a pragmatic position and immediately wanted to know what options they had for a healthy baby moving forward. The reproductive endocrinologist recommended PGT-M, the process that would involve IVF followed by testing the embryos, discarding affected embryos and hoping that there were unaffected embryos to transfer. When Ann realized that there was a possibility that there might not be unaffected embryos and that some embryos might be destroyed, she became acutely anxious and distressed. The treatment team referred her to the infertility counselor, who gave her the opportunity to express her distress and explore her concerns. After a few meetings her anxiety lessened and she felt ready to proceed with the treatment.

Preimplantation genetic testing for monogenic defects

PGT-M, formerly known as PGD, is a widely established procedure for parents with a single-gene disorder to help prevent the risk of having a child with an inherited disorder and has been used for over 100 single-gene mutations [9]. PGT-M was developed to screen for embryos that carried genes for serious childhood-onset diseases (such as cystic fibrosis) but in more recent years the process has been used for serious single-gene diseases such as early-onset Alzheimer disease and Huntington disease [10]. The Ethics Committee of the American Society for Reproductive Medicine posed the arguments for and against the use of PGT-M for serious adult-onset conditions. Arguments offered in support of the procedure included the right to reproductive choice for persons wanting to have children, the medical good of preventing the transmission of genetic disorders, the avoidance of abortion after genetic testing reveals a genetic disorder, and potential societal benefits of reducing the burden of the disease such as costly medical treatments. Arguments against PGT-M included the financial cost, the possibility of misdiagnosis, the unknown risks of the procedure, and the possible negative impact on those living with the disorder, or who have a predisposition to the disorder. The committee agreed that PGT-M for adult-onset conditions is ethically permissible and strongly recommended that a genetics counselor with knowledge of PGT-M counsel patients considering this procedure. The committee also acknowledged the complexity of the scientific, psychological, and social issues involved in this issue [10].

Indications for the use of PGT-M currently cover a much wider spectrum, for example, testing for adult-onset conditions such as Huntington disease, human leukocyte antigen (HLA) tissue matching for stem cell transplants, and sex selection. Needless to say, much has been written about the ethical aspects and concerns of the procedure but little about its psychosocial impact. Pretreatment preparation and guidance are especially vital for those undertaking PGT-M. A clear understanding of the IVF process is the first consideration. Then, does the couple understand the process of PGT-M and are they aware of the risks? Such risks include the possibility that the procedure may result in no embryos at all or only embryos not suitable for testing. Another possibility is that after testing no unaffected embryos will be identified. Or unaffected embryos may be transferred resulting in no pregnancy. There is also the possibility that the embryo may be misdiagnosed and an affected embryo may be transferred or an unaffected embryo may be destroyed. This dizzying list of possible risks coupled with patients who are more than likely already anxious about the procedure is yet another important argument for pretreatment preparation and guidance and posttesting support. These patients may require time to absorb the information and a repeated review of the implications of the testing and the possible options. In one study, patients interviewed after PGT-M stated that they wished they had asked more questions and learned more about the process beforehand. Three women whose embryos had been misdiagnosed stated that they were not given clear instructions about the possibility for misdiagnosis [11].

Couples entering PGT-M must digest a prodigious amount of information about the process. In addition to the aforementioned procedural risks, there are the costs of treatment not always covered by insurance, varying success rates, and the amount of time the cycle demands that patients need to consider. There is also a significant emotional burden that accompanies PGT-M, especially for those patients with a history of reproductive trauma, such as giving birth to a child with a genetic disorder, but all participants may experience the euphoria and dysphoria that accompanies IVF with PGT-M. Many couples struggle with ethical or religious concerns about such issues as testing embryos and destroying affected embryos. In a paper addressing how couples make decisions about PGT-M, Hershberger and Pierce reviewed studies published between 1990 and 2008 of couples who had used, were eligible for, or had contemplated

PGT-M. The authors concluded that how decisions were made about PGT-M was based on cognitive appraisals (such as timing, risks, and costs), emotional responses (such as joy and happiness and pain and suffering), and moral concerns (such as about the status of the embryo) [12].

It is well acknowledged that IVF is emotionally draining, but studies over the years examining the emotional reactions of female IVF patients generally have not shown serious psychiatric morbidity and levels of depression and anxiety were typically within normal limits. Based on what is known about the psychological status of IVF patients, Karatas et al. considered the psychological profiles of 50 Australian women participating in PGT-M. Subjects completed self-administered questionnaires that assessed anxiety, depression, knowledge of technical aspects of PGT-M, expectancy of establishing a pregnancy, and unmet information needs. The authors hypothesized that given the burdens of genetic testing of embryos and the reproductive and genetic circumstances that preceded PGT-M, anxiety levels in subjects would be well above the normal population. Because studies of the psychological state of women entering IVF show that they do not experience greater degrees of depression from the normal population, the authors suggested that depression in these subjects would be within normal limits. Also, that unmet information needs would be associated with higher education levels and because PGT-M patients have been reported as viewing themselves as not infertile [2], their expectations of pregnancy would be higher than the likelihood for pregnancy presented by their clinicians. Results determined that anxiety and depression levels were similar to normal population data. Unmet information needs were indeed positively associated with women's education and their expectancy of pregnancy was above that of the expectancy rate presented by their clinicians [13].

In a review of the literature on the psychological impact of PGT-M, authors observed that most of the studies focus on the women's experience and that less is known about the psychological experience for men [14]. Jarvholm et al., in a more recent study on risk factors of depression and anxiety in men and women planning for PGT-M, reported that men had significantly more symptoms of anxiety than men planning standard IVF, and that having a child with a genetic disease was a significant predictor of anxiety throughout the process [15].

What do we know about pregnancy and maternal–fetal attachment after PGT-M? In a prospective study assessing anxiety, depression, and maternal–fetal attachment in women pregnant as a result of PGT-M, women were tested prior to treatment, following embryo transfer, following the pregnancy test result, and at 24 weeks of pregnancy. As the authors predicted, there were significant fluctuations in women's anxiety scores, anxiety increased following transfer and pregnancy testing. Testing during pregnancy revealed that the anxiety had returned to normal levels and maternal–fetal attachment scores were within normal levels. The authors reported that a subset of women experience a significant emotional burden during PGT-M treatment and that it is "these women who require closer attention and support" [16].

Winter et al. studied 157 couples pregnant through PGT-M, ICSI, or spontaneous conception to determine whether PGT-M couples experience higher levels of stress during pregnancy. Subjects were followed from the first trimester of pregnancy through the third month postpartum. Results showed that scores of depression and anxiety were the same for all groups and there were no differences between groups in parental antenatal attachment. The authors concluded that despite the immensely stressful PGT-M experience, PGT-M couples experienced pregnancy no differently than the control groups [17].

Case Example

Kevin, 40, knew that Huntington disease was part of his family health history. He lost his grandmother to the disease and now his father is afflicted. His sister had been tested and was negative for the gene but Kevin was too frightened to learn his own status. He and his wife wanted to have a baby but did not want to risk the possibility of passing on the gene to a child. After a consultation with the Recreational Equipment, Inc. team to learn about the procedure, Kevin consulted with the infertility counselor try to arrive at a decision. Although he wanted information about the genetic make-up of the embryos he did not want to know whether or not he himself was positive for Huntington disease. Reviewing his concerns in consultation with the counselor, the team was able to devise a strategy which would identify whether the chromosome containing the Huntington gene in each embryo was contributed by Kevin's father or by his mother. Since it was known that his father was the carrier, this made it possible to eliminate any embryo containing a possible Huntington gene without specifically testing the relevant chromosome for the Huntington gene, thereby eliminating the possibility of passing on the gene to his child without determining if he was indeed a carrier.

Preimplantation genetic testing for aneuploidy

PGT-A, formerly known as PGS, seeks to identify embryos with a normal chromosome count and to eliminate embryos with aneuploidy (the presence of one or more extra chromosomes) during IVF [18]. Chromosomal aneuploids are a major cause of infertility, maternal age-related decreased fertility potential, and over 70% of spontaneous miscarriages [19]. The treatment has gained acceptance, particularly for patients with a history of RPL and for those patients with a history of failed IVF implantation. Women of mature reproductive age (typically 38–40), are thought to have a better likelihood of successful implantation and pregnancy with PGT-A. It is thought that one advantage of the treatment is that it encourages single embryo transfer and helps reduce the dilemma of what to do with excess embryos.

The reproductive history of women undergoing PGT-A differs but it is often one that has been stressful. A review of studies of the psychological effects of miscarriage determined that a significant number of women who suffer a miscarriage have a grief reaction that mirrors those of other losses such as the death of a loved one. The grief typically dissipates gradually over time but can be quite distressing while it lasts [20]. A high prevalence of depression and emotional stress was reported in women with RPL where the grief is ongoing and never fully psychologically processed [21]. Women with a history of pregnancy loss who are referred for PGT-A are often overwhelmed by the IVF process and require pre and post genetic counseling and benefit from ongoing psychological support and counseling. Another group under great stress and grieving is women with a history of repeated IVF implantation failure. This group by definition is all too familiar with IVF but they can be confused about the genetic testing and have their hopes raised by the possibility of success and again dashed when that too fails. Women of mature age who have not been able to conceive are also referred for PGT-A. They too may be new to the IVF process and may find themselves hopeful and bewildered if the cycle fails.

Case Example

Jane, 36, had four miscarriages in the first 5 years of her marriage to Joe, 37. Though overcome with sadness after each loss she was determined to keep trying, despite the fact that she was depressed and frequently in tears. Joe was worried about Jane's physical and emotional health and wanted to stop trying, but when they were referred for IVF with PGT-A Jane insisted that they go for the consultation. They met with the reproductive endocrinologist and the genetics counselor, both of whom became alarmed about Jane's psychological state. They referred her to the infertility counselor. The therapist determined that Jane had unresolved grief resulting from her miscarriages that she never adequately processed, pushing herself to continue trying despite her distress. She recommended that Jane continue in counseling and defer treatment until she could come to terms with her grief and was better able to cope with the stress of the proposed treatment.

When the potential for having a child with a genetic disorder is sex-linked, PGT-A is the procedure used to determine the gender of the embryos. The fact that a couple with a sex-linked gene can prevent the familial disorder and have a healthy child with this technology is a benefit of this testing. The issue becomes more controversial when gender selection is done for nonmedical reasons [22]. The practice is banned in many countries, including Australia, Canada, and the United Kingdom, but is legal in the United States. In the United States a growing number of couples seek gender selection for so-called "family balancing," meaning that they may already have one or more children of the same sex and would like to have a child of the opposite sex. The Ethics Committee of the American Society for Reproductive Medicine issued a statement on the use of sex selection for nonmedical reasons and presented arguments for and against. Arguments in support of the procedure are patient autonomy and reproductive liberty. They added that the preference for a particular gender does not necessarily reflect discriminatory attitudes and that parents may have many important reasons for wanting to choose the sex of their offspring. Arguments against the use of preimplantation genetic testing for nonmedical reasons are potential harm to offspring, harm to women, misuse of medical resources for nonmedical purposes, and risks of discrimination and social injustice [23].

Couples considering gender selection may benefit from exploring the process with their infertility counselor, reviewing the pros and cons and specifically noting its potential for disappointment (e.g., hoping for a girl but all embryos are all male).

The role of the infertility counselor

The majority of patients going through PGT-A and PGT-M appear to be psychologically well adjusted but often find the amount of information they have to take in and the uncertainty of whether the cycle will bring success or failure especially anxiety provoking. This is often compounded by a stressful reproductive history which has brought them to this treatment. Karatas et al. recommend routine provision of information about coping strategies and state that "the gold standard of care may involve routine psychological assessment and targeted intervention where required" [13]. The infertility counselor should be competent and well-informed about infertility, its treatments, and its psychological impact on individuals and couples. In addition to being well versed in ART, the counselor should have a clear understanding of reproductive genetic screening and testing and potential psychological issues that may be a part of the process [24].

The ESHRE PGT-M Consortium has extensive guidelines for psychological evaluation of couples seeking PGT-M, for patients with a history of reproductive failure, patients with a history of traumatic experiences; couples about whom the geneticist, gynecologist, or other member of the IVF/PGT-M team has doubts regarding the welfare of existing or future children or about the psychological wellbeing of the future parents, for couples who actively ask for psychological intervention, and for couples undergoing HLA-matching PGT-M. They recommend that counseling should be offered both before and after the PGT-M cycle [25].

Conclusions

The integration of reproductive genetic screening and ART is expanding at an accelerating rate, raising the hopes of many seeking the chance to have a healthy baby. The psychological impact of genetic testing and screening can often be disturbing and stressful, so much so that the addition of a qualified infertility counselor can be an essential addition to the treatment team.

References

[1] Brezina PR, Kearns WG. The evolving world of genetics in reproductive medicine. Obstet Gynecol Clin N Am 2014;41–55.

[2] Kalfoglou AL, Doksum T, Bernhardt B, et al. Opinions about new reproductive genetic technologies: hopes and fears for our genetic future. Fertil Steril 2005;85: 1612–21.

[3] Fransiak JM. Expanded preconception carrier screening for infertile couples. Blog 2018. https://www.ivi-rmainnovation.com/expanded-preconception-carrier-screening-infertile-couples/.

[4] Henneman L, Borry P, Choioshvili DK, et al. Responsible implementation of expanded carrier screening. Eur J Hum Gen 2016;24(6):e1–e12.

[5] Marteau TM, Croyle RT. Psychological responses to genetic testing. BMJ 1998;316(7132):693–6.

[6] Nazareth SB, Lazarin GA, Goldberg JD. Changing trends in carrier screening genetic disease in the United States. Prenat Diagn 2015;35(10):931–5.

[7] Anido A, Carlson LM, Taft L, Sherman SL. Women's attitudes toward testing for fragile X carrier status: a qualitative analysis. J Genet Couns 2005;14:295–306.

[8] Lewis C, Skirton H, Jones R. Can we make assumptions about the psychosocial impact of living as a carrier, based on studies assessing the effects of carrier testing? J Genet Couns 2011;20(1):80–97.

[9] Harper JC, Wilton L, Traeger-Synodinos J, et al. The ESHRE PGT-M Consortium: 10 years of data collection. Hum Reprod Update 2012;18:234–347.

[10] Ethics Committee of the American Society for Reproductive Medicine. Use of preimplantation for monogenic defects (PGT-M) for adult-onset conditions: an Ethics Committee opinion. Fertil Steril 2018; 109:989–92.

[11] Kalfoglou A. PGT-M patients' and providers' attitudes to the use and regulation of preimplantation genetdiagnosis. Reprod BioMed Online 2005;4: 486–96.

[12] Hershberger PE, Pierce P. Conceptualizing couples' decision making in PGT-M: emerging cognitive, emotional and moral dimensions. Patient Educ Couns 2010;81(1):53–62.

[13] Karatas JC, Barlow-Stewart K, Meiser B, McMahon C, et al. Psychological adjustment, knowledge and unmet information needs in women undergoing PGT-M. Hum Reprod 2010;25(6):1481–9.

[14] Karatas JC, Strong KA, Barlow-Stewart K, McMahon C, et al. Psychological impact of preimplantation genetic diagnosis: a review of the literature. Reprod BioMed Online 2010;20:83–91.

[15] Jarvholm S, Broberg M, Thurin-Kjellberg A. Risk factors for depression and anxiety among men and women planning for preimplantation genetic diagnosis. J Genet Couns 2016;34:282.

[16] Karatas JC, Barlow-Stewart K, Meiser B, McMahon C, et al. A prospective study assessing anxiety, depression and maternal-fetal attachment in women using PGT-M. Hum Reprod 2011;26(1):148–56.

[17] Winter C, Van Acker F, Bonduelle M, Van Berkel K, et al. Depression, pregnancy-related anxiety and parental-antenatal attachment in couples using preimplantation genetic diagnosis. Hum Reprod 2016;6: 1288–99.

[18] Hayden H. Preimplantation genetic testing for aneuploidy (PGT-A): The biology, the technology and the clinical outcomes. Aust N Z J Obstet Gynaecol 2019;59 (2):317–24.

[19] Parikh FR, Athalye AS, Naik NJ, et al. Preimplantation genetic diagnosis: its evolution, where are we today? J Hum Reprod Sci 2018;11:306–14.

[20] Brier N. Grief following miscarriage: a comprehensive review of the literature. J Womens Health 2008;17: 451–64.

[21] Kolte AM, Olsen LR, Mikkelsen EM, Christiansen OB, Nielsen HS. Depression and emotional stress in highly

prevalent among women with recurrent pregnancy loss. Hum Reprod 2015;30:777–82.
[22] Sharp RR, McGowan ML, Verma JA, Landy DC, et al. Moral attitudes and beliefs among couples pursuing PGD for sex selection. Reprod Biomed Online 2010;21:838–47.
[23] Ethics Committee of the American Society for Reproductive Medicine. Use of reproductive technology for sex selection for nonmedical reasons. Fertil Steril 2015;6:1418–22.
[24] Patel A, Sharma PSVN, Kumar P. Role of the mental health practitioner in infertility clinics: A review on past, present and future directions. J Hum Reprod Sci 2018;11:219–28.
[25] Thornhill AR, deDie-Smulders CE, Geraedts JP, et al. ESHRE PGT-M Consortium 'Best practice guidelines for clinical preimplantation genetic diagnosis (PGT-M) and preimplantation genetic screening (PGS)'. Hum Reprod 2005;20(1):35–48.

CHAPTER

17

Bioethics in human reproduction (human reproductive genetics)

Heidi Mertes and Guido Pennings

Department of Philosophy and Moral Science, Bioethics Institute Ghent (BIG), Ghent University, Gent, Belgium

Introduction

As the fields of genetics and assisted reproduction are becoming increasingly more intertwined, ever more ethical dilemmas are popping up in the field of reproductive medicine. Whereas until a few decades ago the only way to direct or influence the genetic constitution of our offspring was by the selection of our reproductive partners, we now have numerous tools at hand to avoid the birth of a child with certain genetic conditions and even to select for nonmedical features, such as sex. Specific philosophical and ethical questions following from these new possibilities are, for example, whether there is a moral duty or at least a moral preference to produce the "best possible child" in terms of well-being (and thus avoid the birth of children with disabilities); whether fertility clinics have a responsibility in avoiding the birth of children with genetic abnormalities; whether people who actively choose to have a child with a disability are morally blameworthy; whether public health policies should be aimed at maximizing patient autonomy or at the reduction of the incidence of genetic conditions, etc. For the purpose of this chapter, we focus on three different applications on the crossroads of reproduction and genetics: (1) preconception genetic testing (or carrier screening); (2) preimplantation genetic testing (both preimplantation genetic diagnosis when the parents are carriers of a severe disease and preimplantation genetic screening for the detection of aneuploidies); and (3) prenatal genetic testing (with special attention to cell-free fetal DNA testing, also known as noninvasive prenatal testing or NIPT).

As a preliminary remark regarding terminology, we will use the term "genetic testing" as a broad term that includes both diagnostic testing and genetic screening for risk calculation, both on an individual and on a population level and regardless of whether an a priori elevated risk is present.

Preconception genetic testing

Preconception genetic testing is aimed at determining the carrier status of people who are

Human Reproductive Genetics
DOI: https://doi.org/10.1016/B978-0-12-816561-4.00018-1

planning to reproduce. When such a test reveals that both partners are carriers of the same autosomal recessive disorder, for each child they conceive together there is one chance in four that this child will be affected by that disorder. For X-linked disorders these odds are one in two. Having this knowledge increases the couple's reproductive autonomy as—apart from accepting these odds and conceiving naturally—they have a number of options to avoid the birth of a child affected by this disorder, either by refraining from reproducing, by resorting to third-party reproduction, by using prenatal genetic screening followed by a pregnancy termination in case of an affected fetus, or by using preimplantation genetic diagnosis (PGD, see below) on embryos in vitro in order to select those embryos for transfer that are not homozygous (or compound heterozygous) for the feared condition [1].

Preconception genetic screening is particularly interesting in communities with a relatively high prevalence of certain autosomal recessive disorders. The textbook example is that of the high incidence of Tay-Sachs disease, a lethal neurodegenerative disorder, in the Ashkenazi Jewish population, which has led to a very early widespread implementation of carrier screening programs in that community. This approach reportedly led to a 90% drop in incidence in Canada and the United States between 1970 and 2000 [2]. Similar programs of population-wide screening—either mandatory as a requirement for marriage licenses or voluntary—exist for beta-thalassemia in, for example, several Mediterranean and Arab countries [3]. This kind of preconception carrier testing in high-risk populations has been recommended by several professional societies, although on a voluntary basis [4–6].

The combination of an increased awareness about the reproductive risk of a carrier status and a decrease in the price of genetic testing has led to calls to implement population-wide genetic screening for conditions that are less prevalent, but which—especially when considered as a group—imply a high burden of disease [7]. This type of screening is known as expanded universal carrier screening, whereby "expanded" refers to a combination of several genetic conditions and "universal" to the inclusion of the entire population, regardless of an a priori risk related to ethnic background. Currently, opinions on this option are divided. While an expected decrease in the incidence of serious genetic conditions in the population, better informed reproductive decision-making, and a reduction of stigmatization of specific subpopulations can be considered as positive outcomes of such screening options, concerns are voiced regarding resource allocation, the limited benefit for most people, the provision of sufficient information and counseling for (potential) recipients of screening (especially when test results are delivered direct-to-consumer), test limitations and the accurate communication thereof by healthcare workers, the potential impact on societal views on reproductive responsibility, and stigmatization and discrimination based on genetic traits [8–10]. We discuss some of these issues in more detail below.

First, in terms of health economics, it has proven to be difficult to calculate the cost-effectiveness of population-wide carrier screening programs [11,12]. Moreover, given the continuous evolution in screening methods and their cost, these calculations require constant revisions. While targeted screening—taking ethnic background into account—was traditionally more cost-effective, the added cost of screening for multiple conditions in one test is coming down fast, so that screening for disorders with a very low incidence in the general population can still be cost-effective when "added on" to screening for more common disorders. However, there is more to be considered than the cost of screening alone. The more conditions a carrier screening program screens for, the more pretest counseling is necessary and the more people are likely to test positive and require extensive posttest genetic counseling, even when their partner is not a carrier and a problem therefore does not present itself. It is important to note that a "diagnosis" of carrier status has no clinical significance in itself, yet can be disturbing and confusing for those who receive it. A way to mitigate this problem is by opting for couple-based testing and disclosure, so that a negative result is only obtained when both partners are carriers. The downside of this option, however, is that testing would need to be repeated with a new partner and fewer relatives would be alerted to the presence of a harmful mutation in the family [6]. It is clear that both approaches (individual and couple-based screening) require a thorough communication of the meaning of carrier status: when individual results are given one needs to ensure that the recipient does not overestimate the impact of her carrier status on her health, when couple results are given, one needs to ensure that they understand that their risk may change when they change partners in the future.

This brings us to a second cluster of concerns, related to communication of test limitations and results to the recipients. Expanded carrier screening creates the illusion of risk-free reproduction, while there will always be conditions that are not screened for, disease-associated variants that are not screened for due to technical limitations, harmful mutations that are not yet identified, gonadal mosaicism, and de novo mutations. Apart from that, there are numerous nonhereditary health problems that may present themselves at birth. Again, it is important to convey this information to prospective parents. In order to make this feasible, substantial efforts will have to be made to school more genetic counselors, to increase knowledge about genetic conditions in the primary healthcare setting, with a focus on gynecologists and obstetricians, and in the general population. While information is preferably provided by professionals, making high-quality resources available directly to the general public is important in view of the rise of direct-to-consumer genetic testing, which enables people's access to their carrier status without any contact with healthcare professionals [13].

A third cluster of concerns relates to the societal impact of the implementation of preconception genetic screening. Two recurring themes can be discerned here: (1) a fear for negative consequences for people with disabilities and (2) a fear for an explosion of responsibility and societal pressure on the shoulders of future parents and a de facto limitation of their reproductive autonomy, rather than an expansion of it. Regarding the first, Scully identified three central points in the so-called "disability critique" in relation to genetic testing: (1) selection of offspring based on genetic features is discriminatory and eugenic; (2) the focus on disabilities caused by genetic factors is disproportionate and therefore conceals greater public healthcare needs; and (3) genetics is wrongly used to make a distinction between normality and abnormality [14]. In response to the eugenics reproach, one can observe that the locus of the evil with which we associate eugenics in a historical context is the killing and forced sterilization of people toward the goal of "purifying" the human gene pool, which were clear violations of basic human rights. The new form of eugenics that can be ascribed to expanded carrier screening, known as "new eugenics" or "liberal eugenics" [15,16], in principle reinforces reproductive autonomy, rather than limiting it, and is in that sense in a completely different league than the "old eugenics." However, the old eugenics should serve as a constant reminder that the supposedly morally neutral discipline of genetics can be abused for ideological purposes in order to legitimize discriminatory policies or attitudes toward groups of people based on their genetic features [14,17]. In that respect, it is hardly surprising that disability rights advocates urge for caution when it comes to eugenic interventions. As previously remarked by Adrienne Asch, we do not commonly assume that the suboptimal life prospects generated by characteristics other than genetic "abnormalities" (such as gender or social class) legitimize active prevention of people with such characteristics being born, as we consider this to be discriminatory and stigmatizing. The same could be said about selecting against disabilities that still allow for a reasonable level of welfare.

Besides the disability critique, concerns are commonly voiced regarding the impact on the notion of responsibility in the context of reproduction. The mere availability of preconception carrier screening "is sufficient to impel a person to justify (if not to others, then at least to herself) why she would not make use of it" [18]. This new reality ties in with the so-called "principle of procreative beneficence," which states that when reproducing, one has moral reason to select that child (of all possible children) whose life can be expected to go best (or at least not worse than any of the others) [19,20]. Whether one accepts this principle depends on the relative weight one attributes to the welfare of the future child/the future generation on the one hand and reproductive liberty on the other hand. This tension between the "prevention view" and the "autonomy view" is constantly in the background for all three applications discussed in this chapter [1]. The prevention view takes the prevention of the birth of children with genetic disorders as an explicit aim of genetic testing. The autonomy view considers the goal of genetic testing to be enhancement of the opportunities for meaningful reproductive choice. Whereas especially in preconception genetic testing, oftentimes an explicit reference is made to the prevention view, this is more contentious when prenatal genetic testing is concerned, as in this case "prevention" equals abortion. Especially in recent Western scholarly papers and policy documents, an explicit adoption of the autonomy view, rather than the prevention view is advocated for, mainly because "under the prevention perspective, there is a risk that prospective parents will be expected to make the 'right' decisions and that it will become normal and logical to hold them accountable for the consequences if they do not" [1]. However, in practice it remains a balancing effort, as most would not allow the autonomy view to justify, for example, the deliberate selection of children with disabilities in lieu of a healthy child. Moreover, as mentioned above, in several non-Western societies, policies are adopted that are very directive toward preconception carrier screening.

Preimplantation genetic testing

When, for example, after preconception genetic testing, reproductive partners are aware that there is a substantial risk of conceiving a child with a genetic condition that would have a severely negative impact on the child's and/or the parents' lives, they can opt for in vitro fertilization (IVF) with subsequent genetic testing of the resulting embryos so that only those that are not affected are implanted. This procedure is commonly known as preimplantation genetic diagnosis, or PGD. Another reason why genetic testing is performed on preimplantation embryos is to detect aneuploidies that would make it very unlikely for a particular embryo to result in a healthy live birth. This type of genetic testing used to be known as "preimplantation genetic screening," or PGS, but is now commonly referred to as preimplantation genetic testing for aneuploidy (PGT-A). While we acknowledge that the distinction between both procedures is becoming more and more vague as PGD is moving from targeted to whole-genome technologies, we opt to discuss the ethical implications of both separately below, for clarity's sake.

Preimplantation genetic diagnosis

While PGD has become an acceptable practice in many societies, this has not always been the case and PGD continues to be controversial in several societies due to concerns over the destruction of human embryos, which is inherent to the procedure, and over the message it sends regarding the value of people with disabilities (for the reasons discussed above). Broadly speaking, however, PGD is acceptable as long as it fits within the medical model, that is, PGD as a means to avoid a high risk of having an affected child [21]. Many other applications such as selection of healthy carriers, PGD for risk reduction (not elimination), the selection of savior siblings and selection *for*, instead of *against* disabilities are much more controversial.

Strictly within the medical model, an important problem in the debate on PDG is the range of applications. This problem contains two aspects: the variable expression of genetic mutations and the low(er) penetrance mutations. The first point is linked to the question of the seriousness of the disease. Several committees have tried to compose a list of "serious" diseases for which PGD would be acceptable. However, one soon discovered that this is a very difficult exercise as diseases may impact on multiple aspects of a person's life. Moreover, even if a general consensus on the seriousness could be reached, one may still disagree on the use of PGD because of the percentage of penetrance. In the Netherlands, for instance, there has been a discussion on PGD for BRCA mutations since "only" 80% of women with the mutation will develop breast cancer. A very restrictive position would demand full penetrance of an invariably very serious disorder. Most people are prepared to adopt a more flexible position. It has been argued that the acceptability of PGD for mutations with low(er) penetrance should depend on the balancing of relevant variables such as age of onset, treatability, and effectiveness and burdens of possible treatments [21].

As for preconception and prenatal testing, the ethical questions will change dramatically when whole-genome sequencing is performed on embryos. At the start, PGD was performed for one, or at most a few disorders. This generated a simple binary result: affected or unaffected. Whole-genome sequencing on the contrary can provide information on hundreds of monogenic diseases and on the genetic predisposition for multifactorial diseases such as diabetes. However, given that in each IVF cycle only a limited number of embryos is available, excluding all embryos with abnormalities or genetic risk factors will not work, as no embryo will then be left for transfer. The traditional rule of not transferring an affected embryo will have to be modified too since no embryo will be perfectly healthy. A solution could be that this technology is used in order to ensure that children born after IVF or PGD are at least free from major disorders (selection of "genetically acceptable embryos"), or else to select, from a batch of embryos, the one with the best genetic profile in terms of future health risks (selection of the "genetically best embryo"). When all information is put together, would-be parents will have a hard time deciding which will be the best embryo. Should they go for embryo 1 with a 10% susceptibility for a type of cancer in combination with two relatively minor diseases A and B or for embryo 2 with a 30% risk for autism and a relatively minor disease C? The wealth of information may also challenge the collaborating physicians since they acquire new responsibilities. Conflicts may arise if doctors and patients hold different standards of what is an acceptable disease and what is an acceptable risk [22,23]. Although reproductive autonomy of patients may give patients a large degree of decisional authority, physicians have a responsibility toward the future child that may justify a refusal to participate in a patient's request.

A thrust toward wider testing is already clearly visible. Providing more information rather than less may be regarded as required by the traditional aim of providing options for autonomous reproductive choice to prospective parents, whereas limiting the scope of testing, targeting the analysis, or only disclosing selected information would seem a problematic instance of reproductive paternalism. The ethos of nondirectivity and reproductive autonomy thus seems to align with the technological imperative that "the more testing, the better." It has been argued that "If it is all about choice, then, no option or information potentially relevant to a woman's choice and her decision-making processes should be withheld" [24]. However, "pure autonomy" is not a coherent aim of reproductive testing in a medical context [25]. Moreover, the idea that providing ever more information that might be relevant for choice will eo ipso contribute to reproductive autonomy, ignores the "paradox of choice" [26]. Information overload may actually undermine efforts to provide prospective parents with meaningful options for reproductive choice and render their decision-making vulnerable to the agendas of other stakeholders, despite the rhetoric of nonpaternalism.

Preimplantation genetic testing for aneuploidy screening

While PGD is aimed at contributing to procreative beneficence, PGT-A is aimed at improving the IVF procedure. The hypothesis is that as implantation failure in IVF treatments is oftentimes attributed to aneuploidies in the embryo, selecting euploid embryos for transfer will lead to less implantation failures and miscarriages, and thus to less suffering for the patient and a shorter time to conception (as no time will be wasted on transplanting nonviable embryos). A first version of PGT-A was introduced based on this hypothesis in the mid 1990s, relying on FISH on biopsied day 3 blastomeres. It was first used in poor-prognosis patients, but soon expanded to good-prognosis patients [27]. However, randomized controlled trials that were performed a decade after PGT-A's introduction showed no benefit, but instead a significant decrease in ongoing pregnancy rates [28,29]. Another decade later, a new version of PGT-A is widely used in ART clinics worldwide, this time based on trophoblast biopsy on day 5, using array or massive parallel sequencing technology. There are however, again, a number of concerns associated with PGT-A. First, due to high levels of mosaicism in the embryo, there is no guarantee that the biopsy taken from the outer layer (trophectoderm) of the embryo represents the cells from the inner cell mass, which will develop into the embryo proper [30,31]. That means that a viable embryo is occasionally judged to be nonviable and vice versa, leading to a situation in which viable embryos are sometimes discarded, thus lowering the overall chance of establishing a healthy live birth (given that only a limited number of embryos are available for transfer). Several studies have been published in which—after none of the embryos judged viable led to a live birth—embryos judged to be nonviable were transferred to consenting patients, leading to surprisingly high numbers of healthy live births [32–34]. This has led to the recommendation of using PGT-A primarily as a ranking tool, so that embryos with a euploid biopsy are transferred first, followed by embryos with a mosaic biopsy, going from more euploid to more aneuploid cells [35,36]. Within this whole debate, it is crucial to establish what a mosaic embryo is and how it is diagnosed [37]. Even though PGT-A is widely adopted in fertility clinics around the world, it remains very controversial. While some argue that it is "incumbent on IVF practitioners to try to detect and avoid the transfer and cryopreservation of [aneuploid] embryos using PGS technology" [38], others argue that "after almost

20 years of clinical utilization, and unable to find a clinical purpose for performing PGS/PGT-A, the procedure should be banned outside of clinical study frameworks" [39].

In such an environment, it is very important that information regarding PGT-A aimed at the general public (e.g., hospital websites, test supplier websites, information leaflets and brochures, media reporting, etc.) clearly states which of the benefits attributed to PGT-A are evidence based, which are likely but not (yet) established, and which have turned out to be false or unsubstantiated, so that the patient has a clear and correct view on what the test can and cannot deliver. Informed decision-making is however currently hampered for at least two reasons: (1) the commercial push to adopt PGT-A as widely as possible and (2) the fact that people undergoing fertility treatment are known to be susceptible to the "upselling" of add-on procedures lacking an evidence base, even when they are expensive [40]. It should be clear to practitioners working in the field of reproductive medicine that their duty of care toward the patient should be their primary motivation when deciding to either offer or withhold the option of PGT-A for a specific patient. Any patient opting for PGT-A should therefore be aware that there is great controversy about PGT-A in the scientific community and that PGT-A will involve an extra cost which will not increase their chance of a healthy live birth, but might, for example, spare them a miscarriage or reduce time-to-pregnancy in some groups [37].

Prenatal genetic testing

While preconception and PGS are gaining in popularity, prenatal genetic screening is probably still the most common application of genetic screening in the reproductive context today. During the pregnancy, several tests can be performed for the detection of chromosomal abnormalities in the fetus. Screening tests give an indication of a heightened risk of abnormality and include measurement of nuchal translucency by ultrasound, maternal serum testing, and cell-free fetal DNA testing, more commonly known as non-invasive prenatal testing (NIPT) (noninvasive prenatal screening, NIPS). Diagnostic tests such as chorionic villus sampling (CVS) and amniocentesis can then either confirm or refute that a chromosomal abnormality is in fact present or not. NIPT, CVS, and amniocentesis are genetic tests, respectively analyzing cell-free fetal DNA in the mother's bloodstream, DNA of the placenta, and DNA from fetal cells in the amniotic fluid.

Before discussing some ethical concerns tied to the technicalities of the different methods of prenatal testing, it is important to observe that the most "targeted" condition in prenatal testing is Down syndrome or trisomy 21 (T21) and in the second instance trisomies 13 and 18. The reason for this is not so much the suffering that is associated with these conditions, but the fact that they are easily detected abnormalities. It is therefore hardly surprising that, especially for T21, the above-mentioned disability critique is oftentimes invoked: selecting against Down syndrome is perceived as unduly stigmatizing and discriminatory. While we will not downplay the profound impact that T21 has on daily life, it is important to realize that it presents itself in very variable forms and that an overwhelming majority of people living with Down syndrome report very high levels of well-being and life satisfaction [41]. In addition, great numbers of parents and siblings also report a very positive attitude toward the presence of someone with Down syndrome in their family [42,43]. Taking this into account, it seems that the "welfare of the future child" or the idea that we want to save the next generation from as much suffering as possible is not a straightforward argument in support of T21 screening programs and the associated pregnancy terminations (as opposed to screening and terminations for conditions that cause more suffering). This brings us back to the previously mentioned tension between the prevention and autonomy view on genetic testing in the reproductive context. What is it exactly that we aim to achieve by introducing prenatal genetic testing for chromosomal abnormalities? Do we want to prevent the suffering that is brought about by the birth of disabled children? Do we want to increase reproductive autonomy? Do we want to prevent the loss of healthy pregnancies by reducing the number of invasive tests (see below)? Do we want to save on healthcare costs? Different answers to these questions will justify different policies regarding prenatal testing.

The prenatal screening method that receives most attention at present is noninvasive prenatal testing, made possible by the discovery of the presence of cell-free fetal DNA in maternal plasma and serum in 1997 [44]. The term noninvasive prenatal testing is misleading to the general public in several regards. First "noninvasive" suggests that it is an alternative to invasive prenatal testing—that is, CVS and amniocentesis—which creates the idea that NIPT is also a diagnostic test (detecting an aneuploidy), rather than a screening test (detecting an elevated risk). Second, the word "testing" rather than "screening" reinforces this perception, which is why NIPS has been suggested as a better alternative by the American College of Medical Genetics and Genomics [45]. While it is true that NIPS offers a much better risk calculation than traditional combined first-trimester screening, it is important to keep stressing that this test is not diagnostic, and that the positive predictive value (PPV) is lower than the test's sensitivity and specificity, especially in a low-risk population (e.g., even for the most prevalent condition screened for, trisomy 21, a 25-year-old woman without disturbing sonographic findings and a positive NIPS result has about a 50% chance that her fetus does *not* have trisomy 21). Therefore, when a woman considers a pregnancy termination based on a positive NIPS result, this should always be preceded by follow-up diagnostic testing, preferably by amniocentesis.

Regardless of this caveat though, the higher detection rate that is achieved with NIPS as compared to combined first-trimester screening significantly reduces the overall number of invasive diagnostic tests and the occasional iatrogenic miscarriage that they cause [46,47]. However, this advantage may by undercut by a current trend to expand NIPS to include other, less common abnormalities than trisomies 21, 13, and 18, including sex chromosome abnormalities and clinically significant microdeletions (e.g., DiGeorge). As the PPV for these conditions is much lower, this will again lead to a situation in which women get a risk score that is high enough to worry them, yet low enough to result in numerous cases of unnecessary invasive testing.

Moreover, if in the future NIPS is expanded towards whole-genome NIPS, the informational privacy interests of the future child should also be taken into account [30]. This is a problem that is already present in diagnostic prenatal testing today, especially when a whole genome, rather than a targeted approach, is used. Current recommendations advise against performing predictive genetic testing in minors except when there is a clear potential benefit for the child, in order not to undermine their "right to an open future" and their "right not to know" their genetic risks. These proclaimed rights are commonly grounded in respect for (future) autonomy, respect for privacy, and the best interest of the child [48]. If DNA is sequenced before birth, the future person obviously has no chance to object to the disclosure of this information. Yet, while this is a legitimate aspect to take into account, it is only one of many factors to consider. In this sense, it can lead to a policy not to routinely screen all pregnancies with whole genome sequencing

(WGS), yet allow prenatal arrays or WGS when there is an indication of a genetic abnormality. As mentioned by Laurie in the context of screening of minors, it is preferable to consider these issues "as a matter of discretion for professional judgment and responsibility, rather than an issue of rights" [49].

A related problem in the context of expanded prenatal screening is the potential discovery of incidental findings/secondary findings and/or of variants of uncertain significance. In a clinical setting with adults, the general rule is that secondary findings are reported when they are serious and actionable [50]. However, in the prenatal setting, an additional potential "action" is present, namely pregnancy termination. Therefore, while the reporting of a serious and untreatable condition in an adult may be inappropriate, it may be useful information in the prenatal context [51]. The typical example of a secondary finding of Huntington disease that would not be reported to adults as it is not actionable, presents a major dilemma in the prenatal context. First, it reveals that one of the parents will also develop Huntington disease, information they may not wish to receive. Second, if it is reported and the couple decides not to terminate the pregnancy, this information may place a heavy burden on the life of the parents and the resulting child.

Also, many genetic conditions do not have 100% penetrance. This means that parents may be confronted with odds calculations about different potential diseases their child might develop later in life, or might not. This inevitably leads to the termination of pregnancies which could have resulted in the birth of someone who would never have developed any major health issues and to the birth of children who are labeled from birth as being destined to develop some disability, a phenomenon described as the "healthy ill" [52].

Finally, concerns related to routinization are oftentimes voiced in the context of prenatal screening, as it may undermine informed decision-making [25,53]. While this was already a concern for combined first-trimester screening (a risk score calculation based on maternal age, maternal serum testing, and nuchal translucency), it becomes even more pressing where NIPS is offered to large fractions of, or even all, pregnant women. Ideally, undergoing prenatal screening for fetal abnormalities should be the result of a well-informed choice so that the uptake is limited to those women who would either consider a pregnancy termination in the event of a chromosomal abnormality or who want to prepare (practically and emotionally) for the birth of a child with special needs. The scenario that is to be avoided, though, is that women who do not wish to know any information about the risk of carrying a fetus with a chromosomal abnormality are suddenly presented with this information nonetheless. While the increased acceptance of voluntary pregnancy termination is a positive evolution in terms of reproductive autonomy, we should as a society be wary of the possibility that when abortion of fetuses with chromosomal abnormalities becomes the norm, women may feel pressured into opting for a pregnancy termination while that is not their preferred course of action, which again restricts their reproductive autonomy. As a side-note: prenatal treatments alleviating the symptoms of chromosomal abnormalities are eagerly awaited [54,55]. Once these become available and accessible, the pressure to abort may again lessen.

References

[1] De Wert GM, Dondorp WJ, Knoppers BM. Preconception care and genetic risk: ethical issues. J Community Genet 2012;3(3):221–8.

[2] Kaback MM. Population-based genetic screening for reproductive counseling: the Tay-Sachs disease model. Eur J Pediatr 2000;159(3):S192–5.

[3] Cousens NE, Gaff CL, Metcalfe SA, Delatycki MB. Carrier screening for beta-thalassaemia: a review of international practice. Eur J Hum Genet 2010;18(10):1077.

[4] American College of Obstetrics and Gynecology. Committee Opinion No. 691. Carrier screening for genetic conditions. Obstet Gynecol 2017;129:e41–55.

[5] Edwards JG, Feldman G, Goldberg J, Gregg AR, Norton ME, Rose NC, et al. Expanded carrier screening in reproductive medicine-points to consider: a joint statement of the American College of Medical Genetics and Genomics, American College of Obstetricians and Gynecologists, National Society of Genetic Counselors, Perinatal Quality Foundation, and Society for Maternal Fetal Medicine. Obstet Gynecol 2015;125:653–62.

[6] Henneman L, Borry P, Chokoshvili D, Cornel MC, Van El CG, Forzano F, et al. Responsible implementation of expanded carrier screening. Eur J Hum Genet 2016;24(6):e1.

[7] Blencowe H, Moorthie S, Petrou M, Hamamy H, Povey S, Bittles A, et al. Rare single gene disorders: estimating baseline prevalence and outcomes worldwide. J Commun Genet 2018;9(4):397–406.

[8] Cho D, McGowan ML, Metcalfe J, Sharp RR. Expanded carrier screening in reproductive healthcare: perspectives from genetics professionals. Hum Reprod 2013;28(6):1725–30.

[9] Janssens S, Chokoshvili D, Vears D, De Paepe A, Borry P. Attitudes of European geneticists regarding expanded carrier screening. J Obstet Gynecol Neonat Nur 2017;46(1):63–71.

[10] Van Der Hout S, Holtkamp KC, Henneman L, de Wert G, Dondorp WJ. Advantages of expanded universal carrier screening: what is at stake? Eur J Hum Genet 2017;25(1):17.

[11] Radhakrishnan M, van Gool K, Hall J, Delatycki M, Massie J. Economic evaluation of cystic fibrosis screening: a review of the literature. Health Policy 2008;85 (2):133–47.

[12] Norman R, Van Gool K, Hall J, Delatycki M, Massie J. Cost-effectiveness of carrier screening for cystic fibrosis in Australia. J Cyst Fibros 2012;11(4):281–7.

[13] Howard H, Borry P. Direct-to-consumer genetic testing: more questions than benefits? Pers Med 2008;5:317–20.

[14] Scully JL. Disability and genetics in the era of genomic medicine. Nat Rev Genet 2008;9(10):797.

[15] Agar N. Liberal eugenics: in defence of human enhancement. London: Blackwell Publishing; 2004.

[16] MacKellar C, Bechtel C, editors. The ethics of the new eugenics. New York, NY: Berghahn Books; 2016.

[17] Allen GE. Is a new eugenics afoot? Science 2001;294 (5540):59–61.

[18] Bonte P, Pennings G, Sterckx S. Is there a moral obligation to conceive children under the best possible conditions? A preliminary framework for identifying the preconception responsibilities of potential parents. BMC Med Ethics 2014;15(1):5.

[19] Savulescu J. Procreative beneficence: why we should select the best children. Bioethics 2001;15:413–26.

[20] Savulescu J, Kahane G. The moral obligation to create children with the best chance of the best life. Bioethics 2009;23:274–90.

[21] De Wert G, Dondorp W, Shenfield F, Devroey P, Tarlatzis B, Barri P, et al. ESHRE task force on ethics and law 22: preimplantation genetic diagnosis. Hum Reprod 2014;29(8):1610–17.

[22] Pennings G, Liebaers I, Bonduelle M. Decisional authority and moral responsibility of patients and clinicians in the context of preimplantation genetic diagnosis. Reprod BioMed Online 2003;7(5):509–13.

[23] Hens K. To transfer or not to transfer: the case of comprehensive chromosome screening of the in vitro embryo. Health Care Anal 2015;23(2):197–206.

[24] McGillivray G, Rosenfeld JA, Gardner RM, Gillam LH. Genetic counselling and ethical issues with chromosome microarray analysis in prenatal testing. Prenat Diagn 2012;32(4):389–95.

[25] Dondorp W, van Lith J. Dynamics of prenatal screening: new developments challenging the ethical framework. Bioethics 2015;29(1):ii–v.

[26] Schwartz B. The paradox of choice: why more is less, Vol. 6. New York: HarperCollins; 2004.

[27] Mastenbroek S, Twisk M, Van Der Veen F, Repping S. Preimplantation genetic screening: a systematic review and meta-analysis of RCTs. Hum Reprod Update 2011;17(4):454–66.

[28] Staessen C, Platteau P, Van Assche E, Michiels A, Tournaye H, Camus M, et al. Comparison of blastocyst transfer with or without preimplantation genetic diagnosis for aneuploidy screening in couples with advanced maternal age: a prospective randomized controlled trial. Hum Reprod 2004;19(12):2849–58.

[29] Mastenbroek S, Twisk M, van Echten-Arends J, Sikkema-Raddatz B, Korevaar JC, Verhoeve HR, et al. In vitro fertilization with preimplantation genetic screening. N Engl J Med 2007;357(1):9–17.

[30] Harper JC, Aittomäki K, Borry P, Cornel MC, de Wert G, Dondorp W, et al. Recent developments in genetics and medically-assisted reproduction: from research to clinical applications on behalf of the European Society of Human Genetics and the European Society of Human Reproduction and Embryology Eur J Hum Genet 2018;26:12–33.

[31] Fragouli E, Wells D. Aneuploidy in the human blastocyst. Cytogenet Genome Res 2011;133(2-4):149–59.

[32] Greco E, Minasi MG, Fiorentino F. Healthy babies after intrauterine transfer of mosaic aneuploid blastocysts. N Engl J Med 2015;373(21):2089–90.

[33] Munné S, Blazek J, Large M, Martinez-Ortiz PA, Nisson H, Liu E, et al. Detailed investigation into the cytogenetic constitution and pregnancy outcome of replacing mosaic blastocysts detected with the use of high-resolution next-generation sequencing. Fertil Steril 2007;108(1):62–71.

[34] Spinella F, Fiorentino F, Biricik A, Bono S, Ruberti A, Cotroneo E, et al. Extent of chromosomal mosaicism influences the clinical outcome of in vitro fertilization treatments. Fertil Steril 2018;109(1):77–83.

[35] Maxwell SM, Colls P, Hodes-Wertz B, McCulloh DH, McCaffrey C, Wells D, et al. Why do euploid embryos miscarry? A case-control study comparing the rate of aneuploidy within presumed euploid embryos that resulted in miscarriage or live birth using next-generation sequencing. Fertil Steril 2016;106(6):1414–19.

[36] Preimplantation Genetic Diagnosis International Society. PGDIS position statement on chromosome mosaicism and preimplantation aneuploidy testing at the blastocyst stage, <https://www.pgdis.org/docs/newsletter_071816.html>; 2016 [accessed 28.02.19].

[37] Practice Committee of the American Society for Reproductive Medicine and the Society for Assisted Reproductive Technology. The use of preimplantation genetic testing for aneuploidy (PGT-A): a committee opinion. Fertil Steril 2018;109(3):429–36.

[38] CoGEN (Controversies in preconception, preimplantation and prenatal genetic diagnosis). CoGEN position statement on chromosomal mosaicism detected in preimplantation blastocyst biopsies, <https://ivf-worldwide.com/cogen/general/cogen-statement.html>; 2015 [accessed 28.02.19].

[39] Gleicher N, Kushnir VA, Barad DH. How PGS/PGT—a laboratories succeeded in losing all credibility. Reprod Biomed Online 2018;37(2):242–5.

[40] Harper J, Jackson E, Sermon K, Aitken RJ, Harbottle S, Mocanu E, et al. Adjuncts in the IVF laboratory: where is the evidence for 'add-on'interventions? Hum Reprod 2017;32(3):485–91.

[41] Skotko BG, Levine SP, Goldstein R. Self-perceptions from people with Down syndrome. Am J Med Genet Part A 2011;155(10):2360–9.

[42] Skotko BG, Levine SP, Goldstein R. Having a son or daughter with Down syndrome: perspectives from mothers and fathers. Am J Med Genet Part A 2011;155(10):2335–47.

[43] Skotko BG, Levine SP, Goldstein R. Having a brother or sister with Down syndrome: perspectives from siblings. Am J Med Genet Part A 2011;155(10):2348–59.

[44] Lo YD, Corbetta N, Chamberlain PF, Rai V, Sargent IL, Redman CW, et al. Presence of fetal DNA in maternal plasma and serum. Lancet 1997;350(9076):485–7.

[45] Gregg AR, Skotko BG, Benkendorf JL, Monaghan KG, Bajaj K, Best RG, et al. Noninvasive prenatal screening for fetal aneuploidy, 2016 update: a position statement of the American College of Medical Genetics and Genomics. Genet Med 2016;18:1056–65.

[46] Tabor A, Alfirevic Z. Update on procedure-related risks for prenatal diagnosis techniques. Fetal Diagn Ther 2010;27(1):1–7.

[47] Gil MM, Quezada MS, Revello R, Akolekar R, Nicolaides KH. Analysis of cell-free DNA in maternal blood in screening for fetal aneuploidies: updated meta-analysis. Ultrasound Obstet Gynecol 2015;45(3):249–66.

[48] Borry P, Shabani M, Howard HC. Is there a right time to know? The right not to know and genetic testing in children. J Law Med Ethics 2014;42(1):19–27.

[49] Laurie G. Recognizing the right not to know: conceptual, professional, and legal implications. J Law Med Ethics 2014;42(1):53–63.

[50] Kalia SS, Adelman K, Bale SJ, Chung WK, Eng C, Evans JP, et al. Recommendations for reporting of secondary findings in clinical exome and genome sequencing, 2016 update (ACMG SF v2. 0): a policy statement of the American College of Medical Genetics and Genomics. Genet Med 2017;19(2):249.

[51] Vanakker O, Vilain C, Janssens K, Van der Aa N, Smits G, Bandelier C, et al. Implementation of genomic arrays in prenatal diagnosis: the Belgian approach to meet the challenges. Eur J Med Genet 2014;57(4):151–6.

[52] Hubbard R. Predictive genetics and the construction of the healthy ill. Suffolk Univ Law Rev 1993;27:1209.

[53] Schmitz D, Netzer C, Henn W. An offer you can't refuse? Ethical implications of non-invasive prenatal diagnosis. Nat Rev Genet 2009;10(8):515.

[54] Guedj F, Bianchi DW, Delabar JM. Prenatal treatment of Down syndrome: a reality? Curr Opin Obstet Gyn 2014;26(2):92–103.

[55] Verweij EJT, Oepkes D. Prenatal treatment of genetic diseases in the unborn. Noninvasive prenatal testing (NIPT). Academic Press; 2018. p. 353–67.

CHAPTER

18

The role of genetic counseling in the infertile patient

Josep Pla-Victori
IVI-RMA Global, Barcelona, Catalonia, Spain

Introduction

Genetic counseling

Genetics is a fast-changing landscape. Over the last few decades there has been an exponential development of new technologies and new knowledge in genetics [1–5]. Moreover, everything suggests this fast-paced progress will continue in the years to come, with many new achievements expected and, thus new challenges [6–8].

A genetic diagnosis has a few characteristics that no other medical diagnosis has [9–12]:

- Genetic essentialism: genetic information is unique to each individual (with the exception of monozygotic twins). People tend to feel identified by their genetic information, a concept known as genetic essentialism. Therefore, genetic alterations may be perceived as a fault in one's essence [10,11].
- Given the unique character of an individual's genome, genetic testing also carries many issues of privacy and confidentiality [9].
- Family implications: since genetic traits run in families, a genetic diagnosis usually has implications for other family members [9].
- Complex to communicate: despite most people being exposed to genetic concepts by the media, the nature of genetics is regarded as complex to understand and communicate, both by patients and healthcare professionals [12].

For all this, back in the 1970s, the Medical Genetics Units in the United States started defining a new role and profession: genetic counseling [13]. The National Society of Genetics Counselors defines genetic counseling [14] as the process of helping people understand and adapt to the medical, psychological, and familial implications of the genetic contributions to disease. This process integrates:

- Interpretation of family and medical histories to assess the chance of disease occurrence or recurrence;
- Education about inheritance, testing, management, prevention, resources, and research;

Human Reproductive Genetics
DOI: https://doi.org/10.1016/B978-0-12-816561-4.00019-3

- Counseling to promote informed choices and adaptation to the risk or condition.

The state of the art of genetic counseling worldwide varies greatly, with some countries with well-established professions and national registration systems, while others do not contemplate this profession in their national legislation, as described in Table 18.1 [15].

Psychological and emotional impacts of infertility and/or genetics

The psychological and emotional burden that infertility poses has been long described [16–30]. The infertile patient has been reported to present with higher anxiety, grief, depression, and mood disorder scores; moreover, they present with lower memory,

TABLE 18.1 State of the art of genetic counseling worldwide.

Region	Country	Availability of genetic counseling	MSc training programs	National registration system
Americas	United States	Over 4000 genetic counselors	39 MSc training programs	Yes
	Canada	Approximately 350 genetic counselors	Five MSc training programs	Yes
	Cuba	About 900 genetic counselors	One MSc training program	No
Europe	Belgium	Over 10 genetic counselors	No	Genetic Nurse and Counsellor Professional Branch of the European Board of Medical Genetics Registration System
	Denmark	About 20 genetic counselors	No	
	Finland	Approximately five genetic nurses	No	
	France	Approximately 175 genetic counselors	One MSc training program	
	Ireland	Less than 10 genetic counselors	No	
	The Netherlands	55 genetic counselors	Four MSc training programs	
	Norway	40 genetic counselors	One MSc training program	
	Portugal	Less than 10 genetic counselors	One MSc training program*	
	Romania	About 75 genetic counselors	One MSc training program*	
	Spain	Over 75 genetic counselors	One MSc training program*	
	Sweden	Approximately 40 genetic counselors	No training programs	
	Switzerland	Less than 10 genetic counselors	No training programs	
Middle East	Israel	80 genetic counselors	Three MSc training programs	No
	Saudi Arabia	20 genetic counselors	Two MSc training programs	No

(Continued)

TABLE 18.1 (Continued)

Region	Country	Availability of genetic counseling	MSc training programs	National registration system
Oceania	Australia/ New Zealand	220 genetic counselors	Two MSc training programs	Yes
Asia	China	No	No	No
	India	No	No	No
	Japan	Over 230 genetic counselors	14 MSc training programs	No
	Malaysia	Less than 10 genetic counselors	One MSc training program	No
	Philippines	Approximately 10 genetic counselors	One MSc training program	No
	Singapore	10 genetic counselors	No	No
	South Korea	12 genetic counselors	Two MSc training programs	No
	Taiwan	120 genetic counselors	One MSc training program	No
Africa	South Africa	Over 120 genetic counselors	Two MSc training programs	Yes

*Accredited by the European Board of Medical Genetics Registration System.

concentration, self-esteem, perceived control, and quality-of-life scores. Patients describe recurrent emotions such as feeling defective, inadequate, inferior, useless, ashamed, guilty, anxious, depressed, stressed, distant or conflicted with their partner, family, and/or friends, frustrated, socially pressured, loss of control, failure, low self-esteem, worried, fatigued, disappointed, grieving, and so on. For all this, infertility counseling has become a key point in many assisted reproduction treatments. Infertility counseling has shown improvement in all these feelings and emotions, and even in the treatment outcome.

Similarly, it is well known that both a genetic diagnosis and genetic testing carry a considerable psychological and emotional impact, both in patients and their close relatives [31–39]. Of interest, the psychometric scales that are altered in genetic patients and relatives, as well as the emotions that they report, are very similar to those described in the infertile patient.

Therefore patients undergoing assisted reproduction and genetic testing (with or without a genetic diagnosis) may present with an even higher psychological and emotional burden, derived by the addition of these two stressing factors.

This psychological and emotional impact should not be neglected, and infertility and genetic counseling are appropriate interventions. While infertility counseling and genetic counseling both have specific healthcare professionals trained in these fields, both concepts are described as long-term processes in which any other healthcare professional will be involved. Therefore, it is important that all those professionals involved in assisted reproduction learn some basic concepts of both infertility and genetic counseling.

Karyotype alterations as a cause of infertility

Karyotype alterations have been described as a cause of infertility, both male and female, for a long time [40–44]. These karyotype alterations include sexual chromosome aneuploidies (and their mosaics) and chromosomal structural rearrangements, as well as other chromosomal alterations.

The prevalence of chromosomal alterations is higher in infertile men. The chance of finding a karyotype alteration is inversely proportional to the sperm count: 10%–15% of azoospermic men, 5% of severe oligozoospermic (<5 million/mL) men, and <1% of men with normal sperm counts [40–42].

A relationship between chromosomal alterations and female sterility has also been reported. Between 10% and 15% of women with ovarian failure also have numerical or structural chromosomal alterations [42].

In this section, several karyotype alterations and their involvements in infertility, as well as the basic genetic counseling aspects that should be covered, are described.

Chromosomal heteromorphisms

Chromosomal heteromorphisms are defined as differences in size, shape, or staining properties between homologous chromosomes. Certain chromosomic regions are subject to the presence of heteromorphisms due to their repetitive DNA content [45–47].

The term heteromorphism can be used as a synonym for polymorphism or normal variation. The most common cytogenetic polymorphisms include heterochromatin areas of chromosomes 1, 9, 16, and Y, as well as the short arms, satellites, and stems of acrocentric chromosomes, which appear more prominent than usual [45–47].

Cytogenetic studies in the general population have revealed that 2%–5% of individuals carry one of these findings.

The role of chromosomal heteromorphisms in infertility has been studied. Some studies report a higher incidence of these findings in infertile patients, especially infertile men, but also in infertile women and couples with recurrent pregnancy losses. However, these results have been conflicted by other studies. Therefore, with the current scientific and medical evidence available, the finding of a chromosomal heteromorphism should be considered a normal variant and no additional test should be indicated.

Genetic counseling after the identification of a chromosomal polymorphism should include:

- The finding of a chromosomal heteromorphism, and especially the fact of not modifying the assisted reproduction treatment, may cause anxiety or concern in the individuals in whom they are identified.
- It is important to inform the couple about the high frequency of these findings in the general population (>1%) and that the current evidence regarding their involvement in infertility is very controversial.
- Heteromorphisms may be identified in other family members, so genetic counseling should be advised.

Sex chromosome aneuploides

Sex chromosome aneuploidies are a cause of infertility, both in men and women. These findings are the most frequent chromosomal alterations at birth (1/400, possibly higher due to underdiagnosis).

Sex chromosome aneuploidies include 47,XXY (Klinefelter syndrome), 47,XYY (double Y syndrome), 47,XXX (triple X syndrome), and 45,X (Turner syndrome). The term also includes possible polysomies and mosaics [48–50].

Apart from its implications in infertility, it is important to keep in mind that the presence of an extra chromosome increases the frequency of aneuploid gametes. For this reason, it is important to consider preimplantation genetic testing for aneuploidies (PGT-A) in these patients [51–54].

Genetic counseling:

- A diagnosis of a sex chromosomes aneuploidy may carry an important emotional burden.
- It is important to offer adequate genetic counseling, providing reliable and up-to-date information, making special emphasis on the phenotypic variability of these conditions (large percentage of undiagnosed individuals). When not properly counseled, patients may resort to Internet search engines, with the risk of finding outdated and biased information.
- In those patients where gamete retrieval is possible, PGT-A should be recommended. Embryos conceived by carriers of sex chromosome aneuploidies have a higher incidence of all chromosome aneuploidies.

Structural rearrangements

Reciprocal translocations

Reciprocal chromosome translocations are defined as the reciprocal exchange of genetic material between two chromosomes, with a break point in each of them. This exchange can be balanced, if all chromosomal material is preserved; or unbalanced, if there has been gain and/or loss of chromosomal material in one or both chromosomes involved.

Approximately 1 in 700 people in the general population is a carrier of a balanced reciprocal translocation. This frequency is higher in infertile men (1 in 50 to 1 in 100) and infertile women (1 in 500) [55–57].

Nomenclature in reciprocal translocations is important, and rules are defined by the ISCN: t + open parenthesis + first chromosome + semicolon + second chromosome + close parenthesis + open parenthesis + band in which the break in the first chromosome has occurred + semicolon + band in which the break in the second chromosome has occurred + close parenthesis. For example, t(1;9)(p21;q13) defines a translocation between chromosomes 1 and 9. The break point in chromosome 1 is identified in band p21 of its short arm, whilst the break point in chromosome 9 occurred in band q13 of the chromosome's long arm.

In most cases, being a carrier of a balanced reciprocal translocation has no direct health implications. However, carriers of a balanced reciprocal translocation have some reproduction implications, due to imbalanced gametes:

- *Reproduction issues*:
  - Sterility/infertility;
  - Recurrent pregnancy losses (in 3%–9% of couples with recurrent pregnancy losses).
- *Offspring with an unbalanced translocation*:
  - The risk of live offspring with an unbalanced translocation is supposed to be around 3% when the finding is secondary to infertility, as opposed to approximately 20% if there is a family history of live newborns with the unbalance.
  - The phenotypic implications of the unbalance are highly variable and very hard to predict.

Robertsonian translocations

Robertsonian chromosome translocations are defined as the fusion of the long arms of two acrocentric chromosomes near their centromeric regions. Acrocentric chromosomes are chromosomes 13, 14, 15, 21, 22, and Y. The short arm (p arm) of these chromosomes contains heterochromatic content and, therefore, its loss does not have any phenotypic implication. This type of translocation is always observable on the karyotype, as it involves two whole chromosomes [55–57].

One in 1000 people in the general population carries a Robertsonian translocation, 1 in 100 couples with recurrent loss of pregnancy and 1 in 33 in infertile men. The most common Robertsonian translocation is the one involving chromosomes 13 and 14.

These translocations may be:

- Balanced or unbalanced;
- Heterologous (two different chromosomes) or homologous (two homologous chromosomes).

Nomenclature in Robertsonian translocations is important, and rules are defined by the ISCN: rob or der + open parenthesis + first chromosome + semicolon + second chromosome + close parenthesis + open parenthesis + band in which the break in the first chromosome has occurred + semicolon + band in which the break in the second chromosome has occurred + close parenthesis. For example, rob(13;21)(q10;q10) or der (13;21)(q10;q10) defines a Robertsonian translocation between chromosomes 13 and 21.

In most cases, being a carrier of a balanced Robertsonian translocation has no direct health implications. However, carriers of a balanced Robertsonian translocation have some reproduction implications, due to imbalanced gametes:

- *Reproduction issues*:
  - Sterility/infertility;
  - Recurrent pregnancy losses (in 3%–9% of couples with recurrent pregnancy losses).
- *Offspring with an unbalanced translocation*:
  - Risk of trisomy 13 (Patau syndrome) and 21 (Down syndrome) when the translocation includes chromosome 13 or chromosome 21 [58–62];
  - Risk of imprinting defects when the translocation includes chromosome 14 (Temple and Kagami syndromes) or 15 (Prader-Willi and Angelman syndromes) [63–66].

Inversions

Chromosome inversions are defined as the rearrangement produced by two break-points within the same chromosome, with the subsequent inversion and reinsertion of this fragment.

Chromosome inversions may be:

- *Pericentric*: if the inverted fragment includes the chromosome's centromere;
- *Paracentric*: if the inverted fragment does not include the chromosome's centromere.

The frequency in the general population of chromosome inversions is 1–5 in 10,000 for paracentric inversions and 1–7 in 10,000 for pericentric inversions.

Some inversions are chromosomal heteromorphisms include [57]:

- inv(1)(p11q12);
- inv(2)(p11.2q13);
- inv(3)(p11q11);
- inv(3)(p11q12);
- inv(3)(p13q12);
- inv(5)(p13q13);
- inv(9)(p11q12);
- inv(9)(p11q13);
- inv(10)(p11.2q21.2);
- inv(16)(p11q12);
- inv(16)(p11q13);
- inv(Y)(p11q11).

In most cases, being a carrier of a chromosome inversion has no direct health implications. However, carriers of a balanced Robertsonian translocation have some reproduction implications, due to imbalanced gametes:

- *Reproduction issues*:
  - Sterility/infertility;
  - Recurrent pregnancy losses (in 3%–9% of couples with recurrent pregnancy losses).
- *Offspring with an unbalanced chromosome rearrangement*:

- In unbalanced pericentric inversions: formation of recombinants with deletion and duplication of the inverted segment;
- In unbalanced paracentric inversions: inverted duplications of the segments.

Genetic counseling in structural rearrangements

- Assess family history, with special attention to family members with fertility problems, recurrent pregnancy losses, stillbirth, or offspring with anomalies (congenital conditions, global developmental delay, intellectual disability, etc.).
- Provide information on basic genetics and structural rearrangements.
- Reproduction options include:
  - Spontaneous pregnancy with or without prenatal testing;
  - Preimplantation genetic testing for structural rearrangements (PGT-SR);
  - Gamete donation;
  - Legal adoption.
- In most instances, the identification of a balanced structural rearrangement has no health implications. However, approximately 6% of apparently balanced reciprocal translocations and about 10% of apparently balanced inversions may be associated with phenotypical alterations [67]. Therefore the implications of these findings will vary depending on the setting (prenatal or diagnostic in an individual with phenotypic trait vs an adult with infertility). The presence of phenotypic alterations in apparently balanced rearrangements can be explained by:
  - The rearrangement is, in fact, not balanced: the rearrangement has a size which is not detectable by conventional karyotyping.
  - Cryptic rearrangement in another region of the genome: the cause of the disease/phenotype is not the rearrangement per se but a rearrangement, that is, not being considered.
  - Disruption of dose-sensitive genes in the break point.
  - Gene position effect.
  - Uniparental disomy of a chromosome submitted to imprinting
- The psychological impact of the finding must be addressed, as with any genetic finding.
- The structural rearrangement may be identified in other family members, so genetic counseling is advised.

Small supernumerary marker chromosomes

Small supernumerary marker chromosomes (sSMCs) are abnormal chromosome fragments that can be identified by conventional karyotyping and cannot be completely characterized without further testing. These sSMCs can originate from any of the 24 chromosomes and their frequency in the general population is estimated at approximately 1/2500. However, the incidence increases to 1/800 in infertile couples and they are more commonly found in the male partner [68].

The identification of an sSMC is a challenge for genetic counseling. The majority of cases (70%) occur as de novo events and involve acrocentric chromosomes. In the case of family inheritance, maternal transmission occurs more frequently than paternal transmission. Approximately two-thirds of marker chromosome carriers do not show an identifiable phenotype. The rest exhibit a variety of clinical characteristics, ranging from subfertility, such as azoospermia or oligospermia in men, congenital defects, and/or intellectual disability, including defined syndromes, such as Pallister-Killian syndrome. The identification of an sSMC indicates a risk of segmental aneuploidy (partial trisomy if the extra chromosome has euchromatic content). The prognosis depends on whether there is genetic content and the type of genes included [69–72].

The presence of an sSMC also increases the incidence of aneuploidies in the gametes of carriers. Therefore, PGT-A is advisable when identified in infertile patients [72].

Genetic counseling:

- In order to give an adequate genetic counseling, it is important that the sSMC is characterized with array-CGH or FISH techniques. With these technologies, it is possible to determine whether the sSMC contains euchromatin or heterochromatin.
- The implication of the finding of an sSMC will depend on the context in which the karyotype was requested:
  - In prenatal or postnatal diagnosis of an affected fetus/child, the identification of the euchromatic content of a de novo sSMC may be suspected as the cause of the phenotypic alterations. In contrast, sSMC with heterochromatin may be considered benign variants in these settings;
  - In infertility testing, sSMCs containing both euchromatin or heterochromatin may be considered benign variants. Karyotyping of other relatives may be reassuring in those sSMC containing euchromatin.
- Thirty percent of sSMC are inherited. Therefore, other family members may carry the karyotype alteration and might benefit from genetic counseling and testing.
- PGT-A should be contemplated in carriers of an sSMC with infertility.
- Since in some instances sSMC can be inherited, other family members may benefit from this information and genetic counseling.
- PGT-A is advisable when an sSMC is identified in infertile patients.

Genetic counseling in preimplantation genetic testing

Preimplantation genetic testing (PGT) refers to any genetic test performed on an embryo prior to it being transferred in an in vitro fertilization (IVF) treatment. PGT nomenclature was standardized [73] and categorized in PGT-A, PGT-SR, and preimplantation genetic testing for monogenic conditions (PGT-M).

The PGT procedure usually includes the following steps [74]:

1. In vitro fertilization;
2. Embryos are cultured in the lab to the stage of blastomere (day 3 post-fecundation) or to the stage of blastocyst (day 5 post-fecundation);
3. Embryos are biopsied and embryonic cells are obtained;
4. Embryonic DNA is extracted from the biopsied cells and genetic testing is performed;
5. Genetic testing allows to identify those embryos with the genetic alteration (namely a specific mutation or chromosomal abnormality) and those without it;
6. Those embryos that present the genetic alteration are discarded. Those embryos that do not present the genetic alteration are suitable for transfer.

It is important to note that PGT has some limitations [75–77]:

1. *Mosaicism*: mosaicism refers to two or more cell populations with different chromosomal complements being present within the same embryo. In some instances, embryonic mosaicism between the trophectoderm and the inner cell mass can give rise to false negatives and false positives, which range between 96.6% and 98%.
2. *Embryo viability*: the freezing/thawing process and the biopsy process can affect the embryo availability (survival rates are reported as between 10% and 15%).
3. *Reduce available embryos for transfer*: all aneuploid embryos will be discarded and not used for transfer. This will reduce the number of available embryos to use, and couples should be informed and counseled about this limitation.

4. *Testing objective*: each PGT has a specific testing objective, and couples should understand that any other condition/alteration will not be tested for.

Preimplantation genetic testing for aneuploidies

PGT-A, previously known as preimplantation genetic screening, is defined as genetic testing in embryos to differentiate those that have a normal chromosomal content (euploid embryos) from those that have an abnormal number of chromosomes (aneuploid embryos).

The use of PGT-A, its indications, and its benefits are still being discussed, although most IVF groups agree on its benefits [78,79].

The aim of this chapter is not to evaluate the benefits of PGT-A. PGT-A is generally indicated [80] in advanced maternal age (≥37 years), severe male factor (severe oligozoospermia), repeated implantation failures (≥3 failed transfers of good-quality embryos), and recurrent pregnancy loss (≥3 previous miscarriages). Theoretical benefits of PGT-A include (1) increased pregnancy rate per transfer, (2) increased live birth rates per transfer, (3) decreased rates of spontaneous pregnancy loss per transfer, and (4) decreased incidence of viable trisomies [81].

Preimplantation genetic testing for structural rearrangements

PGT-SR encompasses genetic testing in embryos for carriers of balanced chromosome structural rearrangements (translocations and inversions). PGT-SR enables to detect those embryos with chromosomal imbalances. Carriers of balanced chromosome structural rearrangements have a higher chance of presenting reproduction issues (infertility, subfertility, and recurrent pregnancy losses) and live newborns with congenital alterations and intellectual disability [73].

Preimplantation genetic testing for monogenic conditions

PGT-M refers to genetic testing in embryos to prevent the transmission of a specific genetic condition. Patients with a diagnosis of a genetic condition, or couples with an increased risk for children with a genetic condition may benefit from PGT-M. PGT-M is available for the vast majority of serious genetic conditions, as long as the particular gene mutation(s) in the family has been identified through DNA testing [73].

Legislation regarding PGT-M varies widely worldwide, and thus it may not be available in all countries, or its indications might be restricted to specific conditions [82,83].

Genetic counseling in preimplantation genetic testing

- Benefits, indications, processes, and limitations of PGT should be discussed with patients. Misconceptions and misunderstandings are common in genetics and patients may have false beliefs or expectations about PGT [84].
- Knowledge and understanding about the genetic condition and/or genetic alteration should be assessed.
- Psychological and emotional burden should be addressed. As previously discussed in this chapter, genetics has an important impact on patients.
- If the genetic alteration could have been inherited, other family members may benefit from being informed and they may be advised to seek genetic counseling.

Monogenic causes of infertility

CFTR gene variants as a cause of male infertility

There is a close relationship between obstructive azoospermia caused by congenital bilateral absence of the vas deferens (CBAVD) and the presence of mutations in the cystic fibrosis (CF) gene, called cystic fibrosis transmembrane conductance regulator (*CFTR*). Almost 100% of CF-affected males present with CBAVD and 80% of individuals with CBAVD are carriers of a mutation in the *CFTR* gene. Therefore, *CFTR* genetic testing is advised in all males presenting with CBAVD [85–88].

The *CFTR* gene is one of the most studies genes in the human genome, with over 1000 different mutations having been described. There are two testing strategies in *CFTR*:

- *Targeted panels*: panels that target known mutations, and their implications, in the *CFTR* gene. The most common panel includes 50 known mutations, which are the most prevalent in patients with Caucasian ancestry;
- Whole-gene sequencing.

CFTR mutations can be classified according to their severity. Cystic fibrosis is, nowadays, not considered a single condition, but rather a spectrum of conditions that range from classic CF to male infertility. Part of this variation can be explained by the severity of the mutation (Fig. 18.1).

The *CFTR* gene has a polymorphic region, called the poly T tract. This poly T tract presents different sizes or thymine (T) repetitions; the three most common variants include 5T, 7T, and 9T. Both 7T and 9T are considered benign variants, while the 5T is considered a variant of reduced penetrance. Another polymorphic region lies next to the poly T tract, which is called the TG tract. This tract differs in sizes of a thymine-guanine repetition (TG), with 11TG, 12TG, and 13TG being the most common sizes. A longer TG tract (with lengths of 12 or 13) next to a shorter poly T tract (5T) has the greatest adverse effect [86].

If a mutation in the *CFTR* is identified in a CBAVD male, genetic counseling and testing in the female partner is advised. If both members of a couple are carriers of gene mutations in the *CFTR* gene, their offspring has a 25% chance of inheriting both mutations and, therefore, being at risk for CF; a 50% chance of being healthy carriers of the condition; the other 25% will be healthy noncarriers. If one member of a couple, namely the infertile male, carries two mutations, and the other carries only one, their offspring has a 50% chance of being at risk for CF; the other 50% will be healthy carriers of the condition.

Genetic counseling:

- *CFTR* testing may lead to the diagnosis of a mild form of CF, which can have an emotional impact on the patient.
- Offer an opportunity to give information about the condition, basic genetics, and inheritance pattern.
- The high frequency of carriers in Caucasian ancestry should be addressed. Carrier estimates in these populations range from 1 in 25 to 1 in 30.

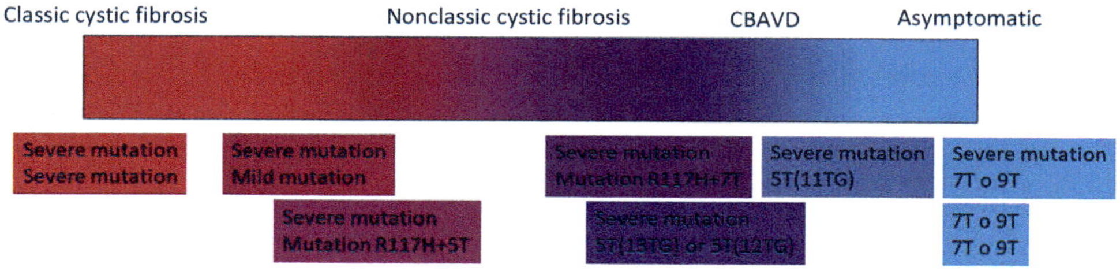

FIGURE 18.1 Representation of phenotypical variation observed in cystic fibrosis, ranging from classic cystic fibrosis to asymptomatic individuals. Genetic contribution, which partly explains this variability, is also depicted.

- Indicate study of the couple's carrier.
  - If both members of the couple are carriers of severe mutations, their offspring would have a chance of 25% of inheriting a classic form of CF. Reproduction options would include PGT.
  - If one member of the couple carries a severe mutation and the other a mild mutation, their offspring would have a 25% chance of inheriting a nonclassic form of CF. Nonclassic CF spans from milder forms of the condition to male infertility. However, the exact phenotype is impossible to predict. Therefore, this uncertainty may cause anxiety in couples. Moreover, PGT may be controverted in these scenarios.
- The identification of a CF mutation in an individual, regardless of being in heterozygosis or homozygosis, will have direct implications for other family members. The siblings of a carrier have a 50% chance of also having inherited the mutation. Given the high frequency of carriers in certain populations, genetic counseling and testing for first-degree family members should be advised.
- Identification of a 5T(11TG) allele in one member of a couple and a classic CF mutation in the other: this combination of variants has never been reported in patients with classic CF. This combination has been described in a varying range of severity, ranging from asymptomatic patients to males with infertility because of CBAVD.
- Identification of a 5T(12TG) or 5T(13TG) allele in one member of a couple and a classic CF mutation in the other: this combination of variants has never been reported in patients with classic CF. This combination has been described in a varying range of severity, from asymptomatic patients to individuals with nonclassic CF symptoms (relatively mild lung and/or pancreatic symptoms).

FMR1 gene variants as a cause of female infertility

Fragile X syndrome is the most common inherited cause of intellectual disability worldwide. The syndrome is caused by a type of mutation, called trinucleotide repeat expansion, in the CGG repeat numbers in the 5′ region of the fragile X mental retardation 1 (FMR1) gene [89,90].

Therefore, alleles of the *FMR1* gene are classified in [91]:

- *Normal allele*: from 5 to 44 CGG repeats. This is the most common allele size in the general population;
- *Intermediate or "gray zone" alleles*: from 45 to 54 CGG repeats;
- *Premutation*: from 55 to 200 CGG repeats;
- *Complete mutation*: more than 200 CGG repeats. Individuals who inherit this allele size will present with the syndrome.

These allele sizes may expand when transmitted from one generation to another; this phenomenon is known as anticipation. Anticipation via maternal transmission is considered to happen more frequently than paternal anticipation [92,93].

Patients with an intermediate allele are not considered at risk of presenting any symptoms related to the syndrome nor transmitting it to their children. However, in approximately 14% of cases [93], the allele may expand when transmitted to their offspring and fall into the premutation range. Again, this is more frequent when it is the mother who transmits the gene to her children. Approximately 1 in 50 people carries an intermediate allele (equivalent to, approximately, 2% of the population).

Patients with a premutation are not at risk of suffering from the condition. However, when a woman transmits the gene to her offspring, it may increase in length and fall in the full mutation range. Therefore, her children would be at risk of inheriting the disease. The chance of expansion to full mutation depends on the size of the maternal allele [94]:

- 55–59 CGG repeats have not been reported to expand to the full mutation;
- 60–69 CGG repeats: 2%;
- 70–79 CGG repeats: 32%;
- 80–89 CGG repeats: 74%;
- 90–99 CGG repeats: 94%;
- 100–200 CGG repeats: 98%.

In most cases, the allele does not increase in length when passed from parents to daughters, so they may also inherit the premutation. Approximately 1 in 150 women and 1 in 450 men are carriers of the premutation.

In addition, it has been described that patients with a premutation have a higher risk of presenting two clinical conditions: fragile X-associated tremor/ataxia syndrome (FXTAS) and FMR1-related primary ovarian insufficiency (POI).

- FXTAS is a neurological condition characterized by tremors, lack of coordination in movements (ataxia), loss of memory, and dementia. It mainly affects males, although it can also affect women, which present milder symptoms. The proportion of males carrying a premutation that will develop FXTAS depends on age. It will affect 17% of males between 50 and 59 years old, 38% between 60 and 69 years old, 47% between 70 and 79 years old, and 75% in men over 80 years.
- POI is defined as the cessation of menstruation at a younger age (before the age of 40). It affects approximately 20% of women who carry an *FMR1* premutation. For this reason, it is important for women carrying a premutation to know their status. This way they will be offered proper genetic counseling, enabling family planning and fertility preservation.

Genetic counseling:

- *FMR1* testing may lead to the diagnosis of an FMR1-related condition, which may have an emotional impact.
- It is important that patients are aware that FMR1 testing may have two implications: (1) explain the woman's POI; (2) reveal a potential risk of offspring with fragile X syndrome. Proper pretest genetic counseling must be provided.
- Offer the opportunity to provide up-to-date and reliable information about the condition, basic genetics, and X-linked inheritance pattern.
- Give and explain the figures for expansion risk associated with premutation allele ranges.
- Assess the emotional impact of the finding.
- The identification of a premutation may have direct implications for other family members. The siblings of a premutation carrier may have inherited the premutation. For this reason, genetic counseling for first-degree relatives is advised.

Genetic counseling in expanded carrier screening

With recent developments in next-generation sequencing, it is now possible to simultaneously detect numerous genetic alterations related to dozens and even hundreds of genetic conditions. This approach can be used to analyze the carrier status for autosomal recessive and X-linked conditions in a preconception setting, allowing for personalized reproductive risk assessment. This type of genetic counseling has been named expanded carrier screening (ECS) [95,96].

ECS genetic panels include two strategies: targeted panels that only study known mutations within the included genes, and complete sequencing of the gene. Both methods have their pros and cons.

ECS is a pan-ethnic approach to carrier screening in which every individual, regardless of their ancestry, is tested for the same conditions. This sort of genetic panel may be attractive to physicians, as it avoids specific protocols for each ethnic group. ECS may also be appealing to patients, as they may feel they are being tested for "everything possible."

However, it is important to note that ECS has important limitations [97–101]:

- In targeted panels, only known mutations are being test. Therefore, the residual risk for the couple will depend on the coverage of the gene.
- In whole-gene sequencing panels, variant interpretation may pose an important challenge to physicians, genetic counselors, and, ultimately, patients.
- There is no consensus on what conditions should be included in these panels and they are often exposed to the misconception of "more is better."
- It is important to note that only autosomal recessive and X-linked conditions are included, and only a selection of these. Even with a negative result, there is still a chance for recessive or X-linked conditions not included in the panel, dominant conditions (with de novo mutations, germline mosaicism, or reduced penetrance/variable expressivity), chromosome alterations, multifactorial conditions, epigenetic disturbances, etc.
- Therefore, a negative result may lead to a false sense of security.

Genetic counseling:

- Discuss the types of conditions that are included in the panel (recessive and/or X-linked), and what criteria have been followed to select them.
- Anticipate possible results, reassuring that, in most instances, being a carrier of a recessive condition has no effect on the carrier's health. Explain the high frequency of carriers in the general population.
- A negative result does not exclude the risk of genetic conditions in the offspring. ECS limitations should be exposed and discussed.
- When both members of a couple are identified as carriers of a genetic recessive condition, or females identified as carriers for a X-linked condition, reproduction options should be discussed.
- When incidental findings are a possibility (e.g., carrier status has some health implications), these should be exposed before ECS is performed.
- Being identified as a carrier of a genetic condition can still have some emotional impact. This should be explored and addressed.
- Since genetic conditions are inherited, other family members may benefit from genetic counseling and testing.

Communication skills in genetics

Taking a family history

One of the pivotal tools in medical genetics and genetic counseling is, beyond any doubt, taking a detailed family history in the form of a genetic pedigree or family tree. The pedigree allows to represent and document a large amount of information related to the transmission of genetic traits in a family in a graphic and intuitive way. In general, it is recommended to document a minimum of three generations for a correct assessment of the family history.

The use of standardized symbology and nomenclature is imperative, as described in the *Standardized Human Pedigree Nomenclature*[102]. Following these guidelines, the interpretation of a pedigree becomes transversal and is not user-dependent. A selection of the *Standardized Human Pedigree Nomenclature* relevant in reproductive genetics is collected in Table 18.2.

Before collecting a family history, it is important to clarify the reason to do so and tell the patients what to expect from it. It is also important to show understanding about patient's not knowing some specific facts. There is no unique order to record a family history, however the following steps may serve as an example (see Fig. 18.2):

1. Ask about your patient's relevant medical history.
2. Proceed by enquiring about their partner and offspring.
3. The following step should be asking about the patient's brothers and sisters.

TABLE 18.2 Selection of relevant pedigree symbols in reproductive genetics, as recommended by the Standardized Human Pedigree Nomenclature.

Symbol description	Symbol		
	Male	Female	Unknown
Individual	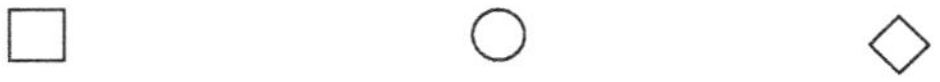		
Affected individual			
Multiple individuals	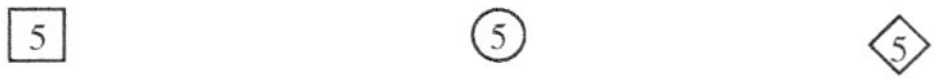		
Multiple individuals, unknown number, or not stated	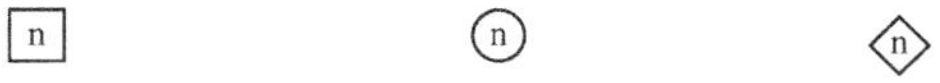		
Deceased individual	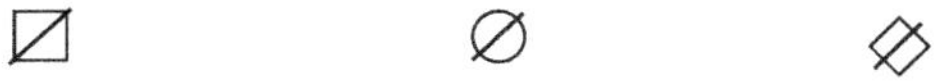		
Consultant			
Stillbirth	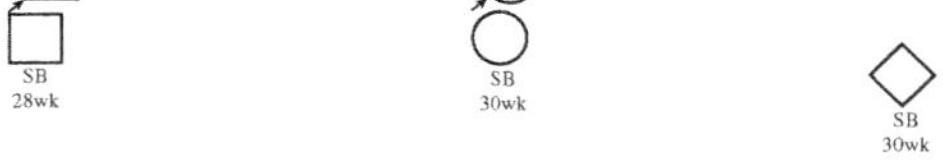		
Pregnancy	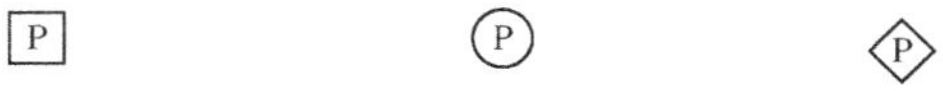		
	Affected		Unaffected
Spontaneous abortion			
Termination of pregnancy			
Relationship			
Relationship lines	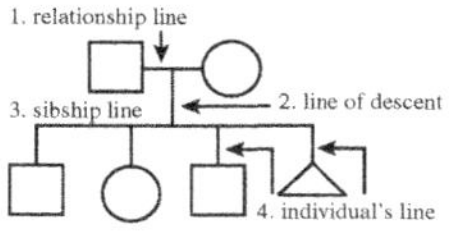		
Broken relationships	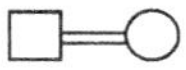		
	Monozygotic	Dizygotic	Trizygotic
Twins	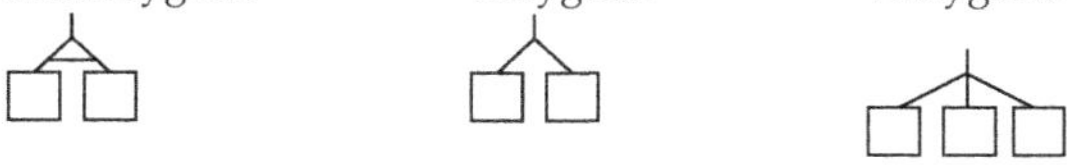		
No children by choice	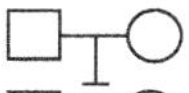		
Infertility	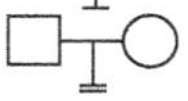		

(*Continued*)

TABLE 18.2 (Continued)

Symbol description		**Symbol**	
	In	Out	By relative
Adoption	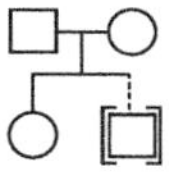	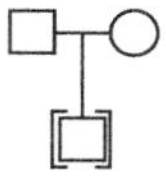	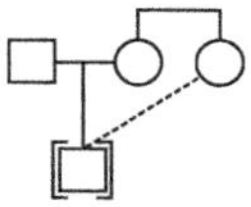
Possible reproductive scenarios			
Sperm donor		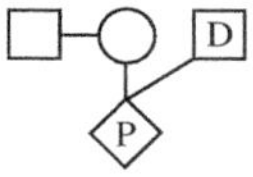	
Ovum donor		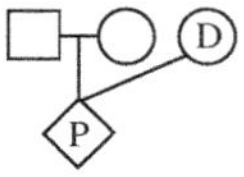	
Surrogate only		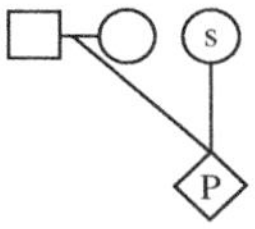	
Surrogate ovum donor		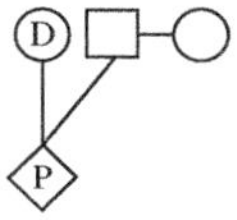	
Planned adoption		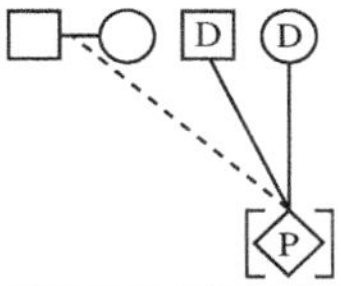	

4. Continue by asking about the siblings' partners and offspring.
5. Ask about the parents of your patient.
6. Start with one side of the family. Ask about siblings first, then about their children, and finally about their parents (the patient's grandparents).
7. Repeat step 6 for the other side of the family.
8. Repeat steps 3–7 with the partner's family.

A selection of important points to cover when taking a family history include:

- Medical conditions that may be related to the condition (congenital abnormalities, intellectual disability, learning difficulties, sensorial disabilities, and so on);
- Age at diagnosis;
- Age at death;
- Whether genetic testing has been performed and its results;
- Ethnic background;
- Presence of consanguinity in the family;
- History of miscarriages or stillbirths;
- Individuals that died at a young age;
- Fertility issues.

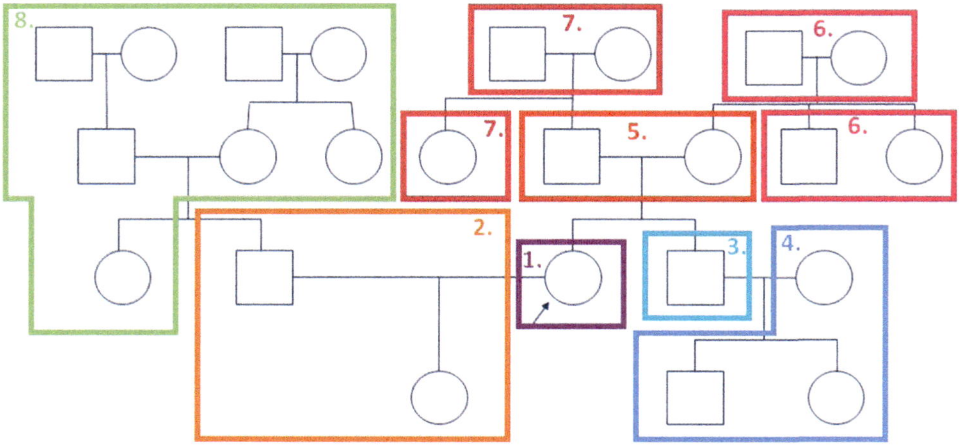

FIGURE 18.2 Recommended questioning order when taking a family pedigree.

Frequent misconceptions about genetics

Genetics can be complex both to the general population and healthcare providers. Regardless, everybody is exposed to genetic concepts via the media. All this leads to frequent misconceptions when discussing genetics [103–108].

- An individual's physical appearance and similarity with other family members can correlate to their risk of developing a condition. For example, taking after the affected parent means that the person has inherited the genetic condition.
- Conditions that are more common in a gender (e.g., breast cancer) can only be inherited through an affected person.
- If a condition only affects individuals from one gender (despite not being X-linked) it will only affect that gender in the family.
- All genetic conditions can be tested for. All genetics conditions have a known cause.
- The identification of a genetic alteration means that the individual will definitely develop the genetic condition.
- Misinterpretations of risks: for example, falsely believing that a 1 in 2 chance means that if a couple already has an affected child, a future child will be healthy.
- There are some common misconceptions about some inheritance patterns. For example, an individual might think that a gene alteration following a dominant inheritance pattern may be "stronger" than the unaltered copy and, thus will be inherited more easily.
- Family history may bias the disease and risk perceptions. The absence of family history may lead to risk underestimation, while severely affected individuals may overestimate the transmission risk.

Delivering genetic information

Regardless of its complexities, there are some strategies than can facilitate communication and understanding in clinical genetics [109–111]:

- Describe medical or genetic terms, while avoiding using too technical concepts. Some concepts such as genes and chromosomes may be familiar to patients, but they may not have a complete understanding of their meaning.
- Provide clear and specific information, in an ordered manner.
- Language commonly used in genetics may be perceived as emotional and judgmental to people who are not familiar with these

concepts (such as, faulty or abnormal genes, mutation, mental retardation, genetic disease, to suffer from, afflicted with, normal, and so on). It is better to use altered gene, intellectual disability, or genetic condition, for example.
- When finishing an information block, assess the patient's understanding and encourage them to ask any questions they may have.

Giving bad news

Bad news in reproductive genetics can include [112]:

- Identification of a carrier status (for autosomal recessive or X-linked conditions, or for chromosomal alterations);
- The reproduction options available to the couple do not meet their expectations.
- Uncertainty following genetic testing (e.g., variants of unknown clinical significance for which their clinical course may not be modified, genetic alterations for which preimplantation testing is not available, or apparently de novo mutations with the possibility of germline mosaicism);
- No embryos available for transfer;
- All analyzed embryos carry the genetic alteration.

It is never easy to give bad news, regardless of the professional's training or expertise. However, there are sensitive ways to give bad news that facilitate coping with the news over time:

- A sensitive and empathic manner is important.
- The news should be given in person and in a direct way. The situation can be prepared by using sentences such as "Unfortunately I have bad news for you," "You may not hear or remember all that I will tell you," "I will repeat it all later," or "Please feel free to ask questions." Avoid euphemisms and false reassuring sentences such as "Next time things may be different," "You are still young," or "I know how you feel." While these expressions come out of good intention, patients may find them annoying and upsetting.
- Silence enables individuals to process the news and respond when they feel ready.
- Emotional reactions are normal and should be allowed and encouraged. These can take the form of distress, blankness, or denial.
- Individuals may appear to be paying attention to information given after being given bad news. However, they might just be shocked or blocked. Written information and ways to recontact should be provided.
- Some coping mechanisms include responding in an intellectual way, while blocking underlying emotions. These should be explored.
- Discussing what will come after the current situation is helpful. Detailing a future plan and providing ongoing support in the interim should always be offered.
- A plan should be put in place for the next contact and provision of ongoing support in the interim, if necessary.
- Encourage a second person, such as their partner, a close friend, or a family member, to be present, if appropriate.

Talking about risks

Discussing genetics usually involves discussion about different types of risk. The term "risk" may carry a negative connotation and sometimes "chance" or "probability" may be a more appropriate term. Many people find the concepts chance or risk confusing and difficult to understand. Sometimes, individuals may think that a risk gives certainty of an event happening, rather than its likelihood [112,113].

There are some common misconceptions about risks or chances. First, risk figures can be misunderstood as excluding options. For example, a one in four chance can be interpreted as meaning once a child is affected, the following three will not inherit the condition. On the contrary, an individual or couple who have experienced an unlikely event can feel susceptible to the event and find it difficult to be reassured that the event is unlikely to happen again [114].

Risk perception varies greatly between individuals. The same figure may appear unacceptable to some, while acceptable to others. For this reason, it is important to explore the individual's reactions and perception to a risk assessment. It is also useful to present figures in different ways [115]:

- Giving a fraction with it is equivalent percentage. For example, a 1 in 4 chance is equivalent to a 25% chance.
- Compare the figure with that observed in the general population. For instance, a *BRCA1* carrier has a life-time risk of developing breast cancer of 60%–80%, as opposed to the 10% of women from the general population.
- Comparison to other individuals with the same test result. For example, of 100 couples with this result, two will have an affected child, whereas the other 98 will have a child without the condition.
- Give relative risks. For example, "Your risk has increased threefold."

References

[1] Harper JC, Aittomaki K, Borry P, Cornel MC, de Wert G, Dondorp W, et al. Recent developments in genetics and medically assisted reproduction: from research to clinical applications. Eur J Hum Genet Engl 2018;26 (1):12–33.

[2] Ormond KE, Mortlock DP, Scholes DT, Bombard Y, Brody LC, Faucett WA, et al. Human germline genome editing. Am J Hum Genet U S 2017;101 (2):167–76.

[3] Joshi N, Chan JL. Female genomics: infertility and overall health. Semin Reprod Med U S 2017;35(3):217–24.

[4] Demain LAM, Conway GS, Newman WG. Genetics of mitochondrial dysfunction and infertility. Clin Genet 2017;91(2):199–207.

[5] Krausz C, Escamilla AR, Chianese C. Genetics of male infertility: from research to inic. Reprod Engl 2015;150 (5):R159–74.

[6] Brunet A, Berger SL. Epigenetics of aging and aging-related disease. J Gerontol A Biol Sci Med Sci 2014;69 (Suppl. 1):S17–20.

[7] Macaulay IC, Voet T. Single cell genomics: advances and future perspectives. PLoS Genet 2014;10(1): e1004126.

[8] Maes E, Kelchtermans P, Bittremieux W, De Grave K, Degroeve S, Hooyberghs J, et al. Designing biomedical proteomics experiments: state-of-the-art and future perspectives. Expert Rev Proteom Engl 2016;13(5):495–511.

[9] Witt MM, Witt MP. Privacy and confidentiality measures in genetic testing and counselling: arguing on genetic exceptionalism again? J Appl Genet Engl 2016;57(4):483–5.

[10] Berryessa CM. Genetic essentialist biases, stigma, and lack of mitigating impact on punishment decisions. J Law Biosci [Internet] 2016;3(2):359–64.

[11] Heine SJ, Dar-Nimrod I, Cheung BY, Proulx T. Essentially biased: why people are fatalistic about genes. Adv Exp Soc Psychol, 55. 2017. p. 137–92.

[12] Lanie AD, Jayaratne TE, Sheldon JP, Kardia SLR, Anderson ES, Feldbaum M, et al. Exploring the public understanding of basic genetic concepts. J Genet Couns U S 2004;13(4):305–20.

[13] Metcalfe SA. Genetic counselling, patient education, and informed decision-making in the genomic era. Semin Fetal Neonatal Med [Internet] 2018;23(2):142–9.

[14] Resta R, Biesecker BB, Bennett RL, Blum S, Hahn SE, Strecker MN, et al. A new definition of genetic counseling: National Society of Genetic Counselors' Task Force report. J Genet Couns 2006;15(2):77–83.

[15] Abacan M, Alsubaie L, Barlow-Stewart K, Caanen B, Cordier C, Courtney E, et al. The global state of the genetic counseling profession. Eur J Hum Genet [Internet] 2019;27(2):183–97.

[16] Newton CR, Hearn MT, Yuzpe AA. Psychological assessment and follow-up after in vitro fertilization: assessing the impact of failure. Fertil Steril 1990;54 (5):879–86.

[17] Demyttenaere K, Bonte L, Gheldof M, Vervaeke M, Meuleman C, Vanderschuerem D, et al. Coping style and depression level influence outcome in in vitro fertilization. Fertil Steril 1998;69(6):1026–33.

[18] Tuschen-Caffier B, Florin I, Krause W, Pook M. Cognitive-behavioral therapy for idiopathic infertile couples. Psychother Psychosom 1999;68(1):15–21.

[19] Lukse MP, Vacc NA. Grief, depression, and coping in women undergoing infertility treatment. Obstet Gynecol 1999;93(2):245–51.

[20] Matsubayashi H, Hosaka T, Izumi S, Suzuki T, Makino T. Emotional distress of infertile women in Japan. Hum Reprod 2001;16(5):966–9.
[21] Lok IH, Lee DTS, Cheung LP, Chung WS, Lo WK, Haines CJ. Psychiatric morbidity amongst infertile Chinese women undergoing treatment with assisted reproductive technology and the impact of treatment failure. Gynecol Obstet Invest 2002;53(4):195–9.
[22] Chen T-H, Chang S-P, Tsai C-F, Juang K-D. Prevalence of depressive and anxiety disorders in an assisted reproductive technique clinic. Hum Reprod 2004;19(10):2313–18.
[23] Cwikel J, Gidron Y, Sheiner E. Psychological interactions with infertility among women. Eur J Obstet Gynecol Reprod Biol 2004;117(2):126–31.
[24] Hammerli K, Znoj H, Barth J. The efficacy of psychological interventions for infertile patients: a meta-analysis examining mental health and pregnancy rate. Hum Reprod Update 2009;15(3):279–95.
[25] Gameiro S, Moura-Ramos M, Canavarro MC, Soares I. Psychosocial adjustment during the transition to parenthood of Portuguese couples who conceived spontaneously or through assisted reproductive technologies. Res Nurs Health 2010;33(3):207–20.
[26] Jongbloed-Pereboom M, Middelburg KJ, Heineman MJ, Bos AF, Haadsma ML, Hadders-Algra M. The impact of IVF/ICSI on parental well-being and anxiety 1 year after childbirth. Hum Reprod 2012;27(8):2389–95.
[27] De Pascalis L, Agostini F, Monti F, Paterlini M, Fagandini P, La Sala GB. A comparison of quality of life following spontaneous conception and assisted reproduction. Int J Gynaecol Obstet 2012;118 (3):216–19.
[28] Reis S, Xavier MR, Coelho R, Montenegro N. Psychological impact of single and multiple courses of assisted reproductive treatments in couples: a comparative study. Eur J Obstet Gynecol Reprod Biol 2013;171(1):61–6.
[29] Rooney KL, Domar AD. The impact of stress on fertility treatment. Curr Opin Obstet Gynecol 2016;28 (3):198–201.
[30] Anderson KM, Sharpe M, Rattray A, Irvine DS. Distress and concerns in couples referred to a specialist infertility clinic. J Psychosom Res 2003;54(4):353–5.
[31] Dinc L, Terzioglu F. The psychological impact of genetic testing on parents. J Clin Nurs 2006;15 (1):45–51.
[32] Bottos AM, Zanon E, Sartori MT, Girolami A. Psychological aspects and coping styles of parents with haemophilic child undergoing a programme of counselling and psychological support. Haemophilia 2007;13(3):305–10.
[33] Wiedebusch S, Pollmann H, Siegmund B, Muthny FA. Quality of life, psychosocial strains and coping in parents of children with haemophilia. Haemophilia 2008;14(5):1014–22.
[34] Galiatsatos P, Rothenmund H, Aubin S, Foulkes WD. Psychosocial impact of lynch syndrome on affected individuals and families. Dig Dis Sci 2015;60 (8):2246–50.
[35] Bancroft EK, Castro E, Bancroft GA, Ardern-Jones A, Moynihan C, Page E, et al. The psychological impact of undergoing genetic-risk profiling in men with a family history of prostate cancer. Psychooncology 2015;24(11):1492–9.
[36] Godino L, Turchetti D, Jackson L, Hennessy C, Skirton H. Impact of presymptomatic genetic testing on young adults: a systematic review. Eur J Hum Genet 2016;24 (4):496–503.
[37] Anderson EE, Wasson K. Personal narratives of genetic testing: expectations, emotions, and impact on self and family. Narrat Inq Bioeth 2015;5(3):229–35.
[38] Quittner AL, Saez-Flores E, Barton JD. The psychological burden of cystic fibrosis. Curr Opin Pulm Med 2016;22(2):187–91.
[39] Richardson E, Spinks C, Davis A, Turner C, Atherton J, McGaughran J, et al. Psychosocial implications of living with catecholaminergic polymorphic ventricular tachycardia in adulthood. J Genet Couns 2018;27 (3):549–57.
[40] Mau-Holzmann UA. Somatic chromosomal abnormalities in infertile men and women. Cytogenet Genome Res 2005;111(3–4):317–36.
[41] Chantot-Bastaraud S, Ravel C, Siffroi JP. Underlying karyotype abnormalities in IVF/ICSI patients. Reprod Biomed Online 2008;16(4):514–22.
[42] Chatziparasidou A, Christoforidis N, Samolada G, Nijs M. Sperm aneuploidy in infertile male patients: a systematic review of the literature. Andrologia 2015;47 (8):847–60.
[43] Hyde KJ, Schust DJ. Genetic considerations in recurrent pregnancy loss. Cold Spring Harb Perspect Med 2015;5(3):a023119.
[44] Page JM, Silver RM. Genetic causes of recurrent pregnancy loss. Clin Obstet Gynecol 2016;59(3):498–508.
[45] Asgari A, Ghahremani S, Saeedi S, Kamrani E. The study of chromosomal abnormalities and heteromorphism in couples with 2 or 3 recurrent abortions in Shahid Beheshti Hospital of Hamedan. Iran J Reprod Med 2013;11(3):201–8.
[46] Sahin FI, Yilmaz Z, Yuregir OO, Bulakbasi T, Ozer O, Zeyneloglu HB. Chromosome heteromorphisms: an impact on infertility. J Assist Reprod Genet [Internet] 2008;25(5):191–5.

[47] Wyandt Golder H.E., Wilson N., Tonk V.S. Human chromosome variation: heteromorphism, polymorphism and pathogenesis. 2nd ed. 2017. Springer Singapore, Singapore.
[48] Hong DS, Reiss AL. Cognitive and neurological aspects of sex chromosome aneuploidies. Lancet Neurol Engl 2014;13(3):306–18.
[49] Printzlau F, Wolstencroft J, Skuse DH. Cognitive, behavioral, and neural consequences of sex chromosome aneuploidy. J Neurosci Res U S 2017;95 (1–2):311–19.
[50] Skuse D, Printzlau F, Wolstencroft J. Sex chromosome aneuploidies. Handbook of Clinical Neurology, 147. Elsevier; 2018. p. 355–76.
[51] Kuo P-L, Guo H-R. Mechanism of recurrent spontaneous abortions in women with mosaicism of X-chromosome aneuploidies. Fertil Steril [Internet] 2004;82(6):1594–601.
[52] Bonomi M, Rochira V, Pasquali D, Balercia G, Jannini EA, Ferlin A, et al. Klinefelter syndrome (KS): genetics, clinical phenotype and hypogonadism. J Endocrinol Invest [Internet] 2017;40(2):123–34.
[53] Ravel C, Chantot-Bastaraud S, Cretet J, Roynard P, Sibony M, Maurin N, et al. Syndrome de Klinefelter: qualité des gamètes et spermatogenèse. Gynécol Obstet Fertil [Internet] 2011;39(9):525–8.
[54] Doğer E, Cakiroglu Y, Ceylan Y, Ulak E, Özdamar Ö, Caliskan E. Reproductive and obstetric outcomes in mosaic Turner's syndrome: a cross-sectional study and review of the literature. Reprod Biol Endocrinol (RB&E) 2015;13::59.
[55] Simpson JL, Bischoff F. Genetic counseling in translocations. Urol Clin North Am 2002;29(4):793–807 vii–viii.
[56] Youings S, Ellis K, Ennis S, Barber J, Jacobs P. A study of reciprocal translocations and inversions detected by light microscopy with special reference to origin, segregation, and recurrent abnormalities. Am J Med Genet A 2004;126A(1):46–60.
[57] Morin SJ, Eccles J, Iturriaga A, Zimmerman RS. Translocations, inversions and other chromosome rearrangements. Fertil Steril 2017;107(1):19–26.
[58] Engels H, Eggermann T, Caliebe A, Jelska A, Schubert R, Schuler HM, et al. Genetic counseling in Robertsonian translocations der(13;14): frequencies of reproductive outcomes and infertility in 101 pedigrees. Am J Med Genet A 2008;146A(20):2611–16.
[59] Kolgeci S, Azemi M, Ahmeti H, Dervishi Z, Sopjani M, Kolgeci J. Recurrent abortions and down syndrome resulting from Robertsonian translocation 21q; 21q. Med Arch 2012;66(5):350–2.
[60] Kolgeci S, Kolgeci J, Azemi M, Daka A, Shala-Beqiraj R, Kurtishi I, et al. Dermatoglyphics and reproductive risk in a family with Robertsonian translocation 14q;21q. Acta Inform Med 2015;178–83.
[61] Yan J, Zhang Q, Chen Y, Chen Z-J. Birth of a mosaic non-Down syndrome offspring to a 45,XY, t(21;21)(q10;q10) homologous Robertsonian translocation carrier: a case report. J Reprod Med 2017;62(5–6):337–41.
[62] Sha J, Liu F, Zhang B, Huang Y, Zhang Q, Juan G, et al. Next-generation sequencing and karyotype analysis for the diagnosis of Robertsonian translocation type trisomy 13: a case report. Iran J Public Health 2017;46(6):848–51.
[63] Casamassima AC, Shapiro LR, Wilmot PL, Smith KB. Prader-Willi syndrome and Robertsonian translocations involving chromosome 15. Clin Genet 1991;39 (4):294–7.
[64] Wenger SL. Robertsonian translocations in Prader-Willi syndrome. Clin Genet 1991;40(6):471.
[65] Yip M-Y. Uniparental disomy in Robertsonian translocations: strategies for uniparental disomy testing. Transl Pediatr 2014;3(2):98–107.
[66] Bertini V, Fogli A, Bruno R, Azzara A, Michelucci A, Mattina T, et al. Maternal uniparental disomy 14 (Temple syndrome) as a result of a Robertsonian translocation. Mol Syndromol 2017;8(3):131–8.
[67] Warburton D. De novo balanced chromosome rearrangements and extra marker chromosomes identified at prenatal diagnosis: clinical significance and distribution of breakpoints. Am J Hum Genet 1991;49 (5):995–1013.
[68] Liehr T. Small supernumerary marker chromosomes (sSMC). 1st ed. Berlin: Springer; 2012.
[69] Liehr T, Kosyakova N. Small supernumerary marker chromosomes (sSMC) - what about the genotype-phenotype correlation? Tsitologiia 2013;55(3):165–6.
[70] Liehr T. Small supernumerary marker chromosomes detected in connection with infertility. Zhonghua Nan Ke Xue 2014;20(9):771–80.
[71] Jafari-Ghahfarokhi H, Moradi-Chaleshtori M, Liehr T, Hashemzadeh-Chaleshtori M, Teimori H, Ghasemi-Dehkordi P. Small supernumerary marker chromosomes and their correlation with specific syndromes. Adv Biomed Res 2015;4:140.
[72] Armanet N, Tosca L, Brisset S, Liehr T, Tachdjian G. Small supernumerary marker chromosomes in human infertility. Cytogenet Genome Res 2015;146(2):100–8.
[73] Zegers-Hochschild F, Adamson GD, Dyer S, Racowsky C, de Mouzon J, Sokol R, et al. The International Glossary on Infertility and Fertility Care. Hum Reprod Engl 2017;32(9):1786–801.
[74] Dahdouh EM, Balayla J, Audibert F, Wilson RD, Audibert F, Brock J-A, et al. Technical update: preimplantation genetic diagnosis and screening. J Obstet Gynaecol [Internet] 2015;37(5):451–63.

[75] Penzias A, Bendikson K, Butts S, Coutifaris C, Falcone T, Fossum G, et al. The use of preimplantation genetic testing for aneuploidy (PGT-A): a committee opinion. Fertil Steril [Internet] 2018;109 (3):429–36.

[76] Imudia AN, Plosker S. The past, present, and future of preimplantation genetic testing. Clin Lab Med 2016;36(2):385–99.

[77] Kuliev A, Rechitsky S. Preimplantation genetic testing: current challenges and future prospects. Expert Rev Mol Diagn 2017;17(12):1071–88.

[78] Kushnir VA, Darmon SK, Albertini DF, Barad DH, Gleicher N. Effectiveness of in vitro fertilization with preimplantation genetic screening: a reanalysis of United States assisted reproductive technology data 2011–2012. Fertil Steril [Internet] 2016;106(1):75–9.

[79] Chang J, Boulet SL, Jeng G, Flowers L, Kissin DM. Outcomes of in vitro fertilization with preimplantation genetic diagnosis: an analysis of the United States Assisted Reproductive Technology Surveillance Data, 2011–2012. Fertil Steril [Internet] 2016;105(2):394–400.

[80] Harper JC, Harton G. The use of arrays in preimplantation genetic diagnosis and screening. Fertil Steril 2010;94(4):1173–7.

[81] Geraedts J, Sermon K. Preimplantation genetic screening 2.0: the theory. Mol Hum Reprod 2016;22 (8):839–44.

[82] Lee VCY, Chow JFC, Yeung WSB, Ho PC. Preimplantation genetic diagnosis for monogenic diseases. Best Pract Res Clin Obstet Gynaecol 2017;44:68–75.

[83] Duguet A-M, Boyer-Beviere B. Preimplantation Genetic Diagnosis: The Situation in France and in Other European Countries. Eur J Health Law 2017;24 (2):160–74.

[84] Quinn MM, Juarez-Hernandez F, Dunn M, Okamura RJ, Cedars MI, Rosen MP. Decision-making surrounding the use of preimplantation genetic testing for aneuploidy reveals misunderstanding regarding its benefit. J Assist Reprod Genet 2018;35(12):2155–9.

[85] Stuhrmann M, Dork T. CFTR gene mutations and male infertility. Andrology 2000;32(2):71–83.

[86] Cuppens H, Cassiman J-J. CFTR mutations and polymorphisms in male infertility. Int J Androl 2004;27 (5):251–6.

[87] Claustres M. Molecular pathology of the CFTR locus in male infertility. Reprod Biomed Online 2005;10 (1):14–41.

[88] Ahmad A, Ahmed A, Patrizio P. Cystic fibrosis and fertility. Curr Opin Obstet Gynecol 2013;25(3):167–72.

[89] Oostra BA, Willemsen R. FMR1: a gene with three faces. Biochim Biophys Acta 2009;1790(6):467–77.

[90] Sullivan SD, Welt C, Sherman S. FMR1 and the continuum of primary ovarian insufficiency. Semin Reprod Med 2011;29(4):299–307.

[91] Saul RA, Tarleton JC. FMR1-related disorders. In: Adam MP, Ardinger HH, Pagon RA, Wallace SE, Bean LJH, Stephens K, et al., editors. GeneReviews (R). Seattle, WA; 1993.

[92] Qin Y, Jiao X, Simpson JL, Chen Z-J. Genetics of primary ovarian insufficiency: new developments and opportunities. Hum Reprod Update 2015;21(6):787–808.

[93] Barasoain M, Barrenetxea G, Huerta I, Telez M, Criado B, Arrieta I. Study of the genetic etiology of primary ovarian insufficiency: FMR1 gene. Genes (Basel) 2016;7(12):123.

[94] Nolin SL, Houck GEJ, Gargano AD, Blumstein H, Dobkin CS, Brown WT. FMR1 CGG-repeat instability in single sperm and lymphocytes of fragile-X premutation males. Am J Hum Genet 1999;65(3):680–8.

[95] Edwards JG, Feldman G, Goldberg J, Gregg AR, Norton ME, Rose NC, et al. Expanded carrier screening in reproductive medicine-points to consider: a joint statement of the American College of Medical Genetics and Genomics, American College of Obstetricians and Gynecologists, National Society of Genetic Counselors, Perinatal Quality Foundation, and Society for Maternal-Fetal Medicine. Obstet Gynecol 2015;653–62.

[96] Lazarin GA, Goldberg JD. Current controversies in traditional and expanded carrier screening. Curr Opin Obstet Gynecol 2016;28(2):136–41.

[97] Henneman L, Borry P, Chokoshvili D, Cornel MC, van El CG, Forzano F, et al. Responsible implementation of expanded carrier screening. Eur J Hum Genet 2016;24(6):e1–e12.

[98] Yao R, Goetzinger KR. Genetic carrier screening in the twenty-first century. Clin Lab Med 2016;36(2):277–88.

[99] Rose NC, Wick M. Carrier screening for single gene disorders. Semin Fetal Neonatal Med 2018;23 (2):78–84.

[100] Gregg AR. Expanded carrier screening. Obstet Gynecol Clin N Am 2018;45(1):103–12.

[101] Dungan J. Expanded carrier screening: what the reproductive endocrinologist needs to know. Fertil Steril 2018;109(2):183–9.

[102] Bennett RL, French KS, Resta RG, Doyle DL. Standardized human pedigree nomenclature: update and assessment of the recommendations of the National Society of Genetic Counselors. J Genet Couns 2008;17(5):424–33.

[103] Surani MA. Genetics: immaculate misconception. Nature 2002;491–3.

[104] Plomin R, Walker SO. Genetics and educational psychology. Br J Educ Psychol 2003;73(Pt 1):3–14.

[105] Mills Shaw KR, Van Horne K, Zhang H, Boughman J. Essay contest reveals misconceptions of high school students in genetics content. Genetics 2008;178 (3):1157–68.
[106] Visscher PM, Hill WG, Wray NR. Heritability in the genomics era—concepts and misconceptions. Nat Rev Genet 2008;9(4):255–66.
[107] Argulian E, Sherrid MV, Messerli FH. Misconceptions and facts about hypertrophic cardiomyopathy. Am J Med 2016;129(2):148–52.
[108] Read CY, Ward LD. Misconceptions about genomics among nursing faculty and students. Nurse Educ 2018;43(4):196–200.
[109] Edwards A, Gray J, Clarke A, Dundon J, Elwyn G, Gaff C, et al. Interventions to improve risk communication in clinical genetics: systematic review. Patient Educ Couns 2008;71(1):4–25.
[110] Paul J, Metcalfe S, Stirling L, Wilson B, Hodgson J. Analyzing communication in genetic consultations—a systematic review. Patient Educ Couns 2015;98 (1):15–33.
[111] Burns C, James C, Ingles J. Communication of genetic information to families with inherited rhythm disorders. Hear Rhythm 2018;15(5):780–6.
[112] Veach PM, Leroy BS, Callanan NP. Facilitating the genetic counseling process: practice-based skills. 2nd ed. Cham: Springer; 2018.
[113] LeRoy BS, Veach PM, Bartels DM. Genetic counseling practice: advanced concepts and skills. 1st ed. Wiley-Blackwell; 2010.
[114] Harper PS. Practical genetic counseling. 7th ed. Hodder Arnold; 2010.
[115] Weil J. Psychosocial genetic counseling. 1st ed. Oxford Universirty Press; 2000.

Index

Note: Page numbers followed by "*f*" and "*t*" refer to figures and tables, respectively.

CPI Antony Rowe
Eastbourne, UK
February 09, 2021